The Future of the Nursing Workforce in the United States

Data, Trends, and Implications

Peter I. Buerhaus, PhD, RN, FAAN
Valere Potter Distinguished Professor of Nursing
Director, Center for Interdisciplinary Health Workforce Studies
Institute for Medicine and Public Health
Vanderbilt University Medical Center

Douglas O. Staiger, PhD
John French Professor in Economics
Dartmouth College
Research Associate
National Bureau of Economic Research

David I. Auerbach, PhD
Principal Analyst
Health and Human Resources Division
Congressional Budget Office

JONES AND BARTLETT PUBLISHERS
Sudbury, Massachusetts
BOSTON   TORONTO   LONDON   SINGAPORE

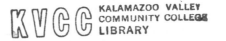

World Headquarters

Jones and Bartlett Publishers
40 Tall Pine Drive
Sudbury, MA 01776
978-443-5000
info@jbpub.com
www.jbpub.com

Jones and Bartlett Publishers
Canada
6339 Ormindale Way
Mississauga, Ontario L5V 1J2
Canada

Jones and Bartlett Publishers
International
Barb House, Barb Mews
London W6 7PA
United Kingdom

Jones and Bartlett's books and products are available through most bookstores and online booksellers. To contact Jones and Bartlett Publishers directly, call 800-832-0034, fax 978-443-8000, or visit our website www.jbpub.com.

Substantial discounts on bulk quantities of Jones and Bartlett's publications are available to corporations, professional associations, and other qualified organizations. For details and specific discount information, contact the special sales department at Jones and Bartlett via the above contact information or send an email to specialsales@jbpub.com.

The authors, editor, and publisher have made every effort to provide accurate information. However, they are not responsible for errors, omissions, or for any outcomes related to the use of the contents of this book and take no responsibility for the use of the products and procedures described. Treatments and side effects described in this book may not be applicable to all people; likewise, some people may require a dose or experience a side effect that is not described herein. Drugs and medical devices are discussed that may have limited availability controlled by the Food and Drug Administration (FDA) for use only in a research study or clinical trial. Research, clinical practice, and government regulations often change the accepted standard in this field. When consideration is being given to use of any drug in the clinical setting, the health care provider or reader is responsible for determining FDA status of the drug, reading the package insert, and reviewing prescribing information for the most up-to-date recommendations on dose, precautions, and contraindications, and determining the appropriate usage for the product. This is especially important in the case of drugs that are new or seldom used.

The views expressed in this book are solely those of the authors and should not be interpreted at those of the Congressional Budget Office.

Production Credits

Executive Editor: Kevin Sullivan
Acquisitions Editor: Emily Ekle
Acquisitions Editor: Amy Sibley
Editorial Assistant: Patricia Donnelly
Production Director: Amy Rose
Associate Production Editor: Wendy Swanson
Associate Marketing Manager: Rebecca Wasley
Manufacturing and Inventory Control Supervisor:
    Amy Bacus

Composition: MacPS, LLC
Cover Design: Kate Ternullo
Cover Images: Left to right—Courtesy of Kate
    Ternullo, © Ryan McVay/Photodisc/Getty Images,
    © 2007 Wes Thomson Photography;
    Background—© Aga/ShutterStock, Inc.
Printing and Binding: Malloy, Inc.
Cover Printing: Malloy, Inc.

Library of Congress Cataloging-in-Publication Data
Buerhaus, Peter I.
  The future of the nursing workforce in the United States : data, trends, and implications / Peter I. Buerhaus, Douglas O. Staiger, David I. Auerbach.
      p. ; cm.
  Includes bibliographical references and index.
  ISBN-13: 978-0-7637-5684-0 (pbk. : alk. paper)
  ISBN-10: 0-7637-5684-9 (pbk. : alk. paper) 1. Nurses—Supply and demand—United States—Forecasting. I. Staiger, Douglas. II. Auerbach, David I. III. Title.
  [DNLM: 1. Nurses—supply & distribution—United States. 2. Forecasting—United States. 3. Nursing—manpower—United States. 4. Nursing—trends—United States. WY 300 AA1 B928f 2009]
  RT86.73.B84 2009
  331.12'91362173—dc22
                            2008004230

6048

Printed in the United States of America
12 11 10 09 08   10 9 8 7 6 5 4 3 2

Contents

SECTION FOUR: SHORTAGES OF HOSPITAL RNs, IMPACT ON QUALITY, AND RN WORKING CONDITIONS

CHAPTER 11: SHORTAGES OF REGISTERED NURSES: THEN AND NOW . . 193

Preface

This book grew out of a collaboration among the three of us that began in the mid-1990s when we were all at Harvard University—David as a doctoral student, Peter as a professor in the School of Public Health, and Doug as a professor at the Kennedy School of Government. Then, our work focused on determining whether there was any evidence that managed care—which was spreading throughout the country—was affecting the wages and employment growth of registered nurses (RNs), licensed practical nurses, and nursing assistants.

In constructing databases on the nursing workforce to conduct our analyses, we noticed that the age composition of the RN workforce was undergoing dramatic change. After completing our initial work on the impact of managed care on the nurse labor market, we turned our attention to trying to identify and understand why the RN workforce was aging so rapidly. We proceeded to develop a model of the nursing workforce that was common in the field of labor economics and used data from the Bureau of Labor Statistics' Current Population Survey rather than relying exclusively on national nursing data provided by the national surveys of RNs that were conducted by the Health Resources and Services Administration—a somewhat novel concept at the time. Our forecasting model turned out to have remarkable predictive ability and led to our publishing a number of journal articles that were the first to project the implications of these age trends into the future. Meanwhile, we continued our analyses of the nurse labor market and other topics, and we continued to monitor economic and noneconomic changes in the RN workforce.

We have been surprised, and gratified, by the positive reaction our publications have received in academic journals and in the popular media, both domestically and internationally. Even more satisfying is to see our body of publications influence public and private policymaking with respect to the nursing workforce. In turn, the positive reception has stimulated our efforts to improve and refine our analyses of the nursing workforce, broaden our thinking, and probe different topics, including the quality of patient care.

Our collaboration has benefited from our common grounding in economics, which allowed us to think about problems in the nursing workforce and communicate with each other using the language and tools of economic analysis. Yet each of us has brought other experiences and perspectives (i.e., as clinician, health-services researcher, policy analyst, economics professor, and health administrator) that have aided our ability to think about the problems and opportunities facing the nursing profession, hopefully in fresh and useful ways.

Because studies by economists, policymakers, and others that have focused on the healthcare workforce have concentrated mostly on physicians and other aspects of the healthcare system and far less on nurses, less objective data or rigorous analyses have been developed on the nursing workforce. Consequently, there is a large gap in understanding the key problems facing the nursing workforce and an even larger gap in high quality data describing the labor market activity of RNs. This book, we hope, will help to fill these gaps in a timely, readable, comprehensive, and focused manner.

We expect the book will be of interest to several audiences. Among nurses, we expect this book will be of interest to undergraduate- and graduate-level nursing students, nurses in clinical practice, managers, policymakers, and leaders in national and state nursing associations. In addition, we have written the book to appeal to the interests of healthcare policymakers, including staffs in state and federal agencies, health legislative aides and committee staff, healthcare labor unions, other professional associations, healthcare foundations, and groups and organizations concerned with quality improvement and patient safety. We also expect this book will be of interest to many researchers, including those in think-tank organizations concerned with national healthcare policy, labor economists, health services researchers, and health policy analysts in academic and nonacademic settings. Finally, we hope that many who are not formally connected with the healthcare sector would nevertheless find this a fascinating account of how the interplay of forces such as social movements, generational trends, family dynamics, and economic incentives are aligning to create a shortage of RNs of unprecedented size beginning in a decade or so.

Acknowledgments

The preparation of any book involves the help of many people who, in their own unique ways, have contributed to making this effort possible. Dr. Buerhaus acknowledges the late Virginia Cleland, Jeptha Dalston, and Frederica Shea who were strong role models and provided early inspiration. He also thanks Lillian Simms, George Zuidema, Joyce Clifford, Eileen Sporing, Yvonne Munn, Jeanette Ives Erickson, Judy Miller, Mary Faye, Colleen Conway-Welch, and Bob Dittus for their support and guidance in critical years. He expresses his gratitude to Bob Blendon and Clarie Fagan for their vision and leadership, to Jack Needleman and Karen Donelan for their research collaboration and friendship over the years, and to Andrea Higham for her generosity and support and that of the Johnson & Johnson Campaign for Nursing's Future for caring enough to get involved to help ensure a strong future for the nursing workforce. Dr. Buerhaus expresses his deepest appreciation to Paul Feldstein, who did more than any other to shape his interest and development in healthcare economics.

Dr. Auerbach gives thanks to the Harvard University PhD program in health policy (and the many wonderful advisors, collaborators, and administrators involved, including David Cutler, Kathy Swartz, Joe Newhouse, Haiden Huskamp, Joan Buchanan, and Joan Curhan) and he thanks AHRQ for partially funding this opportunity. His colleagues at the Congressional Budget Office, particularly James Baumgardner and Bruce Vavrichek, have also been extremely helpful and understanding in allowing him to pursue outside projects such as this one.

Dr. Staiger thanks his early mentors who provided invaluable advice and encouragement, including Gary Gaumer and Mike Keotting, who first introduced him to the field of health policy, and Joe Newhouse who made the initial suggestion to work with Dr. Buerhaus on nurse labor markets. Dr. Staiger also thanks his current and former colleagues and collaborators who have supported this work with their comments and suggestions over the years, including Amitabh Chandra, David Cutler, Tom Kane, Jon Skinner, and Jon Wilwerding.

We especially wish to thank and acknowledge Terrance Keenan at the Robert Wood Johnson Foundation, our long-time supporter and great friend of the nursing profession. We are particularly grateful to the Robert Wood Johnson Foundation for funding early research on the nursing workforce from which this book is partly based. We also thank Brenda Compton and Sarah Beth McLellan for their cheerful and tireless assistance in helping prepare this book.

Finally, we acknowledge the unending support of our families, who have made countless sacrifices over the years to allow our collaboration to grow. Our wives and our children, above all others, are responsible for our ability to come together and produce what we hope will be an insightful and meaningful analysis of a critically important national resource, the RN workforce.

To our families:
Lorraine, John, and Sam Buerhaus
Laura, Ben, and Sam Auerbach
Beth, Katie, John, Kiri, and Mike Staiger

About the Authors

Peter Buerhaus, PhD, RN, FAAN is the Valere Potter Distinguished Professor of Nursing and Director of the Center for Interdisciplinary Health Workforce Studies, Institute for Medicine & Public Health, at Vanderbilt University Medical Center. From 2000 to 2006 he served as the Senior Associate Dean for Research at Vanderbilt University School of Nursing, and from 1992 to 2000, he was an Assistant Professor of Health Policy and Management at Harvard School of Public Health where he developed the Harvard Nursing Research Institute and a postdoctoral program in nursing health services research. During the 1980s Dr. Buerhaus served as assistant to the chief executive officer of The University of Michigan Medical Center's seven teaching hospitals and assistant to the Vice Provost for Medical Affairs, the chief executive of the medical center. Dr. Buerhaus was inducted into the American Academy of Nursing in 1994 and elected into the Institute of Medicine of the National Academies in 2003. Over his career, he has served on a number of governmental and health association boards and committees. Dr. Buerhaus earned his baccalaureate degree in nursing from Mankato State University, a master's degree in nursing health services administration from The University of Michigan, a doctoral degree from Wayne State University, and was a Robert Wood Johnson Foundation faculty fellow in healthcare finance at The Johns Hopkins University (1991–1992).

Douglas Staiger, PhD is the John French Professor in Economics at Dartmouth College, and Research Associate at the National Bureau of Economic Research in Cambridge, Massachusetts. Before coming to Dartmouth, he was Assistant Professor of Economics at Stanford University (1990–1993), and Associate Professor of Public Policy at the Harvard University Kennedy School of Government (1993–1998). Dr. Staiger is a health and labor economist who has worked on topics including nurse labor markets, the quality of medical care, school accountability and school choice programs, and statistical methods in health and economics. Professor Staiger has published numerous peer-reviewed articles in leading journals in the fields of economics, medicine, and education. His work has been supported by grants from government agencies and foundations, including the National Institute of Aging, National Institute of Child Health and Development, Agency for Healthcare Research and Quality, U.S. Department of Education, the Robert Wood Johnson Foundation, and the Spencer Foundation. Dr. Staiger earned his baccalaureate degree in economics and mathematics from Williams College (1984), a doctoral degree in Economics from MIT (1990), and was an NIH postdoctoral fellow at the National Bureau of Economic Research (1994–1995).

David Auerbach, PhD earned his PhD in health policy, with a concentration in economics, from Harvard University in 2002. He then worked briefly with the Research Triangle Institute, working on projects concerning long-term care and has since been Associate then Principal Analyst with the Congressional Budget Office starting in 2003. There, he has researched issues relating to competition in Medicare, health insurance coverage, and geographic variation in healthcare spending—always maintaining an interest in issues surrounding the healthcare workforce. This research at the CBO has resulted in many publications, both in the peer-reviewed literature and on behalf of the CBO, as well as various cost estimates of proposed legislation. He has published numerous papers with Drs. Buerhaus and Staiger over the period from 1999 to 2007.

CHAPTER 1

Introduction and Overview

The nursing workforce comprises registered nurses (RNs), licensed practical nurses (LPNs), and assistants such as aides, orderlies, and personal care attendants. Although there are more than 200 different health professions in the United States, the nursing profession is the largest, and its members are involved in nearly every facet of the healthcare delivery system. In 2004, there were 2.9 million individuals estimated to hold a license to practice as an RN. Approximately 83% of the RNs, or 2.4 million, were employed in nursing with most (1.7 million) working on a full-time basis (U.S. Department of Health and Human Services, Health Resources and Services Administration [HRSA], 2006). The nurse labor market in the United States encompasses all of the major healthcare organizations that employ RNs and other nursing personnel, including both inpatient and outpatient settings that provide a range of healthcare services, spanning preventative, acute, chronic, long-term, and end of life care. Assuring an adequate supply of RNs engaged in producing health care for millions of people each and every day, particularly during periods of nursing shortages, ranks among the most important challenges facing employers, nurses, and nursing educators.

During the past few years, the healthcare industry, media, and policy makers have become increasingly interested in what seems to be a chronic shortage of hospital RNs. Public opinion surveys find that the majority of Americans believe the current shortage is a serious problem and threatens to harm the quality of patient care (Blendon, DesRoches, Brodie, Benson, Allison, Schneider, et al., 2002; Donelan, Buerhaus, DeRoches, & Dittus, 2007). In light of projections of a very large shortage of RNs developing in the years ahead—a topic we will consider in great depth throughout this book—there is a pressing need to act on the knowledge that RNs significantly impact the quality and safety of patient care, assure access to care, and that it might be necessary to intervene to improve the performance of both the nurse labor and education markets. Yet, because studies by economists, policy makers, and others have focused mostly on physicians and the costs of the healthcare system, and far less on nursing, little objective data have been available that provide a comprehensive understanding of

1

the RN workforce. Consequently, there is a large gap in understanding the significance of important changes occurring in the RN workforce and an even larger gap in data describing the performance of the nurse labor market in the United States.

The purpose of this book is to provide a timely, comprehensive, and in-depth understanding of the RN workforce in the United States. Using plain language, we describe key changes in the demand and supply of the RN workforce over the past few decades and discuss the implications for the future. In addition, we discuss policy options that are aimed at hastening the adjustments that health-care organizations (primarily hospitals), RNs, and nursing education programs need to undertake to prepare for the expected challenges that lie ahead.

This book is an outgrowth of a considerable body of research that we have conducted, beginning with analyses of trends in employment and earnings in the nurse labor market during the early 1980s to the late 1990s. This research led to subsequent studies concerned with identifying the reasons for the rapid aging of the population of RNs, examining how RNs impact the quality and safety of patient care, projecting the future age and supply of the RN workforce, and anticipating the implications for employers, educators, and the nursing profession. We have also examined the nature of the nursing work environment, which many RNs believe is the root cause of both previous shortages and the current hospital RN shortage. This body of research has resulted in numerous articles that have been published in various health services research and nursing policy and management journals. However, no one article or combination of articles pulls together the key data on the RN workforce, explains how the RN labor market operates, or dissects the key forces that are expected to shape the future demand and supply of RNs. This book is intended to address these discontinuities by bringing together all of our previous work on the nursing workforce into one coherent and integrated package. In this book we update and extend our earlier research, analyze new data that have become available, add more information on several key issues that were not included in previous publications, and discuss implications and policy options with a fresh perspective and in much greater detail.

FOCUS ON REGISTERED NURSES

For several reasons, most of the content of this book focuses on RNs. First, there are more complete data on RNs versus LPNs and aides, and data are available over a longer number of years. Second, RNs' legal scope of nursing practice entrusts them with greater clinical and ethical responsibilities and the performance of many more nursing activities than either LPNs or aides. Third, there are far more individuals holding a license to practice nursing as an RN than as an LPN. And finally, because of their greater education requirements, legal standing, and capability to perform a greater number and variety of nursing activities and procedures, RNs have a much larger impact on the productivity of the nursing workforce, earn higher wages, and exert a much greater effect on healthcare spending, quality of care, and patient safety. Our focus on RNs is not to imply that the contributions of LPNs and aides are not important; they are. However, given the limited data on LPNs and aides, it is impossible to consider them in this book to the same degree as RNs.

Advance practice nurses (APNs) are an important and growing component of the nursing workforce. An APN is an RN who has completed advanced education and clinical practice in a program of study beyond his or her initial, or basic, nursing education that is required of all RNs. APNs include nurse anesthetists, clinical nurse specialists, nurse practitioners, and nurse midwives. However, because APNs make up only about 8% of the entire RN workforce, and because their nursing practice is more specialized, this book does not focus on APNs.

ECONOMIC PERSPECTIVE

Although we are guided primarily by an economic perspective in our approach to analyzing the RN workforce, the reader does not need to be an economist or have a background in economics to understand the content discussed in each chapter. We specifically attempt to minimize the use of technical terms and economic jargon, trying instead to use ordinary language to describe topics and data presented throughout the book. For the most part, we rely on the economic concepts of demand and supply. These concepts, while rather simple and straightforward, are extremely useful in organizing and describing the wide-ranging forces that are constantly reshaping the composition, size, and impact of the RN workforce. Understanding the forces affecting the demand and supply of RNs also helps to comprehend trends in earnings and employment, the impact of managed care on the nurse labor market, development and resolution of nursing shortages, formation of polices aimed at strengthening the current and future workforce, and the exploration of many other topics that we will address.

OMINOUS OUTLOOK

One of the motivations for writing this book is our concern that the RN workforce, already experiencing troubles today, will be unable to respond effectively to the many challenges that lie ahead, particularly as the healthcare system adjusts to the demands of an aging baby boom generation during the next decade and beyond. As we will see later, and particularly in Chapter 10, in the next 2 decades the supply of RNs in the United States will continue to change dramatically, marked by a rapidly aging RN workforce that will plateau in size as large numbers of RNs retire. Because the demand for RNs is expected to increase steadily over the same period, we expect a very large shortage of RNs to develop in the latter half of the next decade. The implications of doing nothing to mitigate the development of the shortage, or at least better prepare for its consequences, means that patients will have decreased access to health care, receive poorer quality of care, be at greater risk for unsafe care, and be called upon to finance more costly health care. Our hope is that this book provides the data that helps increase the commitment and motivation of those concerned with the well-being of the nursing workforce to act now while it is possible to implement more effective and lower cost strategies to minimize the impact of these expected consequences.

OVERVIEW OF BOOK

We have organized our analysis and discussion of the nursing workforce in the United States into five sections that contain a total of 15 chapters. The sections and the chapters they contain are designed to build logically upon the content presented in previous sections and chapters.

Section One: Introduction and Overview

The purpose of the first section of the book is to provide an overall introduction and overview of the healthcare system, the nursing workforce, and an understanding of basic economic concepts that underpin the performance of the RN labor market. Specifically, in the current chapter, we describe the content that will be presented in each chapter of the book and, following this, conclude by briefly explaining the data sources we used to conduct analyses of the RN workforce and produce the large number and variety of tables and figures showing key data and trends throughout.

Next, in **Chapter 2**, we present an overview of the health delivery system in the United States, including trends in utilization and spending among the major sectors of the healthcare system. We then describe how RNs and the settings in which they work fit into the overall organizations of health care, and then focus on issues relating to RNs specifically, describing employment, earnings, demographic, and educational characteristics of the RN workforce. The characteristics of the healthcare delivery system and of the RN workforce are discussed using both the latest data as well as using data over the last several decades to identify changes over time. We also attempt to place the RN workforce into a broader social context by comparing their education, earnings, and hours in the workforce, to those in other comparable occupations.

In **Chapter 3** we provide a brief primer on demand and supply in a labor market. We begin by focusing on the demand side of the labor market, describing how the wage and other factors influence the hours of work that potential employers want to purchase from the suppliers of labor. We then consider the supply side, discussing how the wage and other factors influence the hours of work that potential employees are willing to provide. The remainder of this chapter puts the two sides of the market together to show how supply and demand interact to determine the wage and employment level in a labor market. Wages play a key role, rising or falling to equalize the employment level demanded by employers with that which employees are willing to provide. In the final section of the chapter, we discuss what happens when the wage fails to adjust, leading to shortages. We urge the reader who is unfamiliar with the concepts of demand and supply in relation to the functioning of a labor market to become familiar with the basic economic concepts contained in this chapter.

Section Two: Factors That Influence the Demand for RNs

The overall purpose of Section Two is to evaluate the likely future demand for RNs in the United States. We begin in **Chapter 4** by identifying and discussing the factors that drive the demand for health care and the demand for RNs, clarifying the economic meaning of demand as opposed to need, and explaining the demand for health and the demand for healthcare services and treatments. Most of the factors that determine the overall growth in the demand for health care—population, income, and technology—are reasonably predictable. The demand for RNs is derived from these factors and is reflected by hospitals' and other healthcare delivery organizations' employment of RNs. Thus, in this chapter we also discuss the economic considerations that hospitals and other healthcare organizations take into account when deciding how many RNs to employ. Following this, we provide a brief discussion of two federal government forecasts of the future demand for RNs through 2020.

Far less is known, however, about how changes in healthcare organization and financing are likely to affect the future demand for RNs. Over the last decade, managed care organizations have come to dominate the healthcare delivery system in the United States and resulted in slowing the rate of growth in employment of RNs in the 1990s, particularly in hospitals. This slow down raises questions concerning the potential implications that managed care organizations will have on the future demand for RNs as these organizations continue to grow and mature. We assess these questions in **Chapter 5**, which begins with some background on the growth and impact of managed care organizations in the United States. We then identify the states that were early adopters of managed care relative to those who lagged behind. Next, we analyze data on employment and earnings of RNs in early adopter states relative to the laggard states to document the link between the spread of managed care and the employment and earnings of RNs. We then identify trends that are currently emerging in states that were early adopters of managed care because they are likely to shed some light on what we can expect in the coming decade. The emerging trends in these states are likely to be an indicator of the next wave of innovation that will impact the RN labor market.

Section Three: Factors That Influence the Supply of RNs

In the five chapters that constitute this section, we provide a comprehensive discussion of the forces that are behind the expected near- and long-term changes in the supply of RNs. As hinted at earlier, unless significant improvements in our long-term assessment of the future supply of RNs are achieved, the expected changes in the age and supply of RNs indicate serious trouble ahead.

We begin in **Chapter 6** by analyzing the short-run labor supply decisions of RNs, which refer to whether currently existing RNs participate in the nursing workforce and the number of hours they are willing to work. We devote a large part of the chapter examining economic and sociodemographic factors that determine existing RNs' employment decisions. When there are shortages of RNs, increasing the supply of RNs can come initially from already existing RNs by inducing some of those who are not working to reenter the workforce or by persuading others who are already employed to work additional hours (switching from part-time to full-time hours, working overtime hours, or working a second job). Because economic factors can be changed in a shorter period of time than noneconomic factors, our discussion in this chapter emphasizes how wages and sources of income unrelated to the RNs' earnings influence labor supply decisions. We then move to illustrate how RN wages and nonwage income have changed when the national economy has experienced periods of rapid and slow growth and the different patterns of RN employment and earnings growth during these boom and bust years. Next, we explain striking changes in RN employment that have occurred in recent years, particularly in hospitals, showing once again how changes in RN wages and nonwage income drive yearly changes in RN employment. Chapter 6 concludes by examining the characteristics of the RNs who have supplied the RN labor market since 2000—

primarily older and foreign-born RNs—an unmistakable signal of how the future RN workforce is evolving.

In **Chapter 7** we shift our attention away from the factors that determine the labor supply decisions and hours of work by existing RNs and focus on the factors that determine the number of RNs that will be available to supply the RN workforce in the future. Among the key factors are the number of women in the United States population between the ages of 20 and 40 that represent the majority of individuals from which nursing education programs draw applicants, and the propensity of people in the potential applicant pools to enter the RN workforce now that there are so many new career opportunities for women. Other factors that exert an important influence on the long-run supply of RNs that we discuss include the affect of age in influencing the number of RNs that enter and leave the workforce over the course of their work life, economic factors that affect the decision to become an RN, alternative sources of RN supply (namely, foreign educated RNs), and problems that constrain the capacity of nursing education programs. We bring the chapter to a close by summarizing projections of the long-run supply of RNs made by the authors in 2000 and by HRSA in 2002.

Chapter 8 concentrates exclusively on one of the factors exerting a disproportionately large effect on the long-run supply of RNs: the declining preference of women for a career in nursing. The aspirations of most people for a particular career or profession are frequently derived from motivations and personal intent unrelated to economic considerations, and during the 1950s, 1960s, and much of the 1970s, nursing was a popular career option for many women. Since the 1980s, however, there has been a declining propensity of younger aged women choosing nursing as a career. In this chapter we assess the changes in society that have altered perceptions of the value of becoming a professional nurse. Using 3 decades' worth of data from college freshman men and women, we examine the increase in women's interest in careers traditionally dominated by men and the consequent decline in career aspirations for nursing. Recent evidence, however, suggests that there might be a resurgence of interest in nursing among young women and, to a lesser extent, young men.

Because there has been a substantial expansion in the number of associate's degree nursing education programs since the 1970s, and because the average age of graduates from these programs is considerably older than baccalaureate degree graduates, some believe that the aging of the RN workforce is due to the growth in the number of associate's degree graduates. The focus of **Chapter 9** is to examine trends in nursing education and age of students and determine, in part, whether there is evidence to support this belief. Findings suggest that the age of graduates from all nursing education programs peaked in 1996 and has been declining thereafter. This finding reflects two ongoing trends. First, the age of graduates increased as the large baby boom cohorts of the 1950s passed through the educational system, but now these cohorts have aged beyond the point where they are populating nursing education programs. Second, the more recent cohorts are much more likely to enter nursing at older ages (late 20s and 30s) rather than entering nursing degree programs directly after high school.

The effect of the trends discussed in Chapters 7, 8, and 9 on the age of the current RN workforce and on the future supply of RNs is the subject of **Chapter 10**. This chapter describes trends in the average age of the RN workforce over the past 2 decades, explains a forecasting model that we have developed, and describes our forecasts of the future age composition and total number of full-time equivalent RNs that will be available over the next 2 decades. We start by explaining how the factors that affect the long-run supply of RNs, as discussed in Chapter 7, are used to develop forecasts of the RN workforce years into the future. Then, we describe the results of these forecasts up to 2025, highlighting recent trends, such as the later age of individuals entering the nursing profession, that have a particularly important impact on our forecasts of the future age and supply of RNs. Our supply projections, when compared to the government's forecasts of the number of RNs who will be required in the future, paint a worrisome picture of the future.

Section Four: Shortages of Hospital RNs, Impact on Quality, and RN Working Conditions

In this section, we describe shortages of hospital RNs, the impact of the current shortage on the quality and safety of patient care, and whether, from RNs' perspective, hospital working conditions have improved or worsened in recent years.

We start in **Chapter 11** by examining shortages of hospital RNs. Using an economic perspective, we describe how shortages develop and are resolved in a competitive and properly functioning labor market and what measures are typically used to indicate a shortage of RNs in hospitals. Next, we examine the development of shortages of hospital RNs over the past 50 years, focusing once again on the key role that wages exert in bringing about a balance between the amount of labor supplied by RNs and the amount demanded by hospitals. We examine shortages in the 1960s and 1970s in which RN wages did not adjust rapidly, shortages in the 1980s when the increase in demand for RNs exceeded the growth in the supply of RNs, and then focus on what happened in the nurse labor market during the 1990s when the rapid spread of managed care slowed the growth in RN demand. Next, we discuss an important change in the nurse labor market in which the current shortage of hospital RNs, which began in

1998 in hospital intensive care units and operating rooms, was driven by changes in the *supply* of RNs. In fact, we compare the development of this shortage with the first light winds blowing onshore from the massive nursing shortage "hurricane" that is rapidly strengthening out to sea, obtaining its energy from the steadily aging RN workforce and expected to reach land in less than 10 years.

Chapter 12 focuses on the impact of the *current* hospital RN shortage on the quality and safety of patient care. We set the stage by first reviewing the major developments of what has now become a serious national effort to improve the quality and safety of health care, noting the activities of key groups who have begun to realize that the current nursing shortage is as much of a quality and safety problem as it is a vexing problem for workforce planners. After briefly reviewing the growing body of research that demonstrates a relationship between hospital nurse staffing and an increasing number of adverse patient outcomes, including mortality, we examine the results of recent national surveys of RNs, physicians, hospital chief executive officers, and hospital chief nursing officers. Survey results reveal how these clinicians and executives perceive the prevalence and severity of the shortage in the communities and hospitals where RNs and administrators work and doctors admit patients. The survey findings provide a sobering picture of how the current shortage has impacted various indicators of hospitals' capacity, care delivery processes, RNs' ability to provide nursing care, and the Institute of Medicine's six aims for improving the quality of healthcare systems: safe, timely, efficient, effective, equitable, and patient-centered care.

But there is some good news contained in **Chapter 13** that focuses on the quality of the hospital workplace environment where RNs provide patient care. Based on three national RN surveys conducted in 2002, 2004, and 2006, we examine whether RNs perceive any changes in the workplace environment and their jobs. We compare RNs' perceptions over the time covered by the three surveys to probe four major themes: extent and severity of the current nursing shortage; causes, effects, and hospitals' responses to the nursing shortage; quality of the hospital work environment, including staffing, hours, and their relationships with nurses, physicians, and managers, etc.; and satisfaction with their current job, decision to become a nurse, and RNs' willingness to recommend the nursing profession to others. We find areas where there has not been much improvement but a good number of areas where there is evidence that the workplace has improved. These survey results are encouraging because they provide evidence that change and improvement in the hospital workplace can occur rapidly during a time of shortage.

Section Five: Implications and Recommendations

Section five brings the book to a close by pulling together the main content of all of the preceding chapters and converging on the many important implications for the future. Failing to anticipate what is likely to develop over the next decade, and failing to act on these implications, will place hospitals, RNs, patients, and nursing education programs in peril. In Chapter 14 we describe the implications of failing to act, and in Chapter 15 we provide suggestions on what strategies we might follow to minimize these implications.

As the demand for RNs continues to grow during the foreseeable future, the RN workforce will become increasingly older and, as large numbers of RNs retire in the years ahead, the future supply of RNs will grow more slowly resulting in large shortages of RNs. In **Chapter 14** we describe how hospitals are likely to respond to the future shortage using economic and noneconomic strategies they have used in the past, but the magnitude of the shortage will be so great that it will take many years before the nurse labor market adjusts and reaches a new equilibrium that eventually resolves the shortage. During this time, we anticipate that the RN workforce will continue to grow older, the number of foreign-born and foreign-educated RNs will increase, and, as real RN wages increase, some hospitals will attempt to substitute LPNs and nursing assistants for RNs. Additionally, during this transition period, patients are likely to bear the costs of lower nurse staffing levels that will result in delays in receiving care, lower quality, decreased safety, and a higher risk of experiencing an adverse outcome. While an older and more experienced RN workforce will help mitigate the threat to quality and safety, the physical demands of nursing will place older RNs at increased risk of injury and promote the withdrawal of some RNs from the workforce. Hospitals will be challenged to find ways to provide nursing care using an older RN workforce, maintain recent gains in improving their workplace environment, and ensure that the quality and safety of patient care does not deteriorate to the point where they risk losing their reputation, accreditation, full payment, and market share. Nursing education programs can anticipate growing pressures to resolve the capacity constraints that are currently causing them to turn away thousands of qualified applicants. They can also expect to modify their curriculum to better prepare RNs for providing nursing care that is delivered predominantly in outpatient and community-based settings and to an increasingly diverse and older population.

Chapter 15, the final chapter of this book, discusses two sets of policies for public and private policy makers that are designed to help guide responses to the implications discussed in Chapter 14. The first set of policies is aimed at helping the RN workforce *transition* through the potentially long period of time required before a new equilibrium is reached in the long-run demand and supply of RNs. These strategies are intended to maximize RNs' ability to endure a future shortage in the least costly way, assure that patients receive high quality and safe nursing care, and protect patients from disruptions in access to care. RNs can be helped through this transition by pursuing actions that involve technology and a better use of personnel, improving the efficiency of systems, implementing work redesign, improving management, and avoiding over-regulation. Transition strategies also should focus on accommodating an older RN workforce, improving working conditions, expanding the capacity of nursing education programs, and informing the public about the opportunities in the nursing profession. Beyond transition policies, we discuss long-run strategies that are aimed at expanding the number of RNs in the labor market. These strategies involve removing barriers to enter the nursing profession and revaluing the social contributions of RNs.

DATA ON THE NURSING WORKFORCE

These 15 chapters provide an abundance of tables and figures showing key data, trends, and implications of the various topics discussed in each chapter. To conduct analyses and produce these figures and tables, we have constructed large and comprehensive data sets on the nursing workforce in the United States. The data come from three major sources: the Current Population Survey (CPS) obtained from the U.S. Census Bureau; the National Sample Survey of Registered Nurses (NSSRN) obtained from the federal government's Health Resources and Services Administration; and national surveys of RNs and other health professions conducted as part of privately funded research projects. Throughout the book, we refer to these data frequently and present figures and tables based on our calculations using these data. We conclude Chapter 1 by briefly describing these data sources and highlighting their major strengths and weakness. A more detailed description of these data is provided in Appendix 1-1.

Current Population Survey (CPS)

The CPS is a household-based survey that is administered monthly by the U.S. Census Bureau. The survey is widely used by researchers and by the U.S. Department of Labor to estimate current trends in unemployment, employment, and earnings. The survey is administered monthly to a nationally representative sample of 60,000 households and obtains data from approximately 100,000 individuals, including RNs, LPNs, and aides. Data on employment and earnings of RNs were derived from individuals in the CPS who reported their occupation as RNs during the period 1973 to 2006 (N = 90,145). CPS data offer several advantages over other data commonly used to analyze the nursing workforce. Specifically, the CPS is the only source of *annual* data for RNs. Annual data derived from consistent surveys allows for more accurate modeling of workforce trends. An additional advantage of CPS data is that we are able to obtain information on virtually the entire U.S. workforce and, therefore, we can examine trends in employment and earnings in nursing and compare them to other professions.

Although the CPS data have many advantages, they have some limitations. First, because the CPS is a general survey of the workforce, it does not ask many of the more detailed RN-specific questions concerning educational preparation, clinical background, and employment settings that are typically asked of RNs in a more focused survey, such as the NSSRN. A second limitation is that the survey instrument used to gather data for the CPS was revised periodically, making it difficult to compare some estimates across years. For example, in January 1994 interviewers began probing more thoroughly for jobs in which the individual worked only a few hours in the week of the survey. This change probably resulted in an increase in the number of nursing personnel who reported being employed, particularly for part-time workers, and might have slightly affected estimates of earnings and occupation. Between 2000 and 2002 the CPS changed the way it reported occupation and industry categories in a way that might have affected the estimated number of auxiliary nursing personnel (LPNs and nurses' aides) and some estimates of RN employment in specific industries such as home health care. On balance, we believe that these changes had little impact on most of the estimates that we report, but some caution must be used when comparing the most recent estimates to those of earlier years.

National Sample Survey of Registered Nurses (NSSRN)

The NSSRN is the most well known and comprehensive source of data on individuals who have active licenses to practice in the United States as RNs whether or not they are actually employed in nursing. The surveys have been conducted every 4 years from 1977 to 2004 and provide information on the number of RNs, their educational background and areas of clinical specialty, employment settings, positions, salaries, geographic distribution, and personal characteristics including gender, racial/ethnic background, age, and family status. We use data from all surveys combined into a single data set of questions that were as consistent as possible, with the total number of RN respondents in all surveys totaling 244,153.

The federal government's surveys of RNs are often considered to be the gold standard in providing descriptive statistics about the characteristics of RNs in the United States and are therefore helpful in identifying trends about nurses over time. Nevertheless, these data are limited because they do not reveal how RNs perceive their experience as nurses. These surveys were not designed to assess, for example, RNs' views about their jobs, the environment where they practice nursing, the impact of nursing shortages, professional relationships, or many other aspects of being a professional nurse that, together with descriptive information, help to provide a more complete picture of the RN workforce. In addition, we note that the NSSRN survey changed its questions about hours worked and earnings between 2000 and 2004 (in contrast to earlier surveys, the 2004 survey only asked about hours worked in the past week and explicitly instructed respondents to include paid on-call hours in their hours totals as well as in their reported earnings). This makes some comparisons over time difficult in certain key employment questions.

In **Figure 1-1**, we present data on RN employment derived from CPS data and corresponding estimates derived from the 1977, 1984, 1988, 1992, 1996, 2000, and 2004 NSSRNs. As can be seen, the estimates derived from these two sources of RNs in the United States are quite similar.

Figure 1-1   Number of Employed RNs Using Current Population Survey (CPS) and National Sample Survey of Registered Nurses (NSSRN), 1977–2006

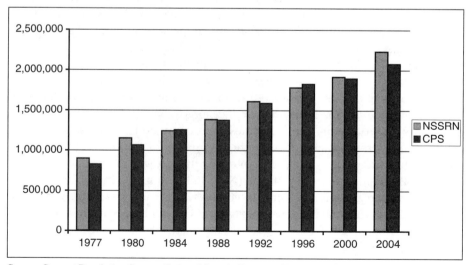

Source: Current Population Survey; National Sample Survey of Registered Nurses

Privately Funded National Surveys

To address some of the limitations of the CPS and NSSRNs, the third source of data we use comes from a family of national surveys conducted as part of a project designed to assess the effectiveness of the Johnson & Johnson Campaign for Nursing's Future. This campaign was launched in February 2002 in response to concerns about the current nursing shortage and projections of an even more severe future shortage. The goals ongoing of this campaign are to raise public awareness of nursing as a career, attract more people into the nursing profession, retain current nurses in clinical care positions, and increase the capacity of the nation's nursing education programs.

Johnson & Johnson engaged a collaboration of researchers from Vanderbilt University and the Massachusetts General Hospital to determine awareness and impact of the campaign.[1] As part of this project, researchers worked with several survey research firms to conduct surveys of various populations, including parents and their teenagers (2003); nursing students (2003); RNs (2004 and 2006); physicians (2004); hospital chief executive officers (CEOs) and hospital chief nursing officers (CNOs; 2005); and the public (2007). Each of the surveys was designed to address unique topics and obtain data tailored specifically to each group. Because many of the same questions were included in each of the surveys, it is possible to compare results among the surveyed populations.

In this book, we use data from only the national random sample surveys of health professionals, which, with the exception of the survey of CEOs, obtained response rates exceeding 50%. The 2004 survey of RNs (N = 1697), 2006 survey of RNs (N = 1392), 2004 physician survey (N = 400), and 2005 hospital CEO (N = 142) and CNO surveys (N = 222) included questions that assessed the following themes: extent and severity of the current nursing shortage; causes, effects, and hospitals' responses to the nursing shortage; characteristics of the nursing work environment, including quality of professional practice and relationships among nurses, physicians, and management; RNs' satisfaction with their current job, satisfaction with their decisions to become nurses, perceptions of the nursing profession, and willingness to recommend nursing as a career to others; and awareness and impact of the Campaign for Nursing's Future. In addition to the surveys that were conducted for this project, we also made use of an earlier 2002 national survey of RNs (N = 4108) conducted by *NurseWeek* and the American Organization of Nurse Executives. This survey was directed by the same Vanderbilt and Massachusetts researchers, and the survey instrument

---

[1] Specifically, Dr. Peter Buerhaus is the principal investigator of this project. The campaign played no role in the design, preparation, or approval of this book.

developed for that project was used, with minor modification, in the subsequent 2004 and 2006 national surveys of RNs.

The chief advantages of these surveys are that they are the most current national data that assess dimensions of the RN workforce in hospitals and other healthcare settings, and they were conducted during the current hospital RN shortage. By using many identical questions, the data permit comparative assessments of RNs, physicians, and hospital executives' perceptions of the prevalence and severity of the current shortage of RNs and whether and how the shortage has impacted the quality and safety of patient care. In the case of RNs, the three surveys permit comparisons across time to determine whether RNs perceive changes in the characteristics of their workplace environment, among other things, from 2002 to 2006. The main disadvantages of these surveys are the sampling and nonsampling errors that affect surveys in general.

A FINAL COMMENT

Throughout this book we will often discuss the RN workforce in terms of changes in employment levels, earnings growth, the presence of a shortage, or other impersonal concepts. While important in understanding certain aspects of the RN workforce, references such as these mask the fact that we are acutely aware that the professional nursing workforce is made up of individual RNs. After investing in a formidable education program to become an RN, these individuals provide nursing services in thousands of settings across the country that make an important difference to hundreds of thousands of people each and every day. We are struck both by the complexity of the healthcare system and how RNs manage to navigate the system in an effort to promote the well-being of patients and protect them from unintended harm when the system falters or breaks down. So much of what RNs do and accomplish is very difficult to measure, let alone describe, and we realize that our attempt to analyze the RN workforce in this book falls well short of providing a comprehensive depiction of the vital importance of these healthcare providers. Nevertheless, we hope that our efforts are helpful in providing information to better guide policy makers and other decision makers to act in ways that benefit and strengthen this national resource.

Next, in Chapter 2, we begin our analysis of key data, trends, and implications for the future of the nursing workforce in the United States. We start by providing an overview of the health delivery system in the United States, which has expanded and changed over the past few decades, and we describe how the RN workforce itself has grown and evolved over time.

Appendix 1-1

Detailed Information About Data Sources

In this appendix we provide a more detailed description of the data sources we used to conduct the various analyses discussed throughout the book as well as produce tables and figures that show key data, trends, and implications for the future. We discuss the Current Population Survey (CPS), National Sample Survey of Registered Nurses (NSSRNs), and various surveys that were conducted for a project evaluating the Johnson & Johnson Campaign for Nursing's Future.

CURRENT POPULATION SURVEY

As mentioned earlier, the CPS is a household-based survey that is administered monthly by the U.S. Census Bureau. The survey is widely used by researchers and by the U.S. Department of Labor to estimate current trends in unemployment, employment, and earnings. The survey is administered monthly to a nationally representative sample of 60,000 households and obtains data from approximately 100,000 individuals, including RNs, LPNs, and aides. Each month one-quarter of the sample (the outgoing rotation group) is asked detailed questions about current employment status, hours worked, earnings, occupation, industry employed, etc. For the research reported in this book, we used data from the CPS Outgoing Rotation Group Annual Merged files.

In addition to demographic information collected in each month of the survey, detailed questions about employment (including occupation and hours worked) have been asked since 1973. Between 1973 and 1978, these questions were asked of all May survey respondents. From 1979 through 2006 (the latest year for which complete data were available), one-quarter of the sample in every month was asked the employment questions. The sample in each year was a representative cross section of individuals, but each housing unit appears in the sample twice (exactly 1 year apart). Thus, some individuals might appear twice in the sample.

Data on employment and earnings of RNs were derived from individuals in the CPS data who reported their occupation as an RN during the period 1973 to 2006 (N=90,145). Hourly wages were calculated as usual weekly earnings divided by usual weekly hours. Wages were adjusted for inflation using the Consumer Price Index for all goods in urban areas (CPI-U) and are usually reported in constant 2006 dollars. Employment was measured as full-time equivalents (FTE; i.e., the number of full-time employees plus one-half the number of part-time employees) where full-time employment is defined as working 30 or more hours per week. In most of our analyses we report data on RNs as FTEs and apply their survey-assigned sampling weights, making estimates representative of the United States noninstitutionalized population.

While national sample surveys of the population of RNs in the United States conducted by HRSA (described below) use the same definition of an FTE, we use "usual hours worked" rather than self-reports of employment status to determine part-time status due to inconsistency in the CPS measure of self-reports of part-time status across years. Our measure produces a similar number of nursing FTEs in 2000 and 2004 as does the national surveys of RNs used by HRSA.

To produce the forecasts of the future age and supply of RNs described in Chapter 10, we restricted the CPS sample to RNs between the ages of 23 and 64 (N = 88,985) to be assured of robust sample sizes at each single year of age. RNs outside of these age ranges generally account for roughly 3% of the workforce, on average, and all supply forecasts are adjusted to account for this exclusion (overall forecasts are adjusted by multiplying the projected RN workforce by 1.03).

Because of the large samples being used in the CPS, all trends reported throughout this book have standard errors of less than 2%. As a result, for example, for all outcome variables reported, one can reject the null hypotheses that there were no changes over time or no differences between high and low HMO enrollment states at the 0.01 level (see Chapter 5).

As noted earlier, the CPS is the only source of *annual* data for RNs, and thus annual data derived from consistent surveys allow for much more accurate modeling of workforce trends—specifically, the forecasts of the future age and supply of the RN workforce described in Chapter 10. A further advantage of CPS data is that we are able to obtain information on virtually the entire United States workforce, which allows us to examine trends in employment and earnings in nursing and compare them to other professions.

The limitations of the CPS primarily involve changes made in January 1994 to the survey instrument that was used to gather data. The revision resulted in interviewers probing more thoroughly for jobs in which the individual worked only a few hours in the week of the survey. This change more than likely led to an increase in the number of nursing personnel who reported being employed, particularly for part-time workers, and might have slightly affected estimates of earnings and occupation. Therefore, one must use some caution when comparing 1994-2001 estimates with those of earlier years. Further revisions were phased in between 2000 and 2002 that changed occupational categories relevant to LPNs and nursing aides in industry settings such as home health care and ambulatory categories. Because of these changes, we do not include detailed estimates for LPNs or aides.

NATIONAL SAMPLE SURVEY OF REGISTERED NURSES (NSSRN)

The NSSRN has been conducted every 4 years during the past 4 decades and provides the most well-known and comprehensive statistics on individuals who have licenses to practice as RNs in the United States whether or not they are actually employed in nursing. The NSSRN provides detailed information on the number of RNs, their educational backgrounds, areas of clinical specialty, employment settings, positions, salaries, geographic distribution, and personal characteristics including gender, racial/ethnic background, age, and family status. A comprehensive technical description of each of the surveys conducted thus far can be found in each of the reports that describe the survey findings. We summarize the main attributes of the surveys in the next four paragraphs using text taken from the report describing the 2004 NSSRN, the most recent survey conducted (HRSA, 2006).

Beginning in the mid-1970s, the federal government's Division of Nursing within the Health Resources and Services Administration (HRSA) has been overseeing the development and administration of the national surveys. Employing various consultants and research and survey firms, the Division of Nursing conducted surveys in 1977, 1980, 1984, 1988, 1992, 1996, 2000, and 2004. Since 2001, HRSA's Bureau of Health Professions (BHPr) began to assume a significantly larger role in the overall conduct of the NSSRN, including leading and directing the 2004 survey, the eighth NSSRN in this series. The BHPr also provides analytic support in assessing the short- and long-term supply of RNs in the workforce and in estimating the nation's requirements for RNs (the federal government prefers to use the term "requirements" rather than "demand" for RNs).

Over the years the surveys have been conducted, a number of improvements in the sampling procedures have been accomplished, as have improvements in follow-up activities to nonresponders. In addition, the questionnaire used to obtain the survey data has been modified slightly from survey to survey. For example, beginning with the 2000 survey, items that assessed RNs' work satisfaction were included in the survey questionnaire. However, as in prior studies, the survey instrument was designed to ensure that the data collected from study to study provide sufficient continuity so that an evaluation can be made of trends in nursing.

With each administration of the survey, the questionnaire is mailed to individuals from samples drawn from each state's list of active licensees (no single list of licensed RNs exits in the United States). Disproportionate sampling across the states was used to provide estimates of the number of nurses in each state, with larger proportions of licensees sampled in states with fewer registrants than in states with more registrants. In the 2000 study, the sampling methodology included oversampling. Because many RNs maintain licenses in more than one state, a weighting procedure was used to account for duplication of licensees from state to state so that estimates could be developed of the number of individuals who hold active licenses to practice as RNs regardless of the number of state licenses they hold.

Most of the surveys have obtained data from a large number of RNs who agreed to respond to the survey. To illustrate, in the 2000 survey, responses from 35,579 RNs were used to derive estimates of the number of RNs in the United States that was estimated at 2,694,540 RNs. With respect to the most recent survey conducted in 2004, the initial sample selection consisted of 56,917 licenses, of which 4250 were identified as duplicates for nurses licensed in other states. After taking account of duplications and sampling frame errors, a total of 50,691 RNs were estimated to be eligible to participate in the survey. A total of 35,724 individual RNs responded to the survey for a final response rate of 70.47%. After weighting these responses, it is estimated that there are 2,909,357 RNs employed or living in the United States, an increase of 7.9% or 212,817 above the 2,696,540 licensed RNs estimated in 2000. Finally, based on the 2004 survey, the estimate of the total RN population in the United States is between 2,897,467 and 2,921,467 RNs at the 95% confidence level, with a margin of error of +/– 0.7%.

As pointed out earlier, between 2000 and 2004, the NSSRN changed its questions about hours worked and earnings (in contrast to earlier surveys, the 2004 survey only asked about hours worked in the past week and explicitly instructed respondents to include paid on-call hours in their hours totals as well as in their reported earnings). This makes some comparisons over time difficult in certain key employment questions; in some cases, 2004 data were not used, and in other cases we attempted to make the comparisons consistent with earlier questions by subtracting out paid on-call hours. Generally, in the analyses described throughout this book, we used data from all NSSRN surveys from 1977 to 2004 combined into a single data set of questions that were as consistent as possible, with the total number of RN respondents in all surveys totaling 244,153.

Although the federal government's surveys of RNs are often considered to be the gold standard in providing descriptive statistics about the characteristics of RNs in the United States and are therefore helpful in identifying trends about nurses over time, nevertheless these data are limited because they do not reveal how RNs perceive their experiences as nurses. These surveys were not designed to assess, for example, RNs' views about their jobs, the environments where they practice nursing, the impact of nursing shortages, professional relationships, or many other aspects of being a professional nurse that, together with descriptive information, help to provide a more complete picture of the RN workforce. In addition, the NSSRNs are not designed to determine how others in society view the nursing profession and who and what influences people to pursue a career in nursing.

NATIONAL SURVEYS CONDUCTED FOR THE JOHNSON & JOHNSON CAMPAIGN FOR NURSING'S FUTURE

To address some of the limitations of the NSSRNs, the third source of data we used came from a family of national surveys conducted for a project designed to assess the effectiveness of the Johnson & Johnson Campaign for Nursing's Future. This campaign was launched in February 2002 in response to the nursing shortage that had begun several years earlier and due to concerns over an even more severe shortage projected to develop in the future. The campaign's goals are aimed at raising public awareness of nursing as a career, attracting more people into the nursing profession, retaining current nurses in clinical care positions, and increasing the capacity of the nation's nursing education programs. The campaign has run national television advertisements about nursing during major media events, produced and distributed a variety of recruitment materials, including more than 10 million brochures, pins, posters, and videos in English and Spanish. These and other materials have been distributed free of charge to 30,000 junior and senior high schools, hospitals, nursing schools, and nursing organizations across the nation. The campaign has also developed a Web site that provides comprehensive information about the nursing profession, organized regional fundraising events that have raised in excess of $10 million for student and faculty scholarships, and produced various media designed to promote the nursing profession, including a feature movie that aired on national television.

To understand whether the campaign is achieving its goals, Johnson & Johnson engaged a collaboration of researchers from Vanderbilt University and the Massachusetts General Hospital to determine awareness and impact of the campaign. As part of this project, researchers worked with several survey research firms to conduct surveys of various populations, including parents and their teenagers; nursing students; RNs; physicians; hospital chief executive officers (CEOs) and hospital chief nursing officers (CNOs); and the public. Each of the surveys was undertaken to obtain data tailored specifically to each group and contained many of the same questions so that it is possible to compare results among the surveyed populations.

In this book, we use data from the surveys of health professionals. In general, the surveys of RNs, physicians, and hospital CEOs and CNOs assessed the extent and severity of the current nursing shortage; causes, effects, and hospitals' responses to the nursing shortage; characteristics of the nursing work environment, including quality of professional practice and relationships among nurses, physicians, and management; RNs' satisfaction with their current jobs, satisfaction with their decisions to become a nurse, perceptions of the nursing profession, and willingness to recommend nursing as a career to others; and awareness and impact of the Campaign for Nursing's Future. In addition to the surveys conducted in this project, we also made use of an earlier national survey of RNs that was conducted in 2002 by *NurseWeek* and the American Organization of Nurse Executives. This survey, which is described in the next paragraph, was directed by the same Vanderbilt and Massachusetts researchers. The survey instrument developed for that project served as the basis for the subsequent 2004 and 2006 national surveys of RNs. Details on each of these surveys follow.

2002 National Survey of RNs

This survey was funded by *NurseWeek*, a national weekly nursing publication and continuing education company, and by the American Organization of Nurse Executives. From October 24, 2001, through March 13, 2002, Harris Interactive mailed the eight-page questionnaire to a nationally representative sample of 7600 RNs who were randomly selected from a list of all RNs licensed to practice in the United States. Response enhancements included continuing education credits valued at $35 and the opportunity to be entered into a lottery drawing for one of three travel vouchers for work-related travel. A total of 4108 RNs completed the survey for a response rate of 55% (177 of the 7600 were determined to be ineligible). The data were weighted by age and region to reflect the distribution of RNs as reported in the federal government's 2000 NSSRN. A total of 1442 hospital-employed RNs who provide direct patient care responded to this survey.

2004 National Survey of RNs

The 2004 national survey of RNs was funded by the Johnson & Johnson Campaign for Nursing's Future and by *Nursing Spectrum*, a national biweekly magazine for nurses (which had acquired *NurseWeek*). The survey contained many of the same questions used in the earlier 2002 survey and included several different questions aimed at exploring new areas and probing certain aspects of the workplace environment in greater depth. From May 11 through July 12, 2004, Harris Interactive mailed the eight-page questionnaire to a random sample of 3500 RNs who were randomly selected from a national database that was compiled from all state board of licensure lists and was developed and maintained by *Nursing Spectrum*. Respondents were given the option of responding at a secure Web site or by mail, and up to five mailings were sent to nonresponders to encourage participation. Response enhancement incentives included 2 hours of continuing education courses valued at $35 and the opportunity to be entered into a lottery drawing for vouchers redeemable for travel to professional conferences. Following the exclusion of cases of retired nurses or those not working at the time of the survey, the researchers obtained a 53% response rate among eligible respondents and 1697 usable responses. The data were weighted by age and region to reflect the distribution of RNs as reported in the federal government's 2000 National Sample Survey of Registered Nurses in the United States. A total of 657 hospital-employed RNs who provide direct patient care responded.

2006 National Survey of RNs

The 2006 survey was funded by the Johnson & Johnson Campaign for Nursing's Future and by *Nursing Spectrum*. From May 24 through July 26, 2006, Harris Interactive mailed the eight-page questionnaire to a random sample of 3436 RNs that were drawn from the *Nursing Spectrum* national database. Given prior low response to the online option in this population, the survey was conducted only by mail. Up to five mailings were sent to nonresponders to encourage participation. Response enhancement incentives included 2 hours of continuing education courses valued at $35 and the opportunity to be entered into a lottery drawing for vouchers redeemable for travel to professional conferences. Following the exclusion of cases of retired nurses or those not working at the time of the survey, a 52% response rate among eligible respondents was obtained, and 1392 responses were usable for analysis.

Data from this survey were not weighted according to the federal government's 2000 NSSRN. The age distribution of respondents reflected differences from the 2000 NSSRN, but it was consistent with an analysis of more recent U.S. Census Bureau data reported by Auerbach, Buerhaus, and Staiger (2007). We determined that it was best not to use weights from previous government national surveys if, in fact, those weights would mask a true change in the characteristics of the nursing workforce (at the time of this analysis, only preliminary findings from the federal government's 2004 NSSRN were available, including information on the weights used by this government survey). A total of 617 hospital-employed RNs who provide direct patient care responded to this survey.

2004 National Survey of Physicians About Nursing

This survey was funded by the Johnson & Johnson Campaign for Nursing's Future, and Harris Interactive was employed to conduct the survey between January 6 and March 5, 2004. The December 2003 American Medical Association (AMA) Physician Masterfile (937,000 AMA members and nonmembers) was obtained to draw a national random sample of 840 primary care and specialty physicians who reported spending more than 20 hours per week in patient care activities, excluding resident physicians and federal employees. The four-page survey instrument contained approximately 60 items intended to be completed in less than 15 minutes. The survey instrument was initially mailed with a check for $25 as an honorarium for completing the survey, and up to five follow-up contacts were made to nonresponders. Of the 840 initial mailings, 20 physicians returned blank questionnaires or cashed the incentive check without completing the survey, and 85 cases were ineligible by reasons of death (10), retirement (7), change in practice or specialty (22), or lost to follow up (46). Of the 765 eligible contacts, 400 physicians completed and returned surveys for a response rate of 53%.

2005 National Survey of Hospital CEOs and CNOs

This survey was funded by the Johnson & Johnson Campaign for Nursing's Future, and Harris Interactive was employed to conduct the survey between January 28 and March 11, 2005. Harris Interactive drew the sample from lists of hospital executives compiled from all United States hospitals and maintained by SK&A Information Services, a firm that specializes in developing lists of healthcare professionals, data, and market research. After an advance letter was mailed to all potentially eligible respondents, the respondent's hospital office was contacted by telephone to establish eligibility, with up to 10 attempts made to speak to eligible respondents. If a direct interview was not accomplished, follow-up attempts by priority mail and facsimile were employed. Respondents were offered a $100 honorarium for their participation, which they could either accept or donate to the American Red Cross. Completed telephone interviews averaged 20 minutes in length. Response rate calculations were made using the Response Rate Calculator version 2.1 developed for telephone surveys by the American Association for Public Opinion Research (AAPOR). The rates we used considered as eligible all respondents for whom contact with an office was established and the respondent's identity was confirmed. Overall, we completed interviews with 222 of 443 eligible CNOs contacted for a response rate of 50%. It was substantially more difficult to establish contact with and interview hospital CEOs. A total of 142 complete responses were obtained from 404 eligible CEOs for a response rate of 31% (AAPOR, Response Rate 3).

RESOURCES

Buerhaus, P., & Staiger, D. (1996). Managed care and the nurse workforce. *The Journal of the American Medical Association, 276*(18), 1487–1493.

Buerhaus, P., & Auerbach, D. (1999). Slow growth in the number of minority RNs in the United States. *IMAGE: Journal of Nursing Scholarship, 31*(2), 179–183.

Buerhaus, P., & Staiger, D. (1999). Trouble in the nurse labor market? Recent trends and future outlook. *Health Affairs, 18*(1), 214–222.

Donelan, K., Buerhaus, P., DeRoches, C., & Dittus, R. (2007). [Preliminary results of a 2007 national public opinion survey of the nursing profession]. Unpublished raw data.

Moses, E. (1986). *The registered nurse population, findings from the National Sample Survey of Registered Nurses, November 1984*. Division of Nursing, Bureau of Health Professions, Health Resources and Services Administration, U.S. Department of Health and Human Services. (NTIS No. HRP-0904551)

Moses, E. (1990). *The registered nurse population, findings from the National Sample Survey of Registered Nurses, November 1988*. Division of Nursing, Bureau of Health Professions, Health Resources and Services Administration, U.S. Department of Health and Human Services. (NTIS No. PB91-145391)

Moses, E. (1994). *The registered nurse population, findings from the National Sample Survey of Registered Nurses, November 1992*. Division of Nursing, Bureau of Health Professions, Health Resources and Services Administration, U.S. Department of Health and Human Services. (NTIS No. PB97-108187)

Moses, E. (1997). *The registered nurse population, findings from the National Sample Survey of Registered Nurses, November 1996*. Division of Nursing, Bureau of Health Professions, Health Resources and Services Administration, U.S. Department of Health and Human Services.

Roth, A., Graham, D., & Schmittling, G. (1978). *1977 National Sample Survey of Registered Nurses and factors affecting their supply*. Kansas City, MO: American Nurses Association. (NTIS No. HRP-0900603)

Spratley, E., Johnson, A., Sochalski, J., Fritz, M., & Spencer, W. (2001). *The registered nurse population, findings from the National Sample Survey of Registered Nurses, March 2000*. Division of Nursing, Bureau of Health Professions, Health Resources and Services Administration, U.S. Department of Health and Human Services.

U.S. Department of Health and Human Services. (1982). *The registered nurse population, an overview from the National Sample Survey of Registered Nurses, November 1980*. Office of Data Analysis and Management, Bureau of Health Professions, Health Resources and Services Administration. (NTIS No. HRP-0904551)

U.S. Department of Health and Human Services, Health Resources and Services Administration.

REFERENCES

American Association for Public Opinion Research. (2006). *Standard definitions: Final dispositions of case codes and outcome rates for surveys* (4th ed.). Retrieved November 19, 2007, from http://www.aapor.org/uploads/standarddefs_4.pdf

Auerbach, D., Buerhaus, P., & Staiger, D. (2007). Better late than never: Workforce supply implication of later entry into nursing. *Health Affairs, 26*(1), 178–185.

Blendon, R., DesRoches, C., Brodie, M., Benson, J., Allison, B., Schneider, E., et al. (2002). Patient safety: Views of practicing physicians and the public on medical errors. *The New England Journal of Medicine, 347*, 1933-1940.

U.S. Department of Health and Human Services, Health Resources and Services Administration. (2006). *The registered nurse population: Findings from the March 2004 national sample survey of registered nurses*. Retrieved November 19, 2007, from http://bhpr.hrsa.gov/healthwork force/rnsurvey04/

CHAPTER 2

Key Trends in the Healthcare Industry and the Nursing Workforce

We begin this book by providing an overview of the healthcare industry in the United States. In 2005, spending on health care comprised 16% of the nation's economy, a higher percentage than any other country in the developed world. Each day thousands of organizations combine people and physical resources to diagnose and monitor illnesses, provide personal healthcare services and treatments, coordinate care, and build, manage, and continuously improve facilities and systems of healthcare delivery. The nursing profession is vital to the operation of this large and complicated enterprise, particularly in the nation's hospitals. Lewis Thomas, in *The Youngest Science*, noted that, "Hospitals are held together, glued together, enabled to function . . . by the nurses" (Thomas, 1983). We assert that this observation reflects not only hospitals but most organizations that provide health care.

In this chapter, we examine the major sectors of the healthcare delivery system and the major organizations within the system that provide health care that are held together by the efforts of the nursing profession in the United States. We focus on registered nurses (RNs), the most highly educated of all those typically referred to as "nurse," and examine how the RN workforce has grown in size and educational attainment, as well as trends in employment and earnings, settings in which RNs work, and other characteristics such as age and racial background during recent decades. We conclude the chapter by attempting to place members of the nursing profession within a broader context by comparing selected trends in education, hours worked, and earnings of RNs with those of other professions.

OVERVIEW OF THE HEALTHCARE SYSTEM AND RN EMPLOYMENT

Total spending on healthcare-related goods and services amounted to $2 trillion and, with the exception of the period from 1992 to 2000, has grown faster than the entire national economy since before 1970. This trend is expected to continue, with health care projected to comprise 20% of the U.S. gross domestic product (GDP, which is a measure of the market value of all final goods and services produced) in 2016, compared to 7% of GDP in 1970 and 16% in 2005. Although the reasons for the relatively high spending on health care in the United States ($5711 per person in 2003, compared to $3847 in Switzerland, the next highest country) have been the subject of long-standing debates, much of the spending in the United States can be attributed to the diffused incentives and limited ability for controlling costs among the many fragmented entities that, together, make up the U.S. healthcare "system," namely individual consumers, providers, health insurers, employers, and government agencies.

While in other countries, healthcare providers are often salaried employees and facilities are often controlled and planned by the regional or central government, providers in the United States act much more closely according to local market principles. Healthcare organizations hire labor and earn salaries based on what the market will allow, maximizing profits or revenues. For these reasons the careers of RNs are constantly changing as the healthcare system interacts with constantly shifting pressures arising from patients, employers (who provide the majority of health insurance in the United States), and state and federal governments.

RN Employment

RNs constitute the largest profession within the largest industry in the United States, and are one of the largest professions in the United States according to the Bureau of Labor Statistics (U.S. Department of Labor, 2007). In 2006, there were roughly 2.3 million full-time equivalent (FTE) RNs working in the United States, roughly 2 million aides (including both nursing aides and home health aides), 900,000 physicians, and roughly 700,000 licensed practical and vocational nurses.[1] As shown in **Figure 2-1**, the total number of RNs has grown considerably over time, from 640,000 to 2.3 million between 1969 and 2006, roughly coinciding with the relative increase in adjusted overall healthcare spending ($900 billion to $2.1 trillion for those same years, expressed in 2006 dollars).[2]

While the underlying relationships between RN supply and national health spending are complex and explored in later chapters (a detailed discussion of drivers of national healthcare spending is beyond the scope of this book), we can learn much about RN employment by understanding trends in the composition

---

[1] As discussed in Chapter 1, full-time equivalents represent the total number of full-time workers plus one-half of the number of part-time workers in any given category of worker.
[2] Dollar figures are adjusted using GDP deflator.

Figure 2-1   National Health Spending and Full-Time Equivalent RNs, 1969–2006

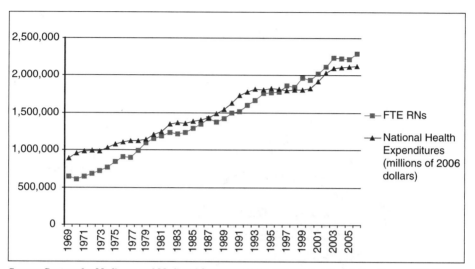

Source: Centers for Medicare and Medicaid Services (CMS) and Current Population Survey, U.S. Census Bureau.
Dollar figures adjusted using GDP deflator.

of the healthcare economy by major sector. **Figure 2-2** shows the sectors that account for the dollars spent on health care in 2005. Of the roughly $2 trillion in total spending, the largest single category of spending was hospital care, accounting for $661 billion, or 30.8%, of spending. Services performed in physicians' offices, ambulatory centers, clinics, and laboratories (including diagnostic testing not performed in hospitals) accounted for $421 billion, or 21.2%. Prescription drugs accounted for roughly 10% of spending, nursing home and home health care together accounted for 8.5%, and other categories, such as administrative costs (7.2%), dental spending (4.4%), and public health activity (2.8%), accounted for the remainder.

Those shares of the national healthcare dollar have been shifting somewhat over the past decades and are projected to continue to adjust in favor of slightly more spending in outpatient settings and on technology and products such as drugs and devices (see **Table 2-1**). The hospital sector has always accounted for the largest share of national health spending, but that share has dropped from nearly 40% in 1980 to just over 30% in 2004. Spending associated with physicians increased from 18.5% in 1984 and has been fairly stable recently at just over 21% in 2004, while spending associated with other personal health care (mainly prescription drugs) has increased from 15.5% to over 20% during this same period. All sectors except for nursing homes have demonstrated (and are projected to

Figure 2-2   National Health Expenditures in 2005, by Sector

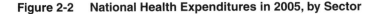

National Health Expenditures

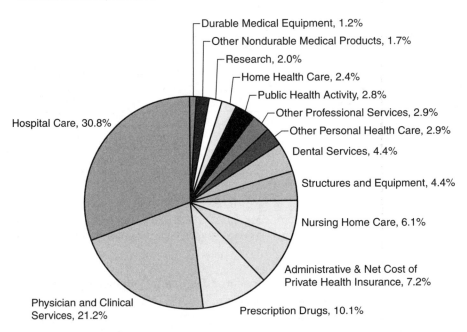

Durable Medical Equipment, 1.2%
Other Nondurable Medical Products, 1.7%
Research, 2.0%
Home Health Care, 2.4%
Public Health Activity, 2.8%
Other Professional Services, 2.9%
Other Personal Health Care, 2.9%
Dental Services, 4.4%
Structures and Equipment, 4.4%
Nursing Home Care, 6.1%
Administrative & Net Cost of Private Health Insurance, 7.2%
Prescription Drugs, 10.1%
Hospital Care, 30.8%
Physician and Clinical Services, 21.2%

Source: National Health Expenditures, Centers for Medicare and Medicaid Services.

continue) substantial increases in inflation-adjusted spending. This is true even for hospitals, despite the fact that spending in that sector has declined as a *percentage* of national health spending.

Not surprisingly, RNs are employed in the more labor-intensive sectors of the healthcare industry. **Table 2-2** offers a detailed breakdown of the employment settings of RNs in 2004 according to the results of the National Sample Survey of Registered Nurses (the NSSRN is described in Chapter 1). Short-term hospitals employ nearly half of all RNs, while long-term, government, and other hospitals employ an additional 10%. The second most common employment setting is in long-term care (nursing homes and home health), followed by physicians' offices and clinics. Significant numbers of RNs are also employed in community and public health roles, schools, nursing education, and in offices that process insurance claims and benefits.

Table 2-1 National Healthcare Spending by Sector for Selected Years, in Millions of 2006 Dollars

	1980		1992		2004		2016 (projected)	
	Spending	% of Total	Spending	% of Total	Spending	% of Total	Spending	% of Total
Hospital Care	$ 479,960	39.8%	$ 627,188	35.3%	$ 641,625	30.5%	$ 807,640	31.1%
Physician and Clinical Services	$ 223,667	18.5%	$ 396,822	22.3%	$ 445,620	21.2%	$ 514,182	19.8%
Home Health Care	$ 11,295	0.9%	$ 38,006	2.1%	$ 48,341	2.3%	$ 69,658	2.7%
Nursing Home Care	$ 90,392	7.5%	$ 129,682	7.3%	$ 130,179	6.2%	$ 132,267	5.1%
Public Health	$ 30,572	2.5%	$ 51,021	2.9%	$ 59,413	2.8%	$ 78,299	3.0%
Other Personal Health Care	$ 187,303	15.5%	$ 275,693	15.5%	$ 430,596	20.5%	$ 561,239	21.6%
Other Health Expenditures	$ 183,344	15.2%	$ 257,550	14.5%	$ 348,192	16.5%	$ 431,166	16.6%
Total	$1,206,533		$1,775,963		$2,103,965		$2,594,452	
% of GDP	9.1%		13.4%		15.9%		19.6%	

Source: National Health Expenditures, Centers for Medicare and Medicaid Services.
Dollar figures are adjusted using GDP deflator.

Table 2-2   Employment Setting of Full-Time Equivalent RNs in 2004

	FTE RN Employment	% of Total
Short-Term Hospital	961,693	47.1%
Long-Term Hospital	87,780	4.3%
Other Hospital	79,261	3.9%
Government Hospital	66,764	3.3%
Nursing Home or Hospice	159,007	7.8%
Home Health/Visiting Nurse	89,701	4.4%
Nursing Education Program	50,558	2.5%
City or State Health Department	49,345	2.4%
Community Clinics and Centers	55,756	2.7%
School Health System	53,942	2.6%
Occupational (Employee) Health Services	19,235	0.9%
Solo and Partnership Physician Practice	43,226	2.1%
Group Physician Practice	44,377	2.2%
Nurse Practice	6,106	0.3%
Group Practice — Mixed Professionals	26,206	1.3%
Freestanding Clinic	13,514	0.7%
Ambulatory/Surgical Center	38,552	1.9%
Dialysis Center	17,431	0.9%
Hospital-Owned Off-Site Clinic	23,032	1.1%
HMO	10,925	0.5%
Insurance Claims/Benefits	40,856	2.0%
Policy, Planning, Regulatory or Licensing Agency	7,850	0.4%
Correctional Facility	15,991	0.8%
Private Duty or Self-Employed Home Work	15,236	0.7%
Other	64,856	3.2%

Source: National Sample Survey of Registered Nurses, 2004.

Over time, RN employment has tended to follow overall trends in health care in general. **Table 2-3** aggregates RN employment settings into categories roughly comparable with those from Table 2-1, which show overall trends in healthcare spending. The percentage of RNs employed in hospitals decreased from 67.5% to 58.6% between 1980 and 2004 (though percentages showed little change between 1980 and 1992) and is similar to the drop in hospital spending as a percentage of total healthcare spending from 39.8% to 30.5% over that same period.[3] Part of this change appears to be related to the shift in the locus of care from hospital to outpatient and office settings, sectors in which both RN employment and total healthcare spending increased. Table 2-3 also shows that the percentage of RNs working in nursing homes has dropped gradually (from 7.6% to 6.4% between 1980 and 2004), while the percentage in home health care has increased (1.5% to 4.7%), both in accord with overall trends in those sectors during this period. There also has been a slight decrease in the proportion of RNs working in educational and school settings and an increase in the proportion working in other settings including administrative and insurance functions.

Table 2-3   Employment Settings of RNs over Time, Selected Years

	1980		1992		2004	
	FTE RNs	% of Workforce	FTE RNs	% of Workforce	FTE RNs	% of Workforce
Hospital Care	713,242	67.5%	1,066,263	67.4%	1,195,498	58.6%
Physician and Clinical Services	76,402	7.2%	118,157	7.5%	233,636	11.4%
Home Health Care	16,033	1.5%	79,476	5.0%	96,818	4.7%
Nursing Home Care	80,313	7.6%	110,782	7.0%	131,518	6.4%
Public Health	58,199	5.5%	76,414	4.8%	133,173	6.5%
Nursing Education	37,081	3.5%	28,125	1.8%	50,558	2.5%
School Settings	30,148	2.9%	33,936	2.1%	53,942	2.6%
Industry/Occupational Settings	26,098	2.5%	17,143	1.1%	60,091	2.9%
Government and Other Settings	18,699	1.8%	50,875	3.2%	85,969	4.2%

Source: National Sample Survey of Registered Nurses.

---

[3] Employment sector trends can also be analyzed using the Current Population Survey, though fewer categories are available, and the smaller sample size makes identification of smaller sectors difficult. The trend in hospital employment of RNs, according to the CPS, mirrors that found in the NSSRN, with hospitals employing just over 70% of RNs in 1983 and approximately 60% in 2006.

Within hospitals, the settings where RN employment has changed mirror changes in the technology of the provision of hospital care. It is difficult to track trends over time because recent changes in care provision have emphasized new categories of care (namely, progressive care and telemetry, radiology, perioperative care, and care across many units) that were not considered categories in earlier NSSRNs. Nevertheless, **Table 2-4** shows care settings within hospitals grouped in a way that permits a consistent comparison across years, and it reveals a trend toward greater specialization: RNs working in labor and delivery, emergency rooms, outpatient departments, and step-down/transitional/recovery units have increased at the expense of general or specialty inpatient units and settings. The percentage of time hospital RNs spend performing direct patient care has hovered around 60% between 1980 and 2004, according to the NSSRN.

LABOR FORCE CHARACTERISTICS OF RNS

RN employment has changed not only in response to specialization, technology, and other factors that affect the nature of nursing practice, but due to important economic and demographic characteristics of RNs. Here we examine several key trends, some of which we will return to and explore in greater detail in subsequent chapters.

Table 2-4   Setting for Majority of Patient Care Within Hospital, 1988 and 2004

	1988		2004	
	FTE RNs	%	FTE RNs	%
Critical Care (ICU)	167,705	20.9%	193,838	19.4%
Emergency Department	56,610	7.0%	98,751	9.9%
Labor/Delivery Room	43,783	5.4%	75,430	7.6%
Operating Room	73,281	9.1%	92,487	9.3%
Outpatient Department	30,275	3.8%	75,541	7.6%
Step-Down/Recovery Department	23,434	2.9%	75,847	7.6%
General/Specialty/Other Inpatient Unit	408,773	50.9%	387,123	38.8%

Source: National Sample Survey of Registered Nurses.

Participation in the Workforce, Hours Worked, and Key Demographic Characteristics

Although the racial and gender composition of the nursing profession has become gradually more diverse, the majority of RNs are white and female, as shown in **Figure 2-3**. The number of male RNs has increased from 15,000 in 1973 to over 200,000 in 2006, which as a proportion of the population of RNs in the workforce represents an increase from just over 2% to 8.9% over those years. Despite this increase, however, men remain significantly underrepresented in nursing when one considers that men constitute 54% of those in the overall national workforce working on a FTE basis.[4]

Growth in the number and proportion of the nursing workforce who are minorities has been stronger than for men, increasing from 11.1% of the RN workforce in 1973 (1 in 9 RNs) to over 20% in 2006 (more than one in five). Breaking down these percentages according to different groups is instructive. Using CPS data, we find that in 1983, 6.5% of RNs in the workforce were black compared to

Figure 2-3   Percent of RNs Who Are Men or Nonwhite, 1973–2005

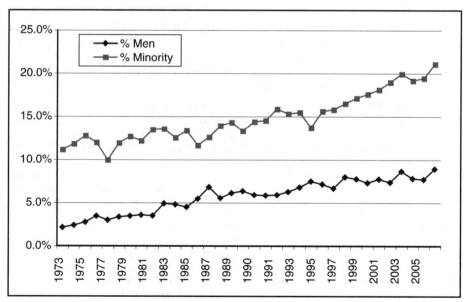

Source: Current Population Survey, U.S. Census Bureau.

---

[4] According to tables based on the Current Population Survey data on employment and earnings compiled by the Bureau of Labor statistics. (see http://www.bls.gov/cps/cpsaat11.pdf).

9.5% of the overall (nonnursing) workforce in the United States at that time. By 2006, the percentage of blacks in the RN workforce had increased to 10%, roughly the same overall percentage of blacks in the national workforce.[5] Hispanics, on the other hand, have always been significantly underrepresented as a percentage of RNs: In 2006, CPS data indicate that Hispanic RNs accounted for just over 4% of the RN workforce compared to nearly 14% of the workforce as a whole.

Beyond changes in the gender and racial composition of the RN workforce, the RN workforce has been aging—the reasons for and implications of a rapidly aging workforce receive extensive analysis and discussion throughout this book. **Figure 2-4** shows the percentages of the RN workforce in different age groups: those under 30, between 30 and 49, and RNs 50 years of age and over. In the 1970s, roughly one in three RNs was under age 30, peaking at 38% in 1978 (nearly as many as the 30 to 49 age group). Since then, the percentage of RNs under age 30 has gradually decreased so that by 2006 less than one RN in eight was under age 30. In the 1970s, one RN in five was age 50 and over, a ratio that held relatively stable until the late 1990s when the number of older RNs began increasing such that today roughly one in every three RNs is older than 50. **Figure 2-5** shows that during most of the 1970s and 1980s, the average age of RNs held steady at roughly 37 years; by the late 1980s, the average age began to increase, and today the average age of RNs in the workforce is 44 years.

Since the time the first NSSRN was conducted in 1977, there has been a trend toward increasing participation in the labor force among RNs and increasing hours worked. **Figure 2-6** displays overall trends in labor force participation

---

[5] Data from the NSSRN are often cited to argue that blacks continue to be underrepresented in nursing because it shows that the proportion of RNs who are black or African American is low and has changed little over the last 20 years. According to the NSSRN, blacks accounted for only 5% of RNs in 1983 and 4.2% in 2004 (a change in the race question might have affected estimates from 2004 somewhat, but estimates in 2000 were similar). Even among RNs graduating since 1990 in the 2004 survey, the NSSRN still estimated that only 4.9% were black. In contrast, the CPS estimates that blacks accounted for over 10% of RNs in 2004, while the National League for Nursing estimates that blacks accounted for over 10% of enrollment in nursing schools since 1990 (National Center for Health Statistics, *Health, United States, 2005*, Table 110, Hyattsville, Maryland, 2005). The NSSRN estimates might be biased downward due to low response rates of minority RNs to the NSSRN survey. Roughly 30% of the NSSRN sample does not respond to the survey (compared to under 10% of the CPS sample), and nonresponse is highest in regions with large minority populations, such as the south and Washington DC (HRSA, *The Registered Nurse Population: Findings from the March 2004 National Sample Survey of Registered Nurses*, Appendix B, Survey Methodology, Washington DC, 2006). As a result, we believe that the NSSRN underestimates the number of black and Hispanic RNs. In contrast, the CPS has a much higher response rate to their survey, and (unlike the NSSRN) has developed sample weights that account for lower response rates among minority populations (BLS, *Current Population Survey: Design and Methodology*, Technical Paper 63RV, Chapter 16, U.S. Census Bureau, Washington DC, March 2002). Therefore, the CPS data are more likely to provide an unbiased estimate of the racial and ethnic makeup of the RN workforce.

Figure 2-4   Percentage of Full-Time Equivalent RNs in Different Age Groups, 1973–2006

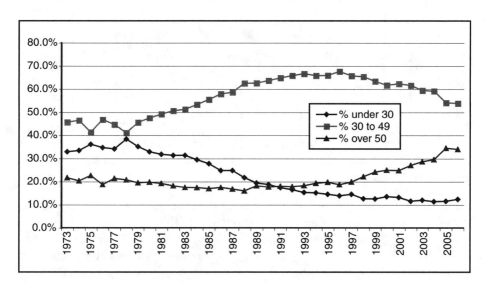

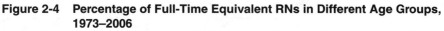

Source: Current Population Survey, U.S. Census Bureau.

Figure 2-5   Average Age of Full-Time Equivalent Registered Nursing Workforce, 1973–2006

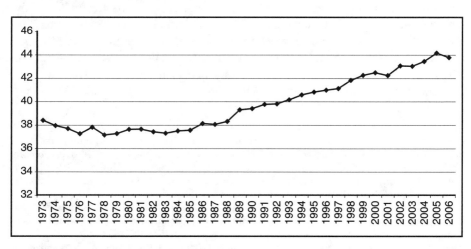

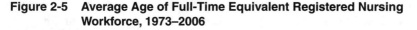

Source: Current Population Survey, U.S. Census Bureau.

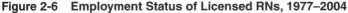

Figure 2-6   Employment Status of Licensed RNs, 1977–2004

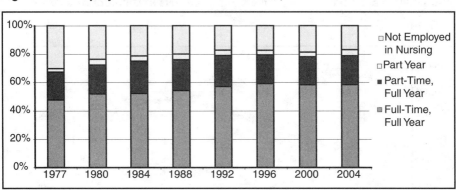

Source: National Sample Survey of Registered Nurses.

among people educated as RNs. Notice that the percentage of RNs who are not employed in nursing (they might be entirely out of the labor force or employed in nonnursing positions) has dropped significantly since 1977, from more than one in four RNs to approximately one in six. Among those working in nursing, the percentage of RNs working full time versus part year or part time has increased slightly from 68% in 1977 to just over 70% in 2004.

The number of hours worked has also increased among RNs who are employed in nursing. According to the CPS, the average number of hours worked by both full- and part-time RNs combined during a given week increased by approximately 6.5% between 1983 and 2006 (see **Figure 2-7**), or from about 35 to 37 hours (this trend is similar in the NSSRN).[6] Average hours for full-time RNs have remained unchanged at roughly 40 hours per week from 1983 to 2006. Thus, the increase in average hours worked is mainly due to an increase in the percentage of RNs working full time. However, at the same time, the percentage of RNs in the CPS who state that they usually work 45 hours per week or more has doubled from 5% in 1983 to over 10% in 2006.

---

[6] Between 2000 and 2004, the question about hours worked in the previous week in the NSSRN changed. In 2004, respondents were explicitly instructed to include paid on-call hours in their total. Respondents in earlier surveys likely did not include those hours in their totals. The data point for 2004 in Figure 2-8 from the NSSRN is constructed by removing those on-call hours, which were broken out separately in subsequent questions and averaged roughly 2 hours per RN. The CPS also asks about "usual" hours worked in a given week—in fact that measure is used as the basis for constructing FTEs that are used in weighting much of the data in this book because it is generally thought to be more reliable and invariant to temporary or seasonal conditions. The trends in usual hours versus hours in the previous week are almost identical in the CPS. The NSSRN, on the other hand, did not ask respondents about usual hours in 2004, and thus, that series was not used in Figure 2-8 in comparison with the CPS.

Figure 2-7   Average Hours Worked in the Previous Week Among RNs, 1983–2006

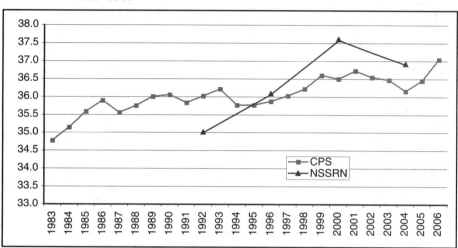

Source: National Sample Survey of Registered Nurses and Current Population Survey.

Earnings of Registered Nurses

There are several ways to analyze the earnings of RNs. According to the NSSRN, gross *annual* earnings for full-time RNs have grown about 35% from roughly $46,000 in 1984 to approximately $62,000 in 2004, in dollars adjusted to 2006.[7] The CPS, which reports *hourly* earnings, shows a smaller increase in earnings, 26%, from 1983 to 2006. The increase in annual earnings measured by CPS data is consistent with the estimates generated by data from the NSSRN when converted to hourly earnings as shown in **Figure 2-8**. The annual data from the CPS also show that the increase in RN earnings was not gradual, and most of the increase occurred between 1983 and 1992—Chapter 11 discusses these earnings increases in the context of significant changes in the demand and supply of RNs in hospitals that were occurring during these same years. From 1992 to 2000, real earnings stagnated or even dipped before growing slightly again after that period. This pattern, incidentally, matches national health spending shown in Figure 2-1, which suggests that the onset of managed care might have had a role in depressing national health spending in part by depressing earnings—these changes are illustrated in Chapter 5, which focuses on the role of managed care on RN earnings and employment.

---

[7] Those amounts do not include earnings reported from "secondary" nursing positions.

Figure 2-8   Hourly Earnings of RNs, in 2006 Dollars, 1983–2006

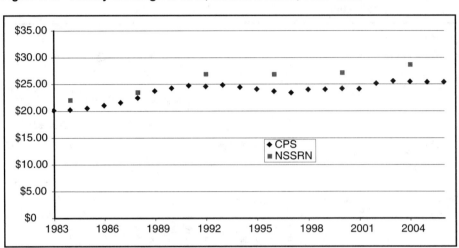

Source: National Sample Survey of Registered Nurses and Current Population Survey.
Dollar figures are adjusted by the Consumer Price Indexes for all goods.

Part of the increase in earnings also might be due to the increased age and experience of RNs in the labor force in recent years. As in most professions, earnings of RNs increase with experience. **Figure 2-9** shows plots of the distribution of earnings of full-time RNs based on how many years it had been since receiving their basic nursing education.[8] For example, the left-most category shows the earnings of RNs with fewer than 10 years since graduating from a basic nursing program. For these RNs, median annual earnings (adjusted for inflation to 2006) were $51,200 (meaning that half of RNs earned more than $51,200 and half earned less than this amount). One-quarter of RNs with this many years since completing their basic nursing education earned less than $42,700, one-quarter earned more than $61,900, and 5% earned more than $80,000. For the next group, those with 10 to 19 years since their basic nursing education, earnings were roughly $5000 higher, except for those at the high end of the distribution, who earned considerably more (5% of RNs with 10 to 19 years since their basic

---

[8] While ideally one would like to know how many years an RN has been working in nursing rather than the number of years since receiving their basic nursing education, that question was only asked as part of the national sample survey in 1980 and 1984. Years since receiving a basic nursing education is a good approximation for years of experience in nursing. (In 1980, the average years since receiving the basic nursing education averaged about 2.5 years higher, mainly differing due to years spent out of the labor force for reasons such as child care. The correlation between the two measures was 0.85 in that year.)

Figure 2-9   Earnings of Full-Time RNs by Years Since Completion of Basic Nursing Education, 2004

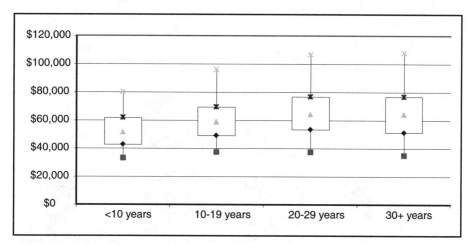

Source: National Sample Survey of Registered Nurses, 2004.
Note: For each category of years of experience, plotted points represent (from bottom to top):
5th percentile, 25th percentile, median, 75th percentile, 95th percentile.
Earnings values expressed in 2006 dollars, adjusted for inflation.

nursing education earned more than $96,000). RNs with another 10 years of experience earned roughly an additional $5000, but earnings appear to plateau at that level. RNs with 30 or more years since receiving their basic nursing education do not earn more than those with 20 to 29 years. Note that the earnings distribution is slightly more spread out among this latter group of most experienced RNs as more RNs earn both higher and lower annual salaries.

That pattern of rising earnings with experience is more pronounced than it was in 1980. In that year, additional experience did not appear to translate into higher earnings for RNs for whom it had been more than 19 years since they had completed their basic nursing education. Even the pattern of earnings and experience observed for 2004, however, would be considered relatively flat compared to many other professions where higher gains in earnings relative to years of experience are expected.

Educational Preparation

There are several educational pathways to becoming an RN. **Figure 2-10** shows the type of education program RNs completed when they first became an RN as well as the highest level of education attained. Under half (46%) of the

Figure 2-10   Educational Preparation of Full-Time Equivalent RNs in 2004

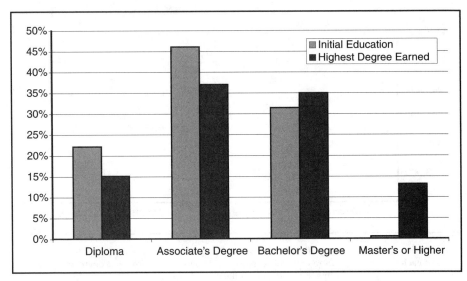

Source: National Sample Survey of Registered Nurses.

workforce in 2004 became RNs by completing associate's degree programs, compared to 32% who received baccalaureate degrees, 22% who had earned a diploma in nursing, and less than 1% who became an RN by completing a master's degree as their initial nursing education. Many RNs go on to receive additional education after their initial education, which is also shown in Figure 2-10. For example, 13% of the 2004 RN workforce (weighted by FTEs) had received a master's degree at some point in their careers, and 35% had received baccalaureate degrees.

Figure 2-10 masks the fact that diploma programs, which are based in hospitals and take 3 years to complete, were the predominant option for becoming an RN decades ago but have dwindled to only a relatively few programs in recent years. **Figure 2-11** reveals trends in basic nursing education over time by showing the type of basic education received by recent RN graduates in 1980, 1992, and 2004 (that is, RNs who completed their basic nursing education in the 4 years leading up to the year of the survey). The percentage of recent graduates earning diplomas fell from 24% in 1980 to just over 2% in 2004, whereas associate's degrees grew to being twice as common a route to becoming an RN as bachelor's degrees in 1992 (60% to 30%) but then declined somewhat so that by 2004 there were roughly three associate's degree graduates for every two baccalaureate (58% versus 39%). One implication of these trends in

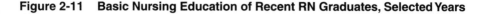

Figure 2-11   Basic Nursing Education of Recent RN Graduates, Selected Years

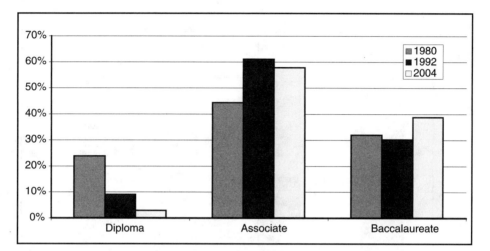

Source: National Sample Survey of Registered Nurses.

educational preparation is that diploma-educated RNs in 2004 are older (52 years), on average, compared to associate's degree graduates (44 years) and baccalaureate degree graduates (41 years), which have been more common among recent cohorts of RNs. An unexpected implication of these trends in nursing education is exposed in Chapter 11 when we explain how the most recent shortage of RNs (that began in 1998) developed.

COMPARING KEY TRENDS BETWEEN RNs AND OTHER PROFESSIONS

To add context to the discussion of earnings and employment characteristics of RNs, we consider the characteristics of other comparable careers and professions, specifically, female teachers of elementary and secondary schools and female managers (defined broadly by the Current Population Survey) with at least some education beyond high school. **Figure 2-12** shows that the educational characteristics of these other groups are not too dissimilar from RNs, but the "manager" includes a wider array of workers with a wider array of educational backgrounds. Teachers have higher average educational levels than

Figure 2-12   Highest Educational Attainment for RNs, Business Managers, and Teachers, 2006

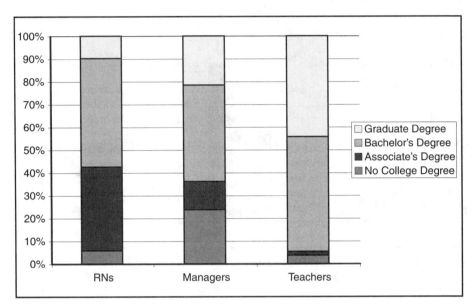

Source: Current Population Survey.

RNs, with close to half (44%) having attained a master's degree or higher compared to only 1 in 10 RNs with a master's degree.

In addition to having fewer years of education, RNs work fewer hours than teachers or managers who are women, yet they earn higher average hourly earnings. In 2006, RNs worked an average of 37 hours per week compared to 41.9 for managers and 40.5 for teachers (however, the number of hours reported for teachers does not consider the time during the summer when they are not working). Nevertheless, earnings are higher for RNs (see **Figure 2-13**). On average, RNs earn about 8% more than managers ($25.19 per hour in 2006 versus $23.34) and 19% more than teachers ($21.14). Not surprisingly, given that teachers are more frequently employed in the public sector and managers in the private sector, with RNs likely to be employed in both sectors, earnings for managers are more variable than for RNs (i.e., more managers earn very high salaries and, at the same time, more managers report earning very low salaries compared to the distribution in earnings for RNs), while earnings for teachers are less variable compared to RNs.

Interestingly, earnings show different patterns with respect to age among the different professions. As noted by others (Iglehart, 1987), earnings of RNs are

Figure 2-13   Average Hourly Earnings for RNs, Business Managers, and Teachers by Age, 2006

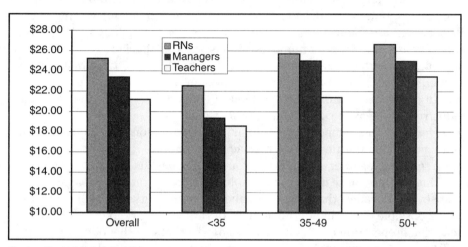

Source: Current Population Survey.

relatively high as RNs start their careers; in fact, the earnings gap between RNs and other professions shown in Figure 2-13 is highest among those under 35 years of age—RNs earn roughly 20% more than women in the other professional groups. In their middle ages, managers experience a steep rise in earnings and nearly catch up to RNs, while teachers experience nearly the same growth in their earnings as RNs. Between the middle years (35-49) and the older working years, RNs experience modest earnings growth, managers experience no growth, on average, and teachers experience the largest earnings growth, though they still remain behind the other two groups. Those patterns can also be explained, to some extent, by the differing public/private sector strategies with respect to compensation among these professions.

The data in Figures 2-12 and 2-13 only capture some of the most basic characteristics of the three professions, yet it is clear that the nursing profession attracts many well-qualified and talented individuals who earn more and work fewer hours, on average, than their counterparts in education and management.

CHAPTER SUMMARY

The healthcare system in the United States has grown rapidly in both size and complexity over the past several decades, and it is expected to continue growing to the point where, in 2020, health care will account for one-fifth of the nation's GDP. As the system has expanded and evolved, so too has the nursing profession. RNs can be found working in virtually every sector of the healthcare system, particularly in healthcare delivery organizations. Although not to as great an extent as a few decades ago, hospitals remain the largest employer of RNs. As these organizations have adopted greater technology and expanded specialty areas, increasing numbers of RNs work in specialty care areas, outpatient care settings, ambulatory, and home healthcare settings that have expanded concurrently. As the healthcare system experienced the shock of the spread of managed care during the 1990s, the overall growth of the healthcare industry slowed, as did the earnings of RNs during this period.

Over time, the composition of the nursing profession has changed, adding more men and minorities. Today, men account for 9% of the RN workforce, and when summed together, all minority groups represent 20% of the RN workforce. Working RNs are more likely to be employed on a full-time basis, and over the past several decades, the average number of hours worked has changed little, with a possible exception of the number of RNs who work long hours. The educational preparation of RNs has experienced a particularly noticeable change as RNs today rarely obtain their nursing education in hospital-based diploma programs but rather in associate's degree community-based colleges or in baccalaureate degree nursing education programs. One in eight RNs eventually receives a master's degree.

Compared to business managers and teachers, RNs work fewer hours (not including summers for teachers), have similar or shorter education requirements, and earn higher salaries on average. RN earnings are particularly high during the start of their nursing careers but do not grow as fast with experience, at least with respect to the earnings of teachers or managers.

Next, in Chapter 3, we complete this introductory section of the book by providing a brief primer on the economic concepts underpinning demand and supply in the labor market for RNs. This discussion will focus on how wages and other factors influence the hours of work that potential employers want to purchase from individuals and how economic factors influence the hours of work that potential employees, including RNs, are willing to provide.

REFERENCES

Iglehart, J. (1987). Problems facing the nursing profession. *The New England Journal of Medicine, 317*(10), 646–651.

Thomas, L. (1983). *The youngest science: Notes of a medicine-watcher.* New York: Viking Press.

U.S. Department of Labor, Bureau of Labor Statistics. (2007). *Career guides to industries.* Retrieved August 30, 2007, from http://www.bls.gov/oco/cg/cgs035.htm

CHAPTER 3

A Brief Primer on Demand and Supply

Throughout this book we rely on the economic concepts of demand and supply. These concepts, while rather simple and straightforward, are extremely useful in organizing and describing the wide-ranging forces that determine earnings and employment in the labor market for RNs. Identifying the forces affecting the demand and supply of RNs will help us to more clearly understand trends in earnings and employment, effects of managed care on the nurse labor market, development and resolution of nursing shortages, formation of polices aimed at strengthening the current and future workforce, and many other topics addressed throughout this book.

In general, economics uses the concept of supply and demand to describe how potential buyers and sellers interact to determine the price and quantity of a good sold in a competitive market. In the labor market, the good being sold is hours of work (which in aggregate is referred to as the employment level), and the price at which it is sold is defined in terms of dollars per hour or per week (and is referred to as the wage rate). Employers are the potential buyers of this good and represent the demand side of the market. Employees are the potential sellers and represent the supply side of the market.

In this chapter, we provide a brief primer on demand and supply in the labor market. We begin our discussion by focusing on the demand side, outlining how the wage and other factors influence the hours of work that potential employers want to purchase. We then consider the supply side, discussing how the wage and other factors influence the hours of work that potential employees are willing to provide. The remainder of this chapter then puts the two sides of the market together to show how supply and demand interact to determine the wage and employment level in the labor market. The wage (which is the price of the good being traded) plays a key role, rising or falling to equalize the employment level demanded by employers with that willing to be provided by employees. In the final section of the chapter, we discuss what happens when the wage fails to adjust, leading to shortages. For now, we will keep our discussion of supply and demand fairly simple and general. In later chapters, we will return to these issues and discuss in much more depth the demand for RNs (Chapter 4) and the supply of RNs (Chapters 6 and 7).

While it is certainly not necessary to be an economist to comprehend the content of this book, it will be helpful to be familiar with the basic economic concepts contained in this chapter. Though not essential, the content of this chapter will help the reader to more fully appreciate later chapters and thereby deepen their overall understanding of the nursing workforce and RN's relationships with employers, patients, and society more generally.

THE DEMAND FOR LABOR

The demand for labor is the total hours of work that potential employers are willing to hire. More specifically, we must define the demand for labor in terms of the amount of a specific type of labor to be hired in a particular market over a specified time interval, for example, the hours of RN time that all employers are willing to hire in the United States during 1 week.

The demand for labor will depend on the wage, just as the demand for other goods depends on their price. An increase in the price of a good usually reduces the demand for that good, a relationship generally referred to as "the law of demand." Similarly, an increase in the wage rate reduces the demand for labor for two reasons. First, employee time is one of many inputs that employers purchase (such as raw materials, equipment, land and structures, etc.) to produce a final product that is sold to consumers. As the cost of any input rises, employers substitute away from that input toward other inputs in an effort to reduce costs. For example, if a hospital has to pay increased wages to obtain more RNs (an input in the production of hospital care), the hospital would face an incentive to substitute away from the more costly RN and employ lower-wage licensed practical nurses. A second reason that an increase in the wage rate reduces the demand for labor is that it raises the cost of the final product to consumers, which can in turn lead to lower demand for the product. The single largest expense for most employers is wages and benefits paid to their employees, accounting for roughly two-thirds of all expenses for the average employer. Thus, an increase in the wage can have a sizable impact on expenses, some of which may be passed along to consumers in terms of higher prices.

In **Figure 3-1** we plot a hypothetical demand curve, which depicts the negative relationship between wages and the demand for labor, holding constant all other things that might affect the demand for labor. As shown in the figure, a rise in the wage from W_1 to W_2 is associated with a decline in demand for labor from E_1 to E_2. This movement along the demand curve captures the negative relationship between the wage and the demand for labor, all else equal.

Figure 3-1   The Labor Demand Curve

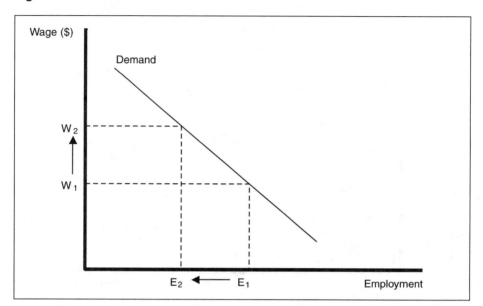

It is standard to use the concept of elasticity to capture how responsive demand is to the wage. The elasticity of demand with respect to the wage (also called the wage elasticity of demand) is defined as the percent change in the demand for labor that is associated with a one percent increase in the wage. The demand curve is referred to as inelastic if the elasticity is less than one in absolute value—that is, if a one percent increase in the wage leads to less than a one percent decline in demand for labor. Thus, an inelastic demand curve is one for which labor demand is not very responsive to the wage (i.e., a steep slope). Similarly, an elastic demand curve has elasticity greater than one (i.e., a flat slope) so that labor demand is more responsive to changes in the wage.

It is important to remember that the demand curve holds constant all other factors influencing labor demand to focus attention on the key role that the wage plays in balancing supply and demand. Nevertheless, many other factors will influence the employer's demand for labor, including the price of other inputs and the number of potential consumers of the employer's final product. When these other factors change, we depict their impact as a shift in the demand curve. In **Figure 3-2** we illustrate an outward shift in the demand curve, as might occur if population growth led to higher demand for the employer's product. For any fixed wage (W_1), the demand for labor has increased (from E_1 to E_2). Thus, while changes in the wage lead to movement along the labor demand curve, changes in other factors lead to a shift in the demand curve.

Figure 3-2   A Shift Outward in the Labor Demand Curve

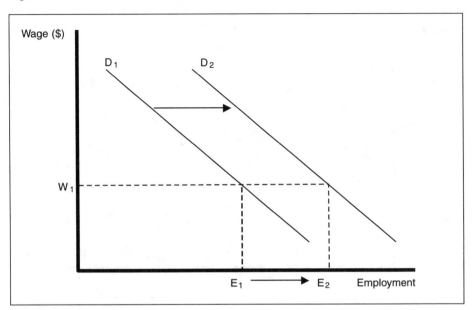

THE SUPPLY OF LABOR

The supply of labor is the total hours of work that potential employees are willing to provide. As was the case with demand, we must define the supply of labor in terms of the amount of a specific type of labor to be provided in a particular market over a specified time interval. For example, we could consider the hours of work that all RNs in the United States are willing to provide during 1 week.

A key factor determining the supply of labor will be the wage. An increase in the price of a good usually increases the supply of that good, a relationship generally referred to as "the law of supply." An increase in the wage rate increases the supply of labor for two reasons. First, in the short run, some individuals who are already working will choose to work more hours (e.g., switching from part time to full time), and others who are not working at all will enter the workforce because of the greater rewards derived from working additional hours. In addition, entry into many labor markets (like RNs) requires that a person first obtain specialized training and education. Higher wages will encourage more individuals to acquire these specialized skills by increasing the return on this investment, leading to additional growth in labor supply in the longer run.

In **Figure 3-3** we plot hypothetical short-run and long-run labor supply curves. These labor supply curves depict the positive relationship between wages and the supply of labor, holding constant all other things that might affect the supply of labor. The short-run labor supply curve illustrates how different wage levels will affect labor supply in the near term, say over the next year or 6 months. The long-run labor supply curve illustrates how the same wage levels will affect labor supply in the longer term after individuals have had time to invest in training and education, say in 4 to 5 years. We assume that wages have been at their current level for many years so that the short-run and long-run supply curves cross at the current wage (W_1). A raise in the wage from W_1 to W_2 will be associated with a larger increase in supply in the long run (from E_1 to $E_{2,LR}$) than in the short run (from E_1 to $E_{2,SR}$), as additional individuals acquire the necessary skills to enter the workforce in the long run. Using the concept of elasticity in a manner analogous to how it was used to describe demand, we would say that long-run labor supply is more elastic than short-run labor supply, that is, a one percent increase in the wage generates a larger percentage increase in labor supply in the long run than in the short run.

As with the labor demand curve, the labor supply curve holds constant all other factors to focus attention on the key role that the wage plays in balancing

Figure 3-3   The Short-Run and Long-Run Labor Supply Curves

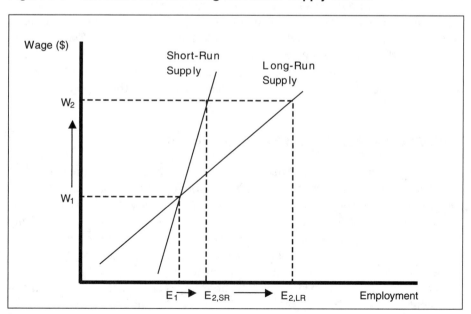

Figure 3-4   A Shift Outward in the Labor Supply Curve

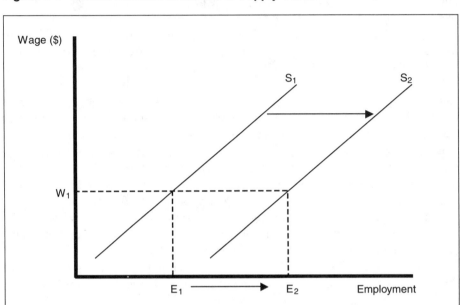

supply and demand. The effect of other factors that influence the supply of labor, such as growth in the working-age population, is seen as a shift in the supply curve. In **Figure 3-4** we illustrate an outward shift in the labor supply curve, as might occur if there was growth in the working-age population. For any fixed wage (W_1), the supply of labor has increased (from E_1 to E_2). As was the case with labor demand, changes in the wage lead to movement along the labor supply curve, while changes in other factors lead to a shift in the supply curve.

EQUILIBRIUM IN A COMPETITIVE LABOR MARKET

We are now prepared to put the two sides of the market together to show how supply and demand interact to determine the equilibrium wage and employment level in a competitive labor market. *The wage plays a key role, adjusting so that in equilibrium the hours of work demanded by employers are equal to the hours of work supplied by employees.* Moreover, competition between employers to hire and competition between employees to get jobs will cause the wage to move toward this equilibrium level where demand and supply are in balance. Thus, competition along with flexible wages ensures that wages and employment are determined by the laws of supply and demand.

Figure 3-5 illustrates how supply and demand interact to determine the wage and employment level. To simplify the figures, we will not distinguish between long-run and short-run supply for the moment, and we will return to this issue later. Because the labor supply curve is upward sloping while the labor demand curve is downward sloping, they will cross at a single point. At the point where demand and supply cross, the wage level (W_1) is such that the supply of labor is exactly equal to the demand for labor at E_1. At any higher wage level, such as W_2, there will be a surplus of workers looking for jobs because the higher wage increases supply while reducing demand. In Figure 3-5 this is seen as the horizontal distance between the supply and demand curves at a wage level of W_2. Competition among the surplus workers to obtain the limited number of jobs will put downward pressure on wages, pushing wages back toward W_1. Similarly, at any wage level below W_1, such as W_3, there will be a shortage of workers as the lower wage reduces supply and increases demand. This shortage is represented in Figure 3-5 as the horizontal distance between the demand and supply curves at a wage level of W_3. Competition among employers to obtain the limited number of workers will put upward pressure on wages, pushing wages again back toward W_1. Thus, the point at which labor supply and labor demand cross determines the unique equilibrium combination of wage and hours of work (W_1 and E_1) that will result in a competitive market.

Figure 3-5   Equilibrium Hours and Employment in a Competitive Labor Market

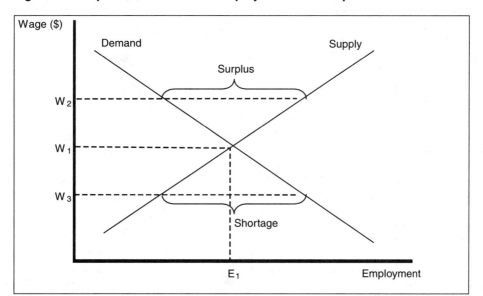

Within this supply and demand framework, we can very simply analyze the changes in equilibrium wages and employment that will result from factors that shift the labor supply curve or the labor demand curve (or both). **Figure 3-6** illustrates what happens to wages and employment when some factor causes the supply of labor to shift outward. Because labor supply has shifted outward, there is now a surplus of labor (supply exceeds demand) at the old equilibrium wage (W_1) and, therefore, wages must decline. The new equilibrium is the point where the new labor supply curve crosses the labor demand curve. At this point, wages are lower (going from W_1 to W_2) and hours of work are higher (going from E_1 to E_2) than in the original equilibrium. Thus, outward shifts in the labor supply curve lead to movements down the demand curve, resulting in lower wages and higher employment. Furthermore, the impact on wages and employment will depend on the elasticity of the labor demand curve, with wages changing less and employment changing more when the labor demand curve is more elastic (i.e., flatter).

A similar analysis can be done to evaluate the impact of an outward shift in the labor demand curve. For this case, it is informative to determine the short-run and long-run impacts by considering both the short-run and long-run labor supply curves. We illustrate the impact of a shift out in the demand curve in **Figure 3-7**. Suppose we begin at a long-run equilibrium wage of W_1, for which the short-run and long-run supply of labor is equal to the demand for labor. In

Figure 3-6   Impact of Outward Shift in Labor Supply on Competitive Equilibrium

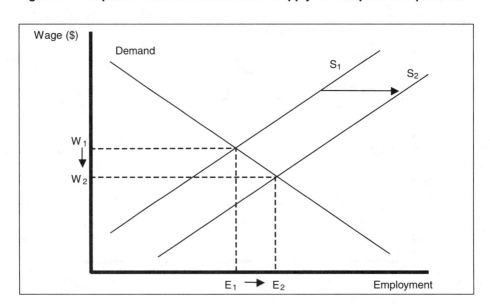

the short run, the outward shift in labor demand leads to a new equilibrium at the point where the new labor demand curve crosses the short-run labor supply curve. This movement along the short-run labor supply curve results in much higher wages ($W_{2, SR}$) ($E_{2, SR}$) and somewhat higher employment in the short run. In the longer run, the new equilibrium will be at the point where the new labor demand curve crosses the long-run labor supply curve. Because long-run supply is more responsive to the higher wage, equilibrium employment will increase more in the long run than in the short run (to $E_{2, LR}$). However, because long-run supply is better able to accommodate the outward shift in demand, equilibrium wages will increase less in the long run than they did in the short run (to $W_{2, LR}$), although they will still be above the original equilibrium wage of W_1. Thus, outward shifts in the labor demand curve tend to primarily increase wages in the short run, while having more of an impact on employment (and less on wages) in the longer run.

Simple supply and demand diagrams such as those in Figures 3-6 and 3-7 are used by economists to evaluate how a wide range of factors will affect the labor market through how these factors lead to shifts in either the labor supply or labor demand curves. For example, population growth is often assumed to shift both labor supply and labor demand outward by a similar amount, leading to a growth in employment but no change in the wage. However, when the working

Figure 3-7   Impact of Outward Shift in Labor Demand on Short-Run and Long-Run Competitive Equilibrium

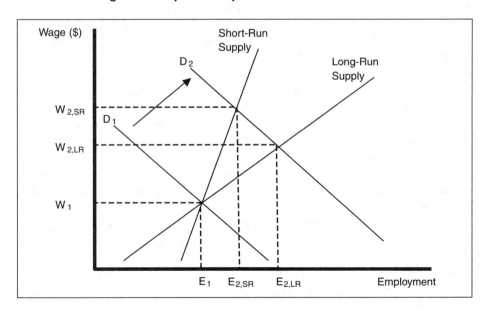

age population grows more slowly than the population of consumers, as is expected in the healthcare sector in the coming decades with the retirement of the baby boomers, we might expect that the labor demand curve will shift out more rapidly than the labor supply curve, leading to growth in both employment and wages in the healthcare sector. Moreover, the impact of this outward shift in the labor demand curve will depend on the elasticity of the long-run labor supply curve. For low-skill occupations such as aides and orderlies, which require very little training or special skills, the long-run labor supply curve is likely to be very elastic—small increases in the wage will encourage many people currently working in other low-skill occupations to become aides and orderlies. In contrast, for high-skill occupations such as doctors and nurses, which require considerable education and special skills, the long-run labor supply curve is likely to be less elastic—it requires a large increase in the wage to encourage people to undertake the years of education required to enter these occupations. Because labor supply is less elastic for high-skilled workers than for low-skilled workers, an increase in labor demand in the healthcare sector is likely to have a larger impact on wages of high-skilled workers while having a larger impact on employment for low-skilled workers.

EQUILIBRIUM WHEN MULTIPLE MARKETS COMPETE FOR THE SAME TYPE OF LABOR

In this book, we will consider many situations where the same type of labor is being used in many different labor markets. For example, RNs work in many different settings, such as hospitals, nursing homes, physician offices, and home health care. Similarly, RNs work in distinct geographic markets. Each of these settings and geographic locations can potentially be thought of as a distinct labor market, with unique factors affecting labor demand and labor supply in each sector or region. For example, demand for RNs will shift outward in regions experiencing rapid growth in their elderly population, placing upward pressure on wages in those regions. Similarly, declining use of inpatient services will shift demand for RNs inward in the hospital sector, placing downward pressure on wages in that market.

However, it is relatively easy and common for RNs to move from one sector to another, or even to migrate from one region to another. Thus, each sector and region must compete with others to attract RNs, and this competition for workers will tend to equalize wages across the markets. For example, suppose there are two labor markets that hire the same type of labor and that workers are able to move freely between the two labor markets. An outward shift in labor demand in one of the markets will increase the wage in that market relative to the other market. The change in relative wages between the two markets will lead workers to move into the market that experienced the outward shift in labor demand—a shift out in the labor supply curve for this market. Correspondingly, the labor supply curve will shift inward in the market that did not experience a change in labor demand as workers move to the other market. In the end, labor supply will shift between the two markets until wages are equalized. Thus, an outward shift in the labor demand curve of one market leads to a shift of employees toward that market and higher wages in both markets.

This simple example illustrates a very general principle. When multiple labor markets compete for the same type of labor, a demand shock (a change in a factor that affects the demand for labor) affecting any one market will affect wages in all markets. An outward shift in demand in any one market will increase wages in all markets, while an inward shift will decrease wages in all markets. A demand shock in any one market might have little impact on the wages of that market relative to the other markets it competes with. Instead, an outward shift in demand in any one market will primarily result in an increase in employment in that market relative to other markets it competes with, while an inward shift will result in a decrease in employment in that market.

LABOR MARKET SHORTAGE AS DISEQUILIBRIUM

What does it mean to say that there is a shortage in a particular labor market? In the popular discussion and in policy debates, people often mean many different things when they refer to a labor shortage depending on their points of view. For example, healthcare policy makers often define a shortage as any time that employment falls below some subjective definition of "requirements" based on what is needed to achieve certain health benchmarks. Alternatively, employers often describe any period of time in which there is upward pressure on wages as a time of labor shortage, reflecting their perception that the labor demand curve has shifted out more than the labor supply curve.

We, however, will define a shortage in the labor market in the way that most economists would. A shortage is a market disequilibrium in which labor demand exceeds labor supply because the wage lies below the equilibrium wage. Thus, when we refer to a shortage in the labor market, we refer to the situation depicted earlier in Figure 3-5 when wages are below the equilibrium wage. We have already discussed how the wage will tend toward its equilibrium level—during a shortage, competition among employers to obtain the limited number of workers will put upward pressure on wages, pushing wages back to their equilibrium level. Thus, shortages should not exist (or at least be short-lived) in a competitive labor market with flexible wages (i.e., when there are no restrictions on the freedom of wages to increase).

Shortages can persist, however, in real-life settings where wages are not perfectly flexible. At the extreme, government wage and price controls (such as those imposed by President Nixon in the early 1970s) can limit the amount that wages can increase. More commonly, labor contracts might set wages a year or more in advance so that unexpected shifts outward in labor demand will lead to temporary shortages until the wage can adjust. Over a period of time when labor demand is growing rapidly, this could lead to a long-lasting shortage. Finally, if an outward shift in the labor demand curve would lead to temporarily high wages in the short run (as we saw in Figure 3-7), employers might be hesitant to raise wages in the short run, knowing that they will have to eventually reduce wages to the long-run equilibrium level. In Chapter 11, Appendix 11-1, we elaborate on why employers, in this case hospitals, are often slow in raising RN wages when they are experiencing a shortage of RNs.

Shortages can also persist in real-life settings where labor markets are not competitive. Rather than competing with each other for scarce workers during a shortage, employers could collude to keep wages low. Of course, such collusion is difficult to maintain when there are many employers in the market because each employer has an incentive to break ranks and offer a slightly higher wage to fill their vacancies. When employers are able to maintain collusion and keep wages below their competitive level, economists say that the labor market is a "monopsony." Monopsony is most likely to occur in labor markets with only a few large employers.

CHAPTER SUMMARY

The economic model of demand and supply is extremely useful in organizing and describing the wide-ranging forces that determine earnings and employment in the labor market. We have seen how wages and employment are determined in a competitive labor market by factors that shift the demand curve for labor and by factors that shift the supply curve for labor. At the same time, the impact these shifts in demand and supply have on the wage and employment will depend on how responsive labor supply and labor demand are to changes in the wage. The next two sections of this book, therefore, investigate in detail the factors that have shifted the demand and supply of RNs over the last 4 decades and that are likely to affect demand and supply into the future. A careful analysis of the forces affecting the demand and supply of RNs will help us to more clearly understand recent trends in earnings and employment, the development and resolution of nursing shortages, and to evaluate polices aimed at strengthening the current and future workforce.

CHAPTER 4

The Demand for Health Care and the Derived Demand for Registered Nurses

When we use the term "demand," we envision an individual willing and able to give up something of value in exchange for a good or service that the individual desires. For example, a person might be willing to give up some of their money (something they value) for a prescription drug (a desired good) or a visit to the chiropractor (a desired service). Demand is an economic concept and refers to an exchange or transaction made between parties. In nursing and throughout the healthcare system, we often hear about an individual's "need" for health care. Need is related to, but differs from, demand. Whereas demand involves an economic exchange, and can thus be observed as in the case of numbers of employed RNs at a given wage rate, need is a concept that is usually used to describe a subjectively determined level of goods or services (housing, food, health care) required to meet some standard that is usually defined without regard to the resources an individual might possess. Different societies might set different standards or definitions of need, ranging from basic survival to a high level of comfort. Thus, the need for health care is generally independent of economic considerations and may or may not involve an economic transaction. In this chapter, we discuss the factors that determine the *demand* for nurses. Although we believe that everyone "needs" a nurse, it is the demand for nurses that is our focus.

The provision of health care consists of products, services, treatments, and personal interventions that promote good health. Health care spans a continuum that covers the life span from birth (even in utero in some cases) to death and involves services and treatments ranging from prevention of illness and disease to providing end of life and palliative care. As we begin to discuss the demand for nurses (more specifically, RNs), it is important to recognize that the demand for RNs is *derived* from society's overall demand for health care. It is society's demand for health care that creates the demand for healthcare institutions and the people they employ, including RNs, who possess unique knowledge and skills that can satisfy this demand. The same can be said of the demand for physicians, pharmacists, physical therapists, and others; the demand for them, like the demand for RNs, is derived from society's demand for health care. Healthcare delivery organizations combine healthcare professionals, equipment, and buildings to produce the goods and services to meet society's demand for health care. Because many organizations require RNs to produce the healthcare services and treatments that people are willing to purchase, organizations are willing to give up something (money in the form of wages) in exchange for the time and services provided by RNs.

With this introduction on the economic meaning of demand, health care, and the role of healthcare delivery organizations, we turn next to examining the factors that determine society's overall demand for health care. Following this, we focus on examining the factors that determine healthcare organizations' demand for RNs. We conclude the chapter by describing the methods and results of different federal government agencies that have recently projected the future demand for RNs.

SOCIETY'S DEMAND FOR HEALTH CARE

Conceptually, we can think about society's demand for health care as arising from the factors that affect individuals' desire to possess good health. People want good health because it allows them to feel better and function at their desired level of performance. Possessing good health enables people to spend more of their time doing the things they desire and that bring them personal satisfaction, such as holding a job and earning money or spending time in leisure activities. Society's demand for health care reflects the sum of every individual's demand for good health. The factors that determine society's overall demand for health care can be grouped into four broad areas: the changes in the health, size, and age composition of the population; sociocultural factors; economic factors; and the organization of the healthcare system. Changes in each of these factors can result in an expansion or contraction in the overall amount of health care demanded by society.[1] With respect to Figure 3-2 in Chapter 3, the factors that affect society's overall demand for health care cause the demand for RNs in the labor market to shift outward and to the right (from D_1 to D_2) or inward and to the left.

---

[1] Throughout this section, it should be noted that the United States has a somewhat unique system of healthcare financing and delivery compared to other developed countries, which tend to treat health care more like we treat education: funded through general taxation and provided to individuals at little or no cost at the time of service. However, many of the concepts are applicable to both systems; demand for different levels of health care in France, for example, is expressed through decisions made by government agencies or officials, whereas many of those decisions are made by individuals, employers, or private insurers in the United States.

Changes in the Health, Size, and Age Composition of the Population

People who are free of disease or illness (physical or mental) are likely to demand less health care than those who suffer from such misfortunes. Many examples illustrate how changes in the incidence of disease impact the demand for health care. Consider how the spread of diseases, the incidence of illnesses due to the exposure to occupational, and environmental hazards, and changing lifestyles that have resulted in substance abuse, obesity, and violence have increased the demand for health care. In contrast, the eradication or reduction of certain communicable diseases through immunization (polio, mumps, tuberculosis, etc.), lessening of air and food contamination, increased fluoridation of drinking water, and improvements in automobile safety have decreased the incidence of diseases and injury and hence the demand for health care. We are all familiar with the efforts to find a cure for cancer, Alzheimer's disease, diabetes, heart disease, and other conditions. If and when cures for these diseases are found, the overall demand for health care may decrease substantially. Over time, the incidence of diseases and illnesses changes, and depending on their effect on increasing or decreasing individuals' stock of good health, such factors will influence society's overall demand for health care.

In addition to the changing incidence and nature of diseases and illness, the demand for health care is related to the size and composition of the nation's population. Growth in the number of people in the United States increases the demand for health care simply by the fact that more people will experience perceived or actual illness and will be willing to purchase services and treatments that prevent disease and illness during their life. Throughout its history, the United States has experienced steady growth in population, and in 2000 the size of the population reached an estimated 282 million (see **Table 4-1**). By 2020, the population is projected to grow to 336 million and reach an estimated 420 million by 2050. Outside of the United States, other countries are projected to experience a different outlook. For example, the population in the European continent, particularly in southern Europe and Italy, is expected to decline by 86 million people between 2000 and 2050. The United States is the only industrialized country expected to rank among the top 10 nations in population by 2050 (Population Resource Center, 2007), and this population growth will positively impact the demand for health care for years to come.

Beyond the increase in size, the population in the United States (and throughout the world) is becoming older at an unprecedented rate. It is well known that the number of people over the age of 65 in the United States has been increasing for many decades (see **Figure 4-1**). Notice that the rate of increase in the elderly is expected to accelerate after 2010. This surge is attributed to the fact

Table 4-1   Projected Population of the United States, by Age and Sex, 2000–2050

(In thousands except as indicated. As of July 1. Resident population.)

Population or percent, sex, and age	2000	2010	2020	2030	2040	2050
POPULATION TOTAL						
TOTAL	282,125	308,936	335,805	363,584	391,946	419,854
0–4	19,218	21,426	22,932	24,272	26,299	28,080
5–19	61,331	61,810	65,955	70,832	75,326	81,067
20–44	104,075	104,444	108,632	114,747	121,659	130,897
45–64	62,440	81,012	83,653	82,280	88,611	93,104
65–84	30,794	34,120	47,363	61,850	64,640	65,844
85+	4,267	6,123	7,269	9,603	15,409	20,861
MALE						
TOTAL	138,411	151,815	165,093	178,563	192,405	206,477
0–4	9,831	10,947	11,716	12,399	13,437	14,348
5–19	31,454	31,622	33,704	36,199	38,496	41,435
20–44	52,294	52,732	54,966	58,000	61,450	66,152
45–64	30,381	39,502	40,966	40,622	43,961	46,214
65–84	13,212	15,069	21,337	28,003	29,488	30,579
85+	1,240	1,942	2,403	3,340	5,573	7,749
FEMALE						
TOTAL	143,713	157,121	170,711	185,022	199,540	213,377
0–4	9,387	10,479	11,216	11,873	12,863	13,732
5–19	29,877	30,187	32,251	34,633	36,831	39,632
20–44	51,781	51,711	53,666	56,747	60,209	64,745
45–64	32,059	41,510	42,687	41,658	44,650	46,891
65–84	17,582	19,051	26,026	33,848	35,152	35,265
85+	3,028	4,182	4,866	6,263	9,836	13,112
PERCENT OF TOTAL						
TOTAL	100.0	100.0	100.0	100.0	100.0	100.0
0–4	6.8	6.9	6.8	6.7	6.7	6.7
5–19	21.7	20.0	19.6	19.5	19.2	19.3
20–44	36.9	33.8	32.3	31.6	31.0	31.2
45–64	22.1	26.2	24.9	22.6	22.6	22.2
65–84	10.9	11.0	14.1	17.0	16.5	15.7
85+	1.5	2.0	2.2	2.6	3.9	5.0
MALE						
TOTAL	100.0	100.0	100.0	100.0	100.0	100.0
0–4	7.1	7.2	7.1	6.9	7.0	6.9
5–19	22.7	20.8	20.4	20.3	20.0	20.1
20–44	37.8	34.7	33.3	32.5	31.9	32.0
45–64	21.9	26.0	24.8	22.7	22.8	22.4
65–84	9.5	9.9	12.9	15.7	15.3	14.8
85+	0.9	1.3	1.5	1.9	2.9	3.8
FEMALE						
TOTAL	100.0	100.0	100.0	100.0	100.0	100.0
0–4	6.5	6.7	6.6	6.4	6.4	6.4
5–19	20.8	19.2	18.9	18.7	18.5	18.6
20–44	36.0	32.9	31.4	30.7	30.2	30.3
45–64	22.3	26.4	25.0	22.5	22.4	22.0
65–84	12.2	12.1	15.2	18.3	17.6	16.5
85+	2.1	2.7	2.9	3.4	4.9	6.1

Source: U.S. Census Bureau. (2004). *U.S. interim projections by age, sex, race, and Hispanic origin.*
Retrieved November 16, 2007, from http://www.census.gov/ipc/www/usinterimproj/
Internet Release Date: March 18, 2004.

Figure 4-1   Growth in Number of Individuals over the Ages of 65 and 85 in the United States, 1990 Projected to 2050

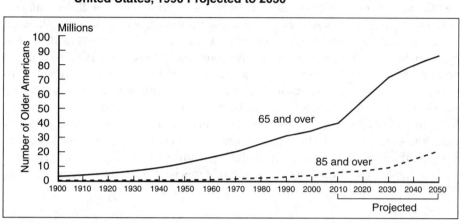

Source: U.S. Census Bureau, Decennial Census and Projections.
Note: Data for 2010–2050 are projections of population.
Reference population: These data refer to the resident population.

that many of the 76 million people born during the baby boom generation (1946–1964) will become seniors starting in 2010 and beyond. In addition, these individuals are expected to live longer than previous generations of older Americans because life expectancy in the United States has increased dramatically during the past century. In 1900, women could expect to live, on average, 48.3 years (46.3 years for men), whereas women born in 2003 can expect to live, on average, 80.1 years (77.5 years for men; National Center for Health Statistics, 2007).

The combination of aging baby boomers and longer life spans, particularly for women, means that the population of Americans over the age of 65 is increasing in absolute size and as a proportion of the total population. U.S. Census Bureau poulation projections show that the number of individuals aged 65 and over will nearly double over the next 25 years and increase by an estimated 127% between 2000 and 2050. By 2030, there will be an estimated 71 million Americans over the age of 65, or about one in five people in the United States (see Table 4-1). Even by 2020 the United States is expected to have 5 million more people over the age of 75 than were alive in 2000 according to HRSA (2003).

These changes in the size and age of the population (achieved in part by the provision of healthcare services) will clearly increase the future demand for health care. As people grow older, their stock of good health will decline, and patterns of morbidity will change from infectious diseases and acute illnesses to chronic diseases and degenerative illnesses. Currently, about 8 in 10 Americans are living with at least one chronic condition (Centers for Disease Control and Prevention, 2007). On a per capita basis, the elderly have more hospital inpatient days, outpatient visits, and emergency department visits. Relative to the nonelderly, they also have more home health visits per capita and are more likely to be in a long-term care facility. Not surprisingly, the cost of providing health care for older people is three to five times greater than the cost for someone younger than 65. As a result of these demographic changes in the United States, by 2030 healthcare spending in the United States is projected to increase by 25% (Centers for Disease Control and Prevention, 2007).

Sociocultural Characteristics

To the extent that people feel there is some value in making additional purchases of healthcare services and treatments in their desire to achieve good health, they will have a greater demand for health care than those who feel there is little value in making additional purchases. The value placed on any good or service, including health care, varies from individual to individual and is influenced by sociocultural beliefs and attitudes and by educational attainment. To resolve a health condition or illness, some people might place a greater value on using home remedies than highly technical treatments, or they might prefer to receive care from nontraditional versus western-oriented providers. As the population in the United States becomes more diverse, cultural differences will increasingly impact the amount of health care demanded, the composition of healthcare services, and the manner in which they are provided. And, as disparities in the use of healthcare services are reduced, we can expect increases in demand among minority populations.

A person's level of education also impacts the demand for health care. Most studies find a negative relationship between education and the demand for health care—as education levels increase, less health care is demanded. According to Feldstein (2005), as education attainment increases, individuals are likely to be more adept at recognizing the early symptoms of illness, resulting in a higher likelihood that they will obtain early treatment or even change their lifestyles to avoid diseases or illnesses. Additional years of education might increase awareness of the need for health care, instill different attitudes, knowledge, and expectations about seeking health care, or promote greater efficiency in purchasing and using healthcare services. Feldstein cites evidence from the Agency for Healthcare Research and Quality showing that people aged 45 to 64 with higher education levels have markedly lower overall medical expenditures than do those of the same age but with lower education. He notes that while people with more education have higher expenditures for physician office visits, these expenditures are offset by lower hospital expenditures and thereby contribute to an overall decreased demand for health care. Growing levels of education in the U.S. population will temper the growth in the demand for health care.

Economic Factors

The demand for health care is also responsive to economic factors. These factors include an individual's income, the price of health care, and the value of an individual's time. With respect to the first of these economic factors, as individuals' *income* increases, they have more resources with which to purchase goods and services. For some goods, less will be purchased as income rises. For example, as individuals' income increases, we might expect them to purchase less fast food or be less likely to rent an apartment. For other goods, however, an increase in income results in an increase in the amount of goods purchased, depending on the individual's unique tastes and preferences—steak or a new house, for example. With more money at their disposal, some people might allocate some of their purchases toward goods and services perceived to be of higher quality or social status, even if they are more expensive, and away from lower priced goods with perceived lower status.

With respect to health care, a positive relationship exists between income and the demand for health care. That is, as incomes increase, we can expect that more health care (perhaps through the purchase of more comprehensive health insurance) will be purchased, on average. This relationship has been verified by numerous studies, though results differ on the degree to which more health care is consumed as income rises. For example, studies find that a 10% increase in income leads to anywhere from a 2% increase in the amount of health care demanded to an increase of greater than 10%.[2] Further, this relationship between income and demand for health care (the income elasticity of demand) varies for different types of health care (e.g., increased use of dental services is more responsive to increases in income than are hospital visits). Returning to our

---

[2] Demand for health care tends to be more responsive to changes in income in the long run, when there has been enough time to develop more healthcare treatments and services. In the short run, one might be limited in the amount of health care available for purchase.

earlier discussion of the aging population, it is important to realize that not only will there be increasing numbers of older Americans in the future who will be living longer. These individuals will, on average, have more income available to spend on health care compared to previous generations of older Americans.

The price of health care also influences the demand for health care. In general, economic theory predicts that when the price of a good falls, more of that good will be purchased, holding all other factors equal (an individual's income, tastes and preferences, and availability and price of substitute goods). How much is actually purchased depends on the size of the price decrease and how sensitive the payer is to the price of the good. For some goods and services, a small change in price might induce a proportionally larger increase in the quantity purchased (the relationship is said to be price "elastic"). For other goods, the same drop in price might result in only a small increase in the quantity purchased (here, the relationship between price and quantity demanded is said to be price "inelastic").

With respect to the demand for health care, the relationship between the use of healthcare services and the price of the service behaves in much the same manner as the purchase of other goods and services. However, most health care is not purchased by the recipient of the care at its full price at the time of use—rather, people generally purchase (or are provided with) insurance to deliberately insulate themselves from those costs. Thus, it is often insurers or government agencies that are directly involved in the relationship between the price of services (for example, specialist physicians who charge high fees) and choosing how much of those and other services are purchased. Consumers might face such choices in the aggregate in selecting different insurance packages that provide more complete coverage of services (e.g., low copayments) in exchange for higher premiums (prices) or on an individual basis when paying for services directly out of pocket (such as certain types of cosmetic surgery, LASIK surgery, etc.) that are not covered by insurance.

Health care is also unique in that certain purchases, such as life-saving treatments, do not follow the usual price-quantity relationship because most people would disregard these costs when confronting a life and death situation. For our purposes, it is important to make the basic point that the price of healthcare services is important in determining the overall demand for health care: As price falls for whatever reason (production costs decrease due to technology innovations; health plans make greater use of nurse practitioners versus physicians; competition among providers grows, forcing reductions in costs or profits; etc.), more health care will be purchased, holding quality and other factors constant. The inverse is also true: When the price of health care increases, holding all else constant, less will be purchased.

One of the most important ways that the price of health care has been reduced for millions of Americans, and hence resulted in increased demand for health care, involves the way the federal government taxes health insurance premiums.[3] Because health insurance premiums paid by the *employer* are excluded from the taxable income of an employee, an individual is better off if the employer spends $5000 on health insurance on that individual's behalf (assuming the individual wants health insurance) rather than giving the individual that money as additional salary, where it would be taxed, and therefore it would amount to, say, $3500, which the individual could use to purchase insurance (or other goods). In addition, employers are able to obtain a lower price for health insurance premiums by purchasing insurance for large groups of people (their employees), whereas individuals on their own would have to pay a larger amount for the same coverage. For these reasons, employees have accepted lower wages in exchange for the purchase of health insurance coverage by their employer, which is exempt from their taxable income.

By permitting employers to purchase health insurance using employees' nontaxable income, however, the price of health insurance has been lowered with the result that the amount of health insurance purchased in the United States has increased more than it would have otherwise. Consequently, many people have obtained very comprehensive healthcare insurance that provides coverage for relatively low cost and predictable events (immunizations, teeth cleaning, etc). Generally, more people have purchased health insurance, and more comprehensive insurance plans, than would have occurred had they been required to buy insurance by themselves using their own money.

With regard to the demand for health care, those with health insurance consume more healthcare services and services of a higher quality. Assuming no change in the law governing the tax treatment of health insurance premiums, and assuming a robust U.S. economy, the demand for privately financed health insurance will continue and further fuel the demand for health care. However, should healthcare reform proposals be enacted that would alter the long-standing tax treatment of employer provided health insurance, then the demand for health care will be altered substantially.

In addition to income and the price of health care, the value of a person's *time* also influences the demand for health care. Time, like the price of a good or the amount of income an individual possesses, acts to constrain the demand for certain goods. This constraint arises from the fact that time is needed to produce or consume a good or service, and thus time has a cost in that the same time

---

[3] For a detailed description of the tax treatment of health insurance, see Chapter 6, "The Demand for Health Insurance" (Feldstein, 2006).

could have been used differently to produce or consume alternative goods and services. With respect to the demand for health care, time is required to travel to a healthcare provider. People who live in rural areas typically have to travel a greater distance and thereby consume more of their time to see a physician or a nurse practitioner than those who live in urban areas. When in the office (or hospital), time is spent waiting to be seen by the provider. And if one engages in preventative behavior, then time is needed to exercise or perhaps cook nutritious meals versus eat at a restaurant.

Each of these examples requires an expenditure of a person's time, which has many alternative uses. Time costs are important generally because they increase the "cost" of health care to consumers. For example, if there is a shortage of RNs, patients might end up spending more time in the hospital during the admission and discharge processes because these processes ultimately depend on the availability of an RN's time. Time costs are more or less important to different people because those who have lower time costs can afford to spend more time waiting for health care than those with higher time costs. For example, if the quantity supplied of medical or nursing services does not increase sufficiently to meet an increased demand for health care (perhaps due to a shortage of nurses), then those who can afford to wait for health care are more likely to receive the care that is available.

Changes in the Organization of the Healthcare System[4]

What amount of health care should be produced? Countries organize their healthcare systems to address three fundamental questions: What is the amount of health care to produce; how best should resources be used to produce health care; and how best should the health care that is produced be distributed throughout the population? The way that the healthcare system in the United States (or in any country) is organized affects the price, quality, and access to health care, as well as how healthcare consumers and providers interact with each other.

Prior to the development of managed care, the healthcare delivery system in the United States grew rapidly, year after year, decade after decade (see Chapter 2 for an overview of these trends). Most individuals and healthcare providers did not face meaningful economic incentives to use and produce health care judiciously. Rather, the incentives that pervaded the healthcare system prior to the 1980s were aligned largely along the principle that "more is better." To some degree no matter what the cost, as long as some treatment or service might help

---

[4] The review of the healthcare system is adapted from Feldstein (2006), Chapter 8, "Market Competition in Health Care."

a patient (even if only a little and at great cost), then healthcare organizations, doctors, and nurses acted to provide it. Because consumers were becoming increasingly well insured via employer paid health plans, people became increasingly shielded from paying out of pocket for health care and were largely unaware of the true costs of the health care they consumed; hence their demand was unchecked by providers who, because they were paid for their costs (fee-for-service), had little incentive to curb a patient's demand or take the time to ensure that they were using the least costly and most appropriate services and treatments.

The Medicaid and Medicare programs were enacted in 1965, and millions of older and poor Americans were provided increased access to health care, mostly acute care services and limited long-term care. Not surprisingly, the growth of these public programs and the limited financial accountability on the part of providers and consumers lead to a steady increase in the amount that society spent on health care. Consequently, throughout the 1970s and 1980s, both federal and state governments attempted to regulate the growth of new healthcare facilities and costly technology, restrict payments to providers, and reduce the rate of growth in overall spending. Among the more important approaches used by regulators included: price controls on the U.S. economy, including health care, imposed by the Nixon administration; comprehensive healthcare planning and Certificate of Need regulations during the 1970s; replacement of the cost-based hospital payment system with a prospective payment system based on Diagnosis Related Groups (DRGs) to curb hospital spending during the 1980s; and a new system to control spending on physicians based on resource-based relative value scales implemented in the 1990s. While the DRG system had some success in limiting the growth of hospital spending within the Medicare program (Medicare now pays hospitals a fixed price for a patient with a certain diagnosis, regardless of the treatment applied; thus, providers are not necessarily rewarded for applying more expensive treatments), these and many other attempts to use a regulatory approach were largely unsuccessful in stemming the rapid annual increase in healthcare spending in the United States.

To combat the high rate of spending, promote more appropriate use of healthcare services, and increase the quality of care, public policy began to promote the application of market forces in health care. Health Maintenance Organizations (HMOs) were embraced as a means to organize health care and to explicitly introduce economic discipline to the delivery of health care. At first, HMOs grew slowly because providers felt threatened and demanded that federal and state governments erect legal and regulatory barriers to stunt their development. But as the high rate of spending continued and the proportion of the gross domestic product (the economic value of all goods and services produced in the United States) devoted to health care rose to double-digit levels, barriers to the growth of HMOs were slowly relaxed. Consequently, during the late 1980s and throughout the 1990s, HMOs and other organizational innovations subsumed under the term "managed care" grew rapidly. This growth was aided by Supreme Court decisions upholding the application of competitive practices (such as advertising) to health care, as well as by the fact that there was an excess supply of physicians and hospital beds in the country (thus, hospitals were willing to lower their prices or enter into arrangements with physicians who would help fill their beds).

Under managed care, providers were paid a predetermined fixed amount for the health care needed by an individual (capitation). By enrolling employees in an HMO that used capitation, employers gave doctors and organizations an economic incentive to find (and use) the least costly way to produce healthcare services because any treatment savings accrue back to the provider (unlike under fee-for-service reimbursement, where higher-cost treatments tend to reward the provider with higher reimbursements). In addition, the rapid adoption of managed care to reorganize the healthcare delivery system had dramatic effects in how health care was delivered. Most HMOs required a patient to get approval from their assigned primary care physician before seeing a specialist physician and often required enrollees to use only those hospitals or physicians in the HMO's network (by driving a large volume of patients to a given provider, the HMO was able to obtain price discounts from that provider). In addition, the pressures to lower costs and retain consumer satisfaction stimulated many managed care organizations to increase employment of nurse practitioners.

The growth of HMOs and managed care organizations slowed the rate of spending on health care in the United States during the mid-1990s. In fact, the rate of increase was the lowest obtained in more than 3 decades. Likewise, annual percentage increases in health insurance premiums fell dramatically from 1993 through 2000. Although many consumers, providers, and the media questioned the incentives and practices of managed care organizations, there is little doubt that this innovation in the healthcare system succeeded at reducing the rate of spending increases and reducing the rapid growth in the demand for health care. (As we will see in Chapter 5, the employment and earnings of RNs and other nursing personnel were affected by the development of managed care.)

Since the late 1990s, however, healthcare costs have resumed their historical rapid rate of annual growth as managed care has lost much of its impact. Providers were unhappy with insurers' involvement in medical practice, and patients objected to the restrictions placed on their choice of provider, to name a few sources of dissatisfaction that have weakened managed care organizations' economic advantage. Preferred Provider Organizations (PPOs) have now become the dominant mode of health insurance. These organizations are a milder form of an HMO because they usually require higher enrollee copayments in exchange for greater choice of providers involving those who are not included in the PPO provider panel. Still, had HMOs and managed care not emerged to reshape the organization of the healthcare system in the United States, the demand for health care would undoubtedly have been higher today, as would the nation's total spending on health.

Looking ahead, managed care organizations will continue to evolve just as other organizational and financing components of the overall healthcare system will and, as they do, they will have an important impact on determining the overall demand for health care in the United States. Current efforts to change health policy at the state or federal level also could influence overall demand for health care. For example, Massachusetts recently enacted legislation to achieve universal health insurance coverage and mandated that all citizens have health insurance coverage. The state is creating mechanisms that make it easier for individuals who are not offered coverage through employers to obtain insurance. Should other states adopt plans to expand health insurance coverage, this would likely increase demand for health care on average (there have already been initial news reports of difficulty finding physicians to treat the influx of newly insured individuals in Massachusetts). At the same time, however, policy makers are well aware of the problem of rising healthcare costs and affordability, and they increasingly seek to couple health insurance expansion proposals with stronger incentives for cost control (such as eliminating the tax exclusion of health insurance purchased by employers, which would dampen demand for health care).

Technology

Before ending our discussion of factors that affect the overall demand for health care, it is important to briefly consider the affect of technology. Broadly speaking, technology with respect to healthcare delivery refers to innovations that make prevention or treatment of a particular health condition more effective, less painful, and possibly less costly in both time and dollars. Technology can affect the demand for care in a number of ways. To the extent that it lowers (or increases) the price of healthcare treatments and services, the demand for health care will be increased (or decreased), other things remaining constant. Technological innovations can also affect demand by altering the patient's time costs. For example, providers are increasingly using the Internet to communicate with patients, visualize their conditions using video cameras, and monitor their conditions using data reported electronically, thereby reducing the frequency of patients traveling to see their providers. This innovation is particularly applicable for people living in rural areas who have to travel considerable distances to see their healthcare providers. The development and increasing use of the Internet have similarly lowered the time costs for people seeking information about health concerns, including obtaining information on the price, quality, and availability of services. In addition, providers use the Internet to transfer radiological images to be read by physicians based in other countries so that results can be obtained quicker and the patients' waiting time is reduced.

Technology also has contributed to expanding the demand for healthcare services as new machines, devices, and instruments are developed that enable the diagnosis, treatment, and monitoring of health conditions more accurately, easily, and more comfortably. For example, the use of nuclear imaging devices, noninvasive surgery, organ transplants (lungs, kidneys, pancreas, heart, etc.), cosmetic implants, and surgery to replace worn out joints and body parts expands the range of healthcare services available to a growing population. Looking to the future, we can anticipate that advances in technology will continue to be developed at a rapid pace and targeted increasingly at health conditions affecting the aging and relatively wealthy baby boom generation, thereby stimulating further increases in demand.

By preventing disease or speeding up healing, certain technological advances can exert a negative effect on the demand for health care. For example, mapping of the genome and related developments in the field of genetics have the potential of preventing many diseases, including some forms of cancer. Similarly, a vaccine for AIDS or virulent strains of influenza would decrease the demand for health care over what would have otherwise been the case. However, technology in these areas has not yet developed to the point where it is clear that these or other similar benefits will actually be achieved in the near future, let alone be offered at a price that enables many people to obtain this technology. Even though some technology will be developed that decreases the demand for health care, on balance, we expect that the rapid pace of technological innovation in other areas of health care will stimulate greater overall demand for health care.

HEALTHCARE ORGANIZATIONS' DEMAND FOR REGISTERED NURSES

With this discussion of the major factors that affect society's overall demand for health care, we now turn our attention to examining the derived demand for nursing personnel, focusing again on RNs for the most part. As noted earlier, when considering the demand for nurses, we indicated that the demand is *derived* from society's overall demand for health care and that healthcare organizations are in business to satisfy society's demand for health care. To produce and deliver health care, organizations combine the time, knowledge, and skills of nurses with other healthcare professionals along with technology, buildings, and other physical assets. To determine the actual demand for nurses, therefore, we must consider the factors that healthcare delivery organizations take into account when they decide how many and which combination of nursing personnel (RNs, LPNs, aides) to employ. The factors include wages, the existing supply of nursing personnel, the output that can be obtained by employing additional nurses, the contributions to quality and safety of employing additional nurses, the relationship between capital and labor, the objective function of healthcare organizations that employ nurses, and budget constraints. Essentially, these factors influence movement along and shifts in the employer's demand curve for nurse labor, as we discussed in Chapter 3.

Factors That Determine Organizations' Demand for RNs

After they have determined the overall demand for health care that exists in their particular markets, organizations obtain the number and type of nursing personnel that are required to provide the health care it expects to deliver by offering nurses compensation in the form of wages and fringe benefits. Employers of RNs are usually willing to vary their wage offerings by the shift and day (nights and weekends pay higher) and by years of experience and educational preparation—more experience and higher education are associated with a more productive employee, who commands a higher wage. The same is true for fringe benefits—employers consider the type and tenure of nurses when offering different combinations of health insurance, vacation time, personal leave days, child care facilities, tuition reimbursements, and any number of other benefits. Thus, at a fundamental level, an organization offers a nurse a compensation package consisting of money income and nonpecuniary benefits, which the nurse either accepts or rejects in exchange for allocating his or her time to providing the employer with the desired nursing services.

As we illustrated in Chapter 3, an inverse relationship exists between *wages* (including the total compensation) paid by the employer and the number of RNs and other nursing personnel that are actually employed. That is, holding other factors constant, as the total compensation an organization must pay an RN *increases*, the organization has an incentive to employ *fewer* RNs. From the organization's perspective, wages are valuable resources that have alternative uses, and when more resources have to be given up in the form of wages, the organization will have less dollars available for other productive uses, such as purchasing equipment, hiring other workers, or developing programs and services to attract patients. On the other hand, the *lower* the amount of compensation required, the organization will have an economic incentive to employ *more* RNs (a movement down its demand curve for RNs). In the past, when the Medicare and Medicaid programs were introduced in the mid-1960s, hospitals faced a large shortage of RNs. Worried that hospitals would not be able to provide all the care to millions of older and poor people who were now far more able to consume hospital care, the Medicare program provided a subsidy to hospitals (cost plus 2%). This subsidy effectively reduced the cost of hiring additional RNs, resulting in increased employment of RNs and a decrease in the number of unfilled RN positions.

A major determinant of the wage level employers have to pay nursing personnel is the *supply* of each type of nursing personnel that is available to the organization at any given period of time. When there is a large supply of RNs or other nursing personnel, organizations will not have to pay as much to employ all the nurses they want, and hence they will demand more nurses than would otherwise be the case. This relationship results from the fact that an RN is more likely to accept a lower wage when there are many RNs available from which the employer is free to select (the opposite exists when the supply of RNs is scarce, in which case the wage rate would be raised). Employers also prefer that a large supply of nursing personnel be available because it gives them greater choices in addition to being able to offer lower relative compensation. For example, an employer might want to hire a certain number of lower wage LPNs, but if they are unavailable due to constrained supply at that particular time, the employer will have to employ higher wage RNs. Thus, the local supply of nursing personnel affects the wages that an organization must pay to employ nurses, and it affects the demand for nurses and other nursing personnel who might be partial substitutes for each other.

Another factor a hospital considers when determining its demand for RNs, and hence the number to employ, is the *additional output*, which can be obtained by employing a particular type of nurse. In other words, a hospital considers more than just the number of hours they will obtain in exchange for hiring an additional RN. The output produced by RNs and nursing personnel can be measured by quantities such as the additional number of treatments and services that can be provided, the additional number of births, emergency visits, surgeries, and the like. Organizations compare the amount of output obtained by employing different types of nursing personnel, for example, an RN versus an additional LPN, or an additional aide versus an RN. Holding all else constant, organizations will employ the type of nursing personnel whose output per wage rate is greater than others. To illustrate, if an organization receives 6 additional units of output (however output might be defined) from an RN at a wage equal to $2 more per hour, the marginal (or additional) product of the RN equals 3. Alternatively, the organization could receive 2 additional units of the same output if it employed an LPN at a wage equal to $1 more per hour; in this case the marginal product would be 2. In this example, the employer who is motivated to increase its overall productivity would hire the RN because it obtains more output per dollar compared to the LPN. In Chapter 11 we examine instances when it was in the hospital's economic interest to employ more LPNs relative to RNs and a different period of time when the hospital employed more RNs relative to LPNs.

As the healthcare system becomes increasingly focused on improving the quality and safety of patient care, we can expect that organizations will consider the *addition to quality and safety* that can be obtained by hiring RNs relative to other nursing and nonnursing personnel. The concern over quality and safety is currently directed at hospitals, which are the largest employer of nurses. From the perspective of hospitals that are facing pressures to improve quality and safety, they will have an economic incentive to hire the type of nurse whose marginal productivity with respect to quality and safety is highest compared to other types of nurses or nonnurses who can substitute for nurses (quality improvement professionals, for example) given the wage they must pay to each. Over time, we expect that organizations will face increasing pressures to demonstrate the quality and safety of the care they provide and even compete for market share based on quality and safety in addition to the price of hospital care. Quality improvement and monitoring organizations are demanding greater public reporting by hospitals, and the Centers for Medicare & Medicaid Services (CMS) and some private payers are taking steps to begin paying hospitals on the basis of quality through so-called "pay for performance." In the future, the demand for RNs and other nursing personnel is likely to be determined more heavily by RNs' productivity to improve quality and safety than it has in the past.

Organizations also consider the changing *relationship between capital (for example, diagnostic imaging machines) and labor* when they determine their overall demand for RNs as well as the mix of nursing personnel to employ. Because the type, amount, and prices of both capital and technology are constantly changing, as well as the type and wages of labor that can be productively combined or substituted for each other, the relationship between capital and labor is not static. Consequently, over time one would expect to observe different amounts and combinations of capital and labor being used by organizations to produce patient care—the combination of resources used to produce health care a decade ago would not produce health care efficiently today. With respect to nursing personnel, the roles and productivity of one type of nurse relative to another (an LPN versus an RN versus a nurse practitioner) have changed markedly over the years due to modifications in state practice acts, changes in institutional policies, changes in knowledge and customs, the emergence of evidence-based practice, and collective bargaining agreements that have expanded or restricted the performance of care-related activities by different types of personnel. At the same time, technology has been rapidly introduced in health care, much of which affects the delivery of nursing care, either directly or indirectly, by changing the practice and relative productivity of physicians, pharmacists, respiratory therapists, and others. As the responsibilities, tasks, and productivity of nonnurses change due to technological innovation and adoption, these changes will similarly impact the responsibilities, tasks, and productivity of RNs as well. In one way or another, employers try to understand these changing relationships and take them into account when considering how many RNs and other nursing personnel to employ.

Yet another factor, the organization's *objective function*, influences the number and combination of nurses to employ. Some organizations are driven by an objective to minimize costs and maximize reimbursements from governments or other payers (which could involve focusing on certain types of care that tend to yield higher margins, such as high-intensity cardiac care), others seek to produce high quality and have highly satisfied patients over anything else, some are in business to satisfy physicians and direct resources toward services and facilities benefiting them, and still other health organizations emphasize building a reputation as an innovator, perhaps by developing programs that better serve the health needs of the community. In reality, organizations simultaneously have multiple objectives that include many of those mentioned. Furthermore, an organization's dominant objective function is likely to change over time as the healthcare environment evolves and new circumstances develop, such as what occurred when managed care developed and spread throughout the 1990s, or with what presently appears to be occurring with respect to improving quality and safety. Thus, this year's cost minimizer might emphasize quality improvement next year, or this year's all-service hospital might decide to limit itself to providing specialty services that it can more profitably produce. As an organization's objective function changes, so too will its demand for the quantity and mix of nursing personnel.

Organizations have a limited amount of financial resources they can spend to employ RNs. The size of their *budget* allocated to nursing varies over time and is subject to factors that are not always under its control, such as when the Medicare and Medicaid programs pay hospitals a fixed price according to DRGs. Some hospitals in certain markets (and states) receive adjustments to help offset higher costs associated with providing care to larger proportions of medically indigent patients or higher labor costs, which in turn affects the size of their budget as well as their demand for nurses. These and many other factors greatly influence organizations' overall operating budgets and result in situations where they might "need" more nurses but do not currently have the amount of dollars in their operating budgets to employ all the RNs they want.

In sum, given the overall demand for health care facing an employer, these factors determine the total employment of nurses at any point in time. While conceptually these factors might seem straightforward, in reality, each is driven by constantly changing forces. Changes in any of the above criteria exert an independent and sometimes interactive effect on the employer's demand for nursing personnel. At different points in time, some criteria might exert a more important impact on decision making than others. Thus, employers' demand for nursing personnel is not the result of a mechanistic application of simple formulas, but it is the result of decisions based on available information about changing, and not always readily visible, forces. Assuming that enough RNs are willing to work at the wages and in the working conditions offered by employers, and taking into account the previously discussed economic criteria, most healthcare organizations seek to employ the number and mix of RNs and other nursing personnel that can most efficiently produce the required treatments and services that are consistent with the organization's objective function, budget, quality standards, and the ways that other healthcare personnel, capital, and technology can be productively combined. Finally, when we consider the impact of the factors that determine society's overall demand for health care, we believe that the combination of population growth, an aging population, growth in income per capita, and increasing technology will lead to growth in the demand for nurses for the foreseeable future.

Now that we have considered the factors that affect society's overall demand for health care and the derived demand for RNs as reflected by the number of RNs employed by employers, we conclude this chapter by examining how forecasters have modeled many of these factors to produce estimates of the future demand for RNs.

PROJECTIONS OF THE FUTURE DEMAND FOR NURSES

In this final section, we briefly examine forecasts of the future demand for nursing personnel provided by two different sources: the Office of Occupational Statistics and Employment Projections based in the Bureau of Labor Statistics (BLS); and the Health Resources and Services Administration (HRSA). Although the projections made by these two agencies differ in their methods and source of data, they are the most widely cited projections. We begin with the BLS projections.

BLS Projections to 2014

We find the BLS projections intriguing for several reasons. First, because they make projections of hundreds of occupations in the U.S. economy, it is possible to compare future employment prospects for RNs to other occupations and industries. Second, estimates are based in part on employer surveys, so they reflect the views of those who are in the industry and are making actual employment decisions. Third, BLS forecasts of future job growth are made more often than other federal agencies that focus on the healthcare workforce. Finally, as discussed later, the BLS forecasts offer a more well-rounded depiction of the healthcare industry, the changes that employers (and nurses) in this industry are facing, and the likely impact of these changes on future employment growth. These attributes of the BLS complement the efforts of others engaged in the difficult task of forecasting the nation's expected demand for RNs and other nursing personnel.

To arrive at their estimates of job growth, the BLS projects changes in three areas: labor force participation rates throughout the U.S. economy using data on age, sex, race, and ethnicity; total economic performance based on assumptions about future growth potential; and industry-level employment based on economic performance, advances in technology, detailed industry trends, and surveys of industries. The occupational projections are based on these overall projections, extended to projections of the demand for workers employed in occupations in each industry. The BLS forecasts focus on the following major occupational groups: management and business and financial operations; professional and related; service, sales, and related; office and administrative support; farming, fishing, and forestry; construction trades and related; installation, maintenance, and repair; production; and transportation and material moving. RNs, LPNs, and aides are included in the professional and related occupational group, as are teachers.

According to BLS projections, job opportunities for RNs in all nursing specialties are described as "excellent." In particular, employment of RNs is expected to grow much faster than average for all occupations through 2014. In fact, projections indicate that the second largest number of new jobs among all occupations will be for RNs partly because thousands of job openings will result from the need to replace RNs who leave the workforce, particularly as the age of the RN workforce continues to rise (a theme we discuss extensively in later chapters). According to the BLS, in 2004 there were 2.4 million RNs employed in the United States, but this number is projected to grow by 703,000 by 2014 (29%), with total RN employment reaching an estimated 3.1 million. Employment growth of retail salespersons was the only occupation forecasted to experience larger job growth during the same period.

The BLS also attributes the faster-than-average growth for RN employment to technological advances in patient care, which permit a greater number of healthcare problems to be treated, and to an increasing emphasis on preventive care. In addition, the BLS recognizes the rapid growth in the number of older people, who are much more likely than younger people to require nursing care. The BLS further indicates that employers in some parts of the country and in certain employment settings are currently reporting difficulty in attracting and retaining an adequate number of RNs, primarily because of an aging RN workforce and a lack of younger workers to fill positions. Enrollments in nursing programs at all levels have increased more rapidly in the past couple of years as students seek jobs with stable employment. However, many qualified applicants to nursing education programs have been, and continue to be, turned away because of a shortage of nursing faculty. The BLS indicates that the need for nursing faculty will increase as a large number of instructors near retirement. Further, the BLS observes that many employers also are relying on foreign-educated nurses to fill open positions for RNs.

Even though employment opportunities for all nursing specialties are expected to be excellent, the BLS indicates that opportunities will vary by employment setting. For example, employment is expected to grow more slowly in hospitals than in most other healthcare sectors. While the intensity of nursing care is likely to increase, requiring more nurses per patient, the number of inpatients (those who remain in the hospital for more than 24 hours) is not expected to grow appreciably. The BLS notes that patients are being discharged earlier, and more procedures are being done on an outpatient basis. Rapid job growth for RNs is expected in hospital outpatient facilities, such as those providing same-day surgery, rehabilitation, and chemotherapy.

Despite the slower employment growth in hospitals, the BLS indicates that job opportunities should still be "excellent" because of relatively high turnover of hospital nurses. RNs working in hospitals frequently work overtime and night and weekend shifts and also treat seriously ill and injured patients, all of which can contribute to job stress and burnout. Hospital departments in which these working conditions occur most frequently—critical care units, emergency departments, and operating rooms—generally will have more job openings than other departments, according to the BLS.

In describing nursing employment opportunities, the BLS notes that more sophisticated procedures, once performed only in hospitals, are being performed in physicians' offices and in outpatient care centers, such as freestanding ambulatory surgical and emergency centers. Accordingly, employment is expected to grow much faster than average in these settings. However, RNs might face greater competition for these positions because they generally offer regular working hours and more satisfying work environments.

Employment in nursing care facilities is expected to grow faster than average because of increases in the number of elderly people, many of whom require long-term care. In addition, the financial pressure on hospitals to discharge patients quickly should produce more admissions to nursing care facilities. Job growth also is expected in units that provide specialized long-term rehabilitation for stroke and head injury patients, as well as units that treat people suffering from Alzheimer's disease.

With respect to home health, RN job growth is expected to increase rapidly in response to the growing number of older people with functional disabilities, consumer preference for care in the home, and technological advances that enable increasingly complex treatments to be administered in the home. The BLS states that the type of care demanded in the years ahead will require RNs who are able to perform complex procedures.

Finally, the BLS suggests that RNs with at least a bachelor's degree will have better job prospects than those without the degree. In addition, all four advanced practice specialties—clinical nurse specialists, nurse practitioners, certified nurse midwives, and nurse anesthetists—will experience high demand, particularly in medically underserved areas such as inner cities and rural areas. Relative to physicians, these RNs increasingly serve as lower-cost primary care providers.

HRSA's Projections Through 2020

A second source of projections for the future demand for RNs in the United States comes from HRSA's forecasts published in 2002 (HRSA, 2002). HRSA collects data on the RN workforce by conducting the National Sample Survey of Registered Nurses (the NSSRN was described in Chapter 1) and maintaining analytic models to project RN supply and demand (HRSA's supply model is described briefly in Chapter 7).

HRSA's demand model projects state level demand for full-time equivalent (FTE) RNs, LPNs and vocational nurses, and nurse aides/auxiliaries and home health aides through 2020. For RNs, the model projects demand in healthcare employment settings that employ the majority of RNs. HRSA defines the demand for RNs as the number of FTE RNs whom employers are willing to hire given population needs, economic considerations, the healthcare operating environment, and other factors. In the description that follows, we focus on demand projections for RNs only.

Changing demographics are a key determinant of HRSA's projected demand for FTE RNs, particularly the growth of older Americans who have much greater per capita healthcare needs compared with the nonelderly (as we discussed earlier). The rapid growth in demand for nursing services is especially pronounced in long-term care settings that predominantly provide care to the elderly.

In addition to considering demographic changes, the forecasting model extrapolates the expected use (demand) of healthcare services by combining national health care use patterns and state population projections by age and gender. The model then adjusts these extrapolations for each state to account for factors that cause the use of healthcare services to deviate from expected levels (e.g., state-level managed care enrollment rates). Next the model projects nurse staffing intensity (e.g., FTE RNs per hospital inpatient days) as a function of current staffing intensity and trends in major determinants of nurse staffing intensity. Combining projected health care use with projected nurse staffing intensity produces projections of demand for FTE RNs by setting, state, and year.

Table 4-2 shows the results of HRSA's projected demand aggregated to a national level and by major employment setting in 5-year increments through 2020. These projections indicate that the total national demand for FTE RNs will increase by 41% (or about 819,000) between 2000 and 2020. This rate of growth translates into an annual rate of growth of 1.7%, which HRSA states is a rather moderate rate of growth compared to the estimate of 2.3% estimated by the BLS. According to HRSA's projections, the fastest growth in FTE RN demand will occur in settings that predominantly serve the elderly; home health will grow by 91% and nursing facilities by 73%. RNs employed in hospitals and nursing education settings will both experience a projected growth of 40%, with smaller growth projected for RNs in ambulatory care settings (23%), occupational settings (12%), schools (8%), and all other settings (17%). Public health settings are the only employment setting that is projected to decrease (–4%) over the forecast period.

CHAPTER SUMMARY

In our examination of the demand for RNs, we began by noting that demand is an economic concept different from need and that the demand for RNs is derived from society's overall demand for health care. The forces that determine society's demand for health care are driven by changes in the incidence of diseases and illnesses, the size, age composition, wealth, and education level of the population, sociocultural attitudes and beliefs, economic factors, the way that the healthcare system is organized, and growth of technology. At any point in time, these societal forces interact to determine the total amount of health care demanded in the United States.

Table 4-2   Health Resources and Services Administration's 2002 Projections of the Demand for Full-Time Equivalent RNs, 2000–2020

Employment Setting	2000	2005	2010	2015	2020	Increase from 2000–2020
Total Demand	1,999,950	2,161,831	2,344,584	2,562,554	2,810,414	41%
Hospitals	1,242,831	1,339,493	1,451,083	1,588,828	1,741,639	40%
Nursing Homes	168,529	194,219	223,193	254,718	291,513	73%
Public Health	95,360	94,328	93,226	92,297	91,360	– 4%
Ambulatory Care	160,911	169,329	178,272	187,348	196,399	23%
Home Health	130,288	152,622	177,583	209,192	248,848	91%
Occupational Health	20,040	20,984	21,826	22,241	22,390	12%
Nursing Education	45,815	49,521	53,640	58,517	64,055	40%
School	57,638	59,657	60,419	61,060	62,244	8%
Other	78,537	81,678	84,872	88,354	91,966	17%

Source: Health Resources and Services Administration. (2004). *Projected supply, demand, and shortages of registered nurses. 2000–2020.* U.S. Health and Human Services, Bureau of Health Professions, National Center for Health Workforce Analysis. Retrieved October 31, 2007, from http://www.ahca.org/research/rnsupply_demand.pdf

Healthcare delivery organizations are in the business of producing goods and services to satisfy society's demand for health care. Producing many of these goods and services requires RNs and other nursing personnel. The number and type of nursing personnel demanded by healthcare organizations are, in turn, determined by the total compensation needed to attract RNs, the available supply of nursing personnel, the productivity of each type of nurse relative to others, the contribution to patient care quality and safety of each type of nurse (RN, LPN, aide, nurse practitioner), the employer's objective function, and the size of the budget available to spend on nursing. Efforts by the BLS and HRSA to quantitatively estimate the societal and organizational factors affecting the demand for RNs indicate much faster than average growth in the number of new jobs for RNs through 2014 and that the total growth in demand for RNs over the period 2000 to 2020 will increase by more than 800,000 FTE RNs.

Whether there is an adequate supply of RNs to match the projected growth in the demand for RNs is another question, and it is one that is discussed extensively in later chapters. But in Chapter 5 we focus more closely on how changes in the organization of the healthcare system—adopted more rapidly in some states than others—impacts the growth in the employment and earnings of RNs and what implications this might have for the future.

REFERENCES

Centers for Disease Control and Prevention. (2007). *The state of aging and health in America 2007 report*. Retrieved July 3, 2007, from http://www.cdc.gov/aging/saha.htm

Feldstein, P. (2005). *Health care economics* (6th ed.). Clifton Park, NY: Thomson Delmar Learning.

Health Resources and Services Administration. (2003). *Changing demographics and the implications for physicians, nurses, and other health workers*. Retrieved November 19, 2007, from http://bhpr.hrsa.gov/healthworkforce/reports/changingdemo/aging.htm

Health Resources and Services Administration. (2002). *Projected supply, demand, and shortages of registered nurses. 2000–2020*. U.S. Health and Human Services, Bureau of Health Professions, National Center for Health Workforce Analysis. Retrieved Oct 31, 2007, from http://www.ahca.org/research/rnsupply_demand.pdf

National Center for Health Statistics. (2007). *Life expectancy at birth, at 65 years of age, at 75 years of age, by race and sex: United States, selected years 1900–2004*. Retrieved November 19, 2007, from http://www.cdc.gov/nchs/data/hus/hus06.pdf#027

Population Resource Center. (2007). *World population trends*. Retrieved July 3, 2007, from http://www.prcdc.org/summaries/worldpop/worldpop.html

U.S. Census Bureau. (2004). *U.S. interim projections by age, sex, race, and Hispanic origin*. Retrieved July 3, 2007, from http://www.census.gov/ipc/www/usinterimproj

CHAPTER 5

Managed Care and the Nurse Labor Market

One of the primary goals of this book is to evaluate the likely future demand for nurses in the United States. Most of the factors that determine the growth in demand for RNs over the next 2 decades are reasonably predictable. The current age structure of the population ensures that, barring an unprecedented decline in birth rates or rise in death rates, the U.S. population will grow by about 8% per decade for the next 50 years, while the population over age 65 will grow at more than twice this rate. Income per capita has increased at an annual rate of between 1% and 3% in each of the last 6 decades, and it can be expected to increase the growth in demand for nurses by perhaps 1% per year over the next few decades. Finally, technological change in medicine and health care can be expected to contribute another 1-2% to the annual growth rate in demand, as it has done in the United States and other developed countries since the 1940s. Taken together, a conservative estimate suggests that these three factors will lead to growth in the demand for RNs of at least 3% per year for the foreseeable future. In comparison, forecasts of demand for RNs by HRSA and BLS that were discussed in Chapter 4 are fairly conservative, predicting an annual growth rate in demand of about 2% over the coming decades.

Far less is known, however, about how changes in healthcare organizations and financing are likely to affect the future demand for RNs. Over the last decade, managed care organizations have come to dominate the healthcare delivery system in the United States, and, as we saw in Chapter 2, this was a decade of unusually slow growth in employment for RNs, particularly in hospitals. But was this slowdown in demand for RNs the result of managed care, and what impact, if any, will these managed care organizations have on the future demand for RNs as they continue to grow and mature? In this chapter, we first provide some background on the growth and impact of managed care organizations in the United States, and then we discuss the impacts that managed care has had on the nurse labor market and the likely implication for the future.

OVERVIEW OF MANAGED CARE

Traditional health insurance pays for health care on a fee-for-service (FFS) basis, reimbursing patients (or healthcare providers directly) for the cost of all covered services. In these traditional FFS plans, patients may choose to receive care from any licensed healthcare provider and are reimbursed for any service provided by a licensed healthcare provider with no third-party oversight by the insurer. Because the patient does not pay directly for the cost of care, there is a tendency by patients to overuse services and thereby increase the costs of care (a problem referred to as "moral hazard" by healthcare economists). Traditional fee-for-service plans discourage such overuse with copayments and deductibles, making patients pay for at least some portion of their care. In the 1970s, over 95% of private insurance coverage and all public insurance coverage (Medicare for the elderly and Medicaid for the poor) were structured on the fee-for-service model.

Managed care organizations are health insurance plans that provide care through a network of healthcare providers, and typically they require patients to obtain prior approval from their primary care physician or some other third party to receive full reimbursement for certain services. Thus, in contrast to traditional fee-for-service plans, managed care organizations attempt to actively participate in patient care decisions to improve quality of care and control costs. There are three types of managed care organizations: Health Maintenance Organizations (HMOs) are the oldest and least flexible, requiring all care to be provided by network providers and to be approved by the primary care provider; Preferred Provider Organizations (PPOs) have grown in popularity since the 1980s and are more flexible, providing patients with a discount (e.g., lower copayment) if they receive care from a network provider but otherwise placing few limits on patient care; and Point Of Service (POS) plans arrived on the scene in the early 1990s and are a blend of HMO and PPO plans, expanding the traditional HMO model to include partial coverage (with higher copayments and deductibles) for out-of-network providers and nonapproved care.

Figure 5-1 shows recent enrollment trends in HMO, PPO, POS, and FFS plans among workers covered by employer-provided health insurance (accounting for roughly 73% of all insured and 88% of all privately insured individuals). Between 1988 and 2002, fee-for-service plans went from the dominant form of health insurance (73% of coverage) to virtually disappearing (4% of coverage). While all forms of managed care grew over this period, PPOs had become the dominant form by 2002. Similar trends, though not as dramatic, are seen in managed care enrollment in Medicare and Medicaid, as shown in **Figure 5-2**. Over half of Medicaid enrollees are now covered by managed care, while Medicare enrollment in managed care rose from just 5% in 1990 to over 16% by 1999.

Figure 5-1   Enrollment Trends in HMO, PPO, POS, and FFS Plans Among Workers Covered by Employer-Provided Health Insurance, Selected Years

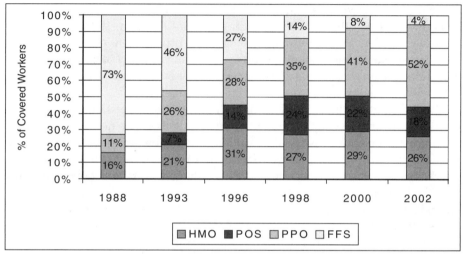

Source: Centers for Medicare and Medicaid Services. March 24, 2003. *Health Care Industry Market Update: Managed Care.*

Figure 5-2   Managed Care Enrollment Trends in Medicare and Medicaid, 1991–2002

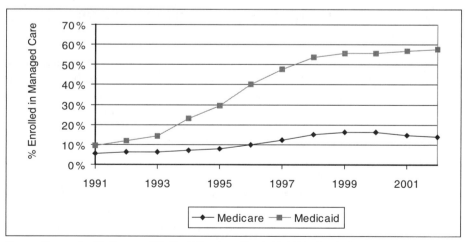

Source: Centers for Medicare and Medicaid Services. March 24, 2003. *Health Care Industry Market Update: Managed Care.*

There is a large amount of literature suggesting that managed care plans reduce healthcare spending and utilization by 10-20% among their members and that these reductions are concentrated in hospital settings (Luft, 1981; Miller & Luft, 2002). Similarly, growth in managed care penetration in a market has been associated with lower spending and utilization in aggregate (Anderson & Kohn, 1996; Baker, 1997; Baker, 1999; Chernew, 1995; Robinson, 1996; Tussing and Wojtowycz, 1994). However, managed care and other recent cost-containment techniques tend to have a one-time effect: reducing the *level* of healthcare costs and utilization but not having any long-term effect on the *growth rate* (Schwartz, 1987; Newhouse, 1992).

Taken together, the existing evidence suggests that the shift from a healthcare system dominated by FFS plans in the late 1980s to one dominated by managed care by the late 1990s should have reduced healthcare costs and utilization by between 10% and 20% relative to what they would have been if this shift toward managed care had not occurred. This reduction, spread out over a decade, would have temporarily slowed the growth rate of healthcare costs by between 1% and 2% per year and, correspondingly, slowed the growth in the demand for nurses. In fact, the annual growth rate of real healthcare costs per capita during the 1990s was about 2% below what it was during the 1980s (3.3% versus 5.4%) and, as we saw in Chapter 2, nurse employment grew particularly slowly during the mid-1990s. However, by the late 1990s and early 2000s, as the spread of managed care slowed down, this evidence would suggest a return to historical growth rates in demand for health care.

THE IMPACT OF MANAGED CARE ON THE DEMAND FOR REGISTERED NURSES

So far in this chapter we have focused on indirect evidence suggesting that managed care led to a temporary slowdown in demand for health care in the 1990s—and by implication, a temporary slowdown in the demand for RNs. But is there any direct evidence of the effects of managed care on the demand for nurses during the 1990s or of the likely effect that managed care or more recent innovations in healthcare organization will have on the demand for RNs in the coming decades? In the remainder of this chapter, we provide direct evidence on these questions based on a simple comparison of employment and earnings for RNs in states that were early adopters of managed care to states that lagged behind. The purpose of this analysis is twofold. The first is to document the link between the spread of managed care and the employment and earnings of RNs: Did the slowdown in employment growth occur earlier in states that were early adopters of managed care? The second purpose of this analysis is to identify trends currently emerging in states that were early adopters of managed care as a useful guide to what we can expect in the coming decade: Has employment growth picked back up since managed care has matured in these states? Emerging trends in these states are likely to be an indicator of the next wave of innovation that will hit the nurse labor market.

Identifying States That Are Early Adopters of Managed Care

As with any innovation in health care, managed care disseminated slowly and unevenly throughout the country.[1] The growth in managed care followed the typical diffusion pattern, with slow adoption initially followed by more rapid adoption after passing a threshold in the neighborhood of 15-20% adoption. But this aggregate pattern of adoption hides considerable variation across states in the timing and rate of adoption. In the language of Rogers (1995), some states are early adopters while others are laggards. Midway through the process of adopting a new innovation such as managed care, the innovation will be widespread among the early adopters yet largely unknown among the laggards. Moreover, geographic areas that are early adopters of one innovation tend to be early adopters of other innovations. For example, Skinner and Staiger (2007) find that the same states that were early adopters of hybrid corn and tractors in the 1930s also tended to be early adopters of beta blockers (a highly effective drug treatment for heart attacks) in the 1990s. Thus, areas that are early adopters of one form of managed care are likely to also be early adopters of the next innovation in healthcare delivery, and trends emerging in these states are likely to be good leading indicators of national trends in the next decade.

We identify states as early adopters of managed care based on a high proportion of citizens enrolled in HMOs in 1994. We focus on HMO enrollment in 1994 for a number of reasons. First, as we saw in Figure 5-1, 1994 lies near the midpoint of the diffusion of managed care, and the midpoint of a diffusion process is when the differences in adoption are likely to be most pronounced between the early adopters and the laggards. Second, state-level data from the 1990s are primarily limited to information on HMO enrollment, and 1994 was a year in which HMOs were still the leading form of managed care. Finally, this division of states into early adopters and laggards is consistent with our earlier analyses of nurse employment and earnings trends (Buerhaus & Staiger, 1996, 1999).

---

[1] See Berwick (2003) for an excellent summary of the challenges to the diffusion of innovations in health care, and see Rogers (1995) for a comprehensive textbook on the subject.

Table 5-1 lists the states that we identify as early adopters based on high HMO enrollment in 1994. These 16 states and the District of Columbia contain approximately one-half of the U.S. population and had an average HMO enrollment nearly three times higher than the 34 low enrollment states in 1994 (24% versus 9%). Virtually all of the growth in HMO enrollment between 1990 and 1994 occurred in the early adopter states. Since 1994, enrollment in HMOs and other forms of managed care has grown in all states.

Table 5-1   States with the Highest Percentage of Enrollment in HMOs in 1994

State	Percent of Population Enrolled in HMO in 1994
Arizona	22.6
California	34.5
Colorado	26.5
Connecticut	19.9
District of Columbia	93.4*
Florida	16.5
Hawaii	21.2
Maryland	21.0
Massachusetts	34.5
Michigan	17.7
Minnesota	16.3
New Mexico	16.3
New York	21.2
Oregon	30.2
Pennsylvania	18.8
Washington	16.5
Wisconsin	20.2
Mean for all high managed care states	24.2
Mean for all other states	8.8

Source: Interstudy, Bloomington, Minnesota, written communication, February, 1995.
*HMO enrollment for the District of Columbia is overstated because it is based on place of employment, while population is based on place of residence.

Trends in personal healthcare spending in the early adopter states have closely reflected the diverging trends in HMO enrollment, as can be seen in **Figure 5-3**. Personal healthcare expenditures grew at similar rates in early adopter and laggard states until 1990. They grew about 1% per year more slowly in early adopter states between 1990 and 1996, and they grew at a similar rate in the two groups of states after 1996 (albeit with early adopters at a lower level than they had begun, relative to late adopters).

Trends in the Employment and Earnings of Nurses in Early Adopter and Laggard States

In **Figures 5-4** and **5-5** we compare trends in total employment and earnings of RNs between states with high HMO enrollment in 1994 (the "early adopter" states) and states with low HMO enrollment in 1994 (the "laggard" states). Figure 5-4 plots cumulative growth in employment since 1983 for RNs, while Figure 5-5 contains similar plots of the cumulative growth in real wages (adjusted for inflation) since 1983. We compare cumulative growth since 1983 in the high HMO and low HMO states. As we did in Chapter 2, we are plotting cumulative growth over time to emphasize the divergent trends in the two types of states.

Figure 5-3   Total Personal Health Spending in States That Were Early Adopters of Managed Care (High HMO Enrollment Rates in 1994) Versus Other States, 1985–2004

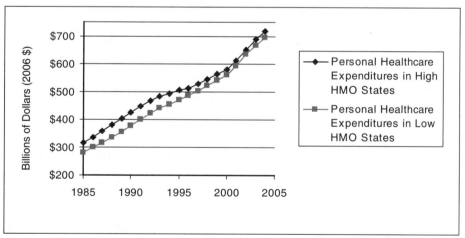

Source: Centers for Medicare and Medicaid Services. *Health expenditures by state of provider, 1980–2004 (Final, February 2007).* Retrieved November 16, 2007, from http://www.cms.hhs.gov/NationalHealth ExpendData/downloads/provider-state2004.zip

Figure 5-4   Cumulative Growth in Employment Since 1983 for RNs in States with High and Low HMO Enrollment in 1994, 1983–2006

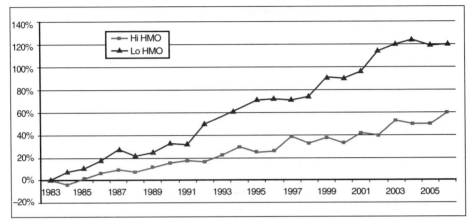

Source: Current Population Survey.

Figure 5-5   Cumulative Growth in Real Wages Since 1983 for RNs in States with High and Low HMO Enrollment in 1994, 1983–2006

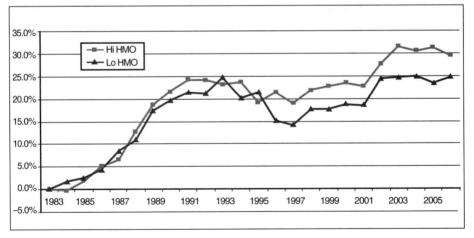

Source: Current Population Survey.

For example, in Figure 5-4 we see that the employment of RNs grew by 120% between 1983 and 2006 in the states with low HMO enrollment, while employment of RNs grew by only 60% over the same time period in states with high HMO enrollment.

The most striking difference between high and low HMO states has been in the employment trends for RNs. As can be seen in Figure 5-4, beginning around 1990 there was a dramatic slowdown in the employment of RNs in the high HMO states. Between 1990 and 1995, RN employment grew less than 2% per year in the high HMO states, while RN employment in the low HMO states grew more than 5% per year. This slowdown in employment occurred precisely at the time that HMOs were experiencing rapid growth in the high HMO states (but not in the low HMO states), suggesting that the growth in HMOs was causing this slowdown in RN employment. If managed care in fact caused this slowdown, then we would expect that the slowdown would have continued in the high HMO states (as managed care continued to spread throughout the 1990s) and also would begin to appear in the remaining states (as managed care began to spread in these states after 1994). In other words, trends that were first observed in states that were early adopters of managed care should be indicative of what happens later in other states (and the country as a whole) as managed care spread.

This is precisely the pattern observed in Figure 5-4. The slowdown in employment growth, which occurred around 1990 in states with high HMO enrollment, occurred in the low HMO states roughly 5 years later beginning around 1995. Between 1995 and 2000, RN employment growth in the low HMO states slowed to about 2% per year, while RN employment in the high HMO states continued to grow at under 2% per year. RN employment growth finally resumed in the high HMO states starting around 2000, growing at an average annual rate of just over 3% between 2000 and 2006 (about the same rate as in the late 1980s). Meanwhile, employment growth in the low HMO states picked up a bit but remained at around 2.5% per year since 2000. Taken as a whole, this evidence suggests that emerging trends in the high HMO states are useful leading indicators of trends that are likely to emerge nationwide within 5-10 years. Thus, the recent increase in the growth of RN employment observed in the high HMO states since 2000 suggests that overall demand for RNs is likely to grow at a robust 3% per year in the near term.

Taken together, these employment trends suggest that the spread of managed care has affected nurse employment in two waves. First, there was a slowdown in demand for RNs that occurred in the high HMO states in the early 1990s and in the rest of the country in the mid 1990s. More recently, as managed care became fully diffused, growth in the demand for RNs in high HMO states has returned to the historical (pre-HMO) level of 3% per year. If the high HMO states continue to serve as a reliable guide, we would expect similar growth rates in the demand for RNs to soon be observed in all states.

Despite the apparent negative impacts of managed care on the employment of RNs, there is little evidence that wage growth for nurses was depressed in the high HMO states that were early adopters of managed care. If anything, as can be seen in Figure 5-5, wages tended to grow more rapidly in the high HMO states during periods when employment was growing relatively slowly. Wages of RNs grew a bit more rapidly in the high HMO states during the early 1990s and then remained about 5% above the low HMO states through 2006.

While we might have expected the growth of managed care to depress wages of RNs in the high HMO states, there are a number of good reasons to think that this would not occur. First, the market for RNs is a national market, which makes it difficult for employers in one region to reduce their wages below that paid in other regions. Thus, while demand for nurses might be determined locally, wages are largely determined nationally. In this type of market, as was discussed in Chapter 3, the growth of managed care might depress wages nationally, but it is unlikely to reduce wages in one state relative to another. In fact, RN wages declined in all states in the mid-1990s just at the time that managed care was slowing demand growth in all states.

A second reason that we might expect wages to actually rise when employment growth slows is a shift in the composition of the nurse workforce toward more experienced (and hence higher paid) RNs during periods of slow employment growth. This "composition bias" has been found to be an important factor in the economy as a whole, leading to higher wages during recessions (when unemployment is high and job growth is low) because higher paid workers are more likely to keep their jobs (Bound & Solon, 1999).

Trends in the Employment of RNs by Sector in Early Adopter and Laggard States

Managed care has not only affected the overall employment picture for nurses, it has also affected the settings in which nurses are employed. The most important distinction for nurses is between employment in the hospital sector and employment outside the hospital sector because hospitals have traditionally employed roughly two-thirds of all RNs. Both the hospital and nonhospital sectors have experienced large impacts of managed care on their demand for nurses. Trends in the employment growth of RNs are shown in **Figure 5-6** for the hospital sector and in **Figure 5-7** for the nonhospital sector, which includes all employment settings of RNs other than hospitals. As in the previous figures, these figures compare cumulative growth in employment since 1983 in the high HMO and low HMO states.

Hospitals continue to be the primary employer of RNs, so it is not surprising that the trends in hospital employment in high HMO and low HMO states are similar to the trends in overall employment in these states. However, the slowdown in hospital employment was much more dramatic than the overall slowdown in

Figure 5-6   Cumulative Growth in Employment in the Hospital Sector Since 1983 for RNs in States with High and Low HMO Enrollment in 1994, 1983–2006

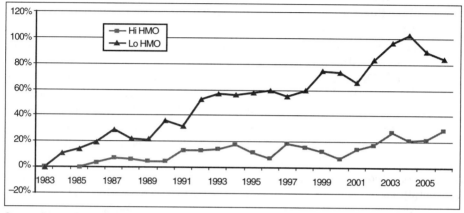

Source: Current Population Survey.

Figure 5-7   Cumulative Growth in Employment Outside the Hospital Sector Since 1983 for RNs in States with High and Low HMO Enrollment in 1994, 1983–2006

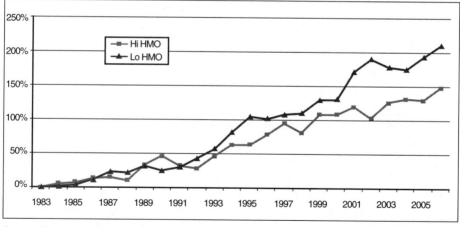

Source: Current Population Survey.

employment. The number of RNs employed in hospitals did not grow at all between 1990 and 2000 in the high HMO states, while the number of RNs employed in hospitals grew less than 1% per year between 1994 and 2001 in the low HMO states. Thus, nearly all of the slowdown in RN employment growth that was associated with managed care appears to have occurred in the hospital setting, leading to the steady shift toward employment in nonhospital settings among RNs that was discussed in Chapter 2. Since 2000, RN employment in hospitals has grown more than 3% per year in the high HMO states, while RN employment in hospitals has grown by more than 2% per year in the low HMO states since 2001.

Until recently, nonhospital employment was growing rapidly for RNs in both the low HMO and the high HMO states. Between 1983 and 2000, nonhospital employment of RNs grew at an annual rate of about 5% per year in both the low HMO and high HMO states. Since 2000, however, there was a sharp slowdown in nonhospital employment growth of RNs in the high HMO states relative to the low HMO states, with nonhospital employment growing at an annual rate of about 3% per year in the high HMO states while growth has continued at over 5% per year in the low HMO states. In fact, what we have seen since 2000 for nonhospital employment is reminiscent of what was seen in the early 1990s for hospital employment: A slowdown in employment growth occurring first in the high HMO states. Thus, it seems that a slowdown in employment growth outside of hospitals might be an emerging trend.

CHAPTER SUMMARY

The evidence in this chapter suggests that the rapid spread of managed care in the 1990s had clear and profound impacts on the demand for RNs. In particular, it appears that initially, managed care reduced the growth in demand for RNs in hospitals. Most recently, there has been an apparent reappearance of growth in demand for RNs in hospitals and a slowdown in demand for RNs in nonhospital settings associated with managed care.

What does this evidence imply for the growth in demand for nurses over the coming decades? Perhaps the simplest lesson is that, despite the rapid rise of managed care and the negative impacts this had on employment growth, RN employment still managed to grow nearly 30% between 1990 and 2000. While managed care might reduce demand somewhat, the impact has been small relative to the other forces that are driving growth in demand for nurses.

Recent employment trends in the states that were early adopters of managed care provide a more detailed guide to likely developments in the demand for RNs in the near future. While demand growth for RNs in hospitals has resumed in these states since 2000, demand growth outside of hospitals has declined. Meanwhile, total employment growth of RNs in these states has returned to about 3% per year—levels that were seen in the 1980s before the growth of managed care. This evidence suggests that we can expect robust growth of 3%

per year in the demand for nurses over the coming decades in both hospital and nonhospital settings. Thus, in the long run, the most important impact of managed care on the demand for nurses is in the shift toward nonhospital settings rather than lasting impacts on employment growth.

The fact that managed care now accounts for over 95% of private health insurance coverage suggests that its impacts on nurse employment might be over, and we can now expect strong growth in demand over the coming decades unless some new innovation to healthcare finance appears on the horizon. Over the last few years, the most important innovation that has begun has been the development of plans for universal health insurance coverage in a number of states. Massachusetts passed a universal coverage law in 2006 that will come into effect in 2008, while California appears likely to enact legislation in 2008. Note that these states that are early adopters of universal coverage are the same states that were early adopters of managed care. Thus, the next wave of innovation in healthcare financing appears to be on the horizon. Unfortunately, it is too early to see the impact that these new innovations will have on nurse employment. Because the uninsured account for less than 20% of the population (and even less in the states that are likely to be the first adopters of universal coverage), we might expect the impacts of universal coverage to be small relative to the spread of managed care unless universal coverage states adopt other policies at the same time (such as a single payer system) that have a broader impact. However, whatever the impact will be, we can expect to see an early indication to emerge first in the employment trends of the early adopter states.

REFERENCES

Anderson, G., & Kohn, L. (1996). Hospital employment trends in California, 1982-1994. *Health Affairs*, *15*(1), 153–158.

Baker, L.C. (1997). The effect of HMOs on fee-for-service health care expenditures: Evidence from Medicare. *Journal of Health Economics, 16*(4), 453–481.

Baker, L.C. (1999). Association of managed care market share and health expenditures for fee-for-service Medicare patients. *Journal of the American Medical Association, 281*(5), 432–437.

Berwick, D.M. (2003). Disseminating innovations in health care. *The Journal of the American Medical Association*, 289, 1969-1975.

Bound, J., & Solon, G. (1999). Double trouble: On the value of twins-based estimation of the return to schooling. *Economics of Education Review, 18*(2), 169–182.

Buerhaus, P., & Staiger, D. (1996). Managed care and the nurse workforce. *The Journal of the American Medical Association, 275*(18), 1487–1493.

Buerhaus, P., & Staiger, D. (1999). Trouble in the nurse labor market? Recent trends and future outlook. *Health Affairs, 18*(1), 214–222.

Chernew, M. (1995). The impact of non-IPA HMOs on the number of hospitals and hospital capacity. *Inquiry*, Summer, 143–154.

Luft, H. (1981). *Health maintenance organizations: Dimensions of performance*. New York: John Wiley.

Miller, R., & Luft, H. (2002). HMO plan performance update: An analysis of the literature, 1997–2001. *Health Affairs, 21*(4), 63-86.

Newhouse, J. (1992). Medical care costs: How much welfare loss? *Journal of Economic Perspectives, 6*(3), 3–21.

Robinson, J.C. (1996). Decline in hospital utilization and cost inflation under managed care in California. *Journal of the American Medical Association, 276*(13), 1060–1064.

Rogers, E.M. (1995). *Diffusion of innovations* (4th ed.). New York: The Free Press.

Skinner, J., & Staiger, D.O. (2007) Technology adoption from hybrid corn to beta blockers. In Ernst R. Berndt & Charles R. Hulten (Eds.), *Hard-to-measure goods and services: Essays in honor of Zvi Grilliches*. Chicago, IL: University of Chicago Press.

Schwartz, W.B. (1987). The inevitable failure of current cost-containment strategies. Why they can provide only temporary relief. *Journal of the American Medical Association, 257*, 220–224.

Tussing, A.D., & Wojtowycz, M.A. (1994). Health maintenance organizations, independent practice associations, and cesarean section rates. *Health Services Research*, April, 75–93.

CHAPTER 6

The Short-Run Supply
of Registered Nurses

When thinking about the supply of RNs, it is useful to differentiate between the short- and long-run supply of RNs. The *short-run* supply of RNs refers to individuals who currently hold a license to practice as an RN and their decisions to participate in the labor market and how many hours to spend working. As discussed in Chapter 2, if we are interested in increasing the supply of RNs to help resolve an existing shortage of RNs, then any increase in the supply of RNs will come initially from stimulating the number of currently available RNs to participate in the workforce or, if they are already working, increase the number of hours they are willing to work (or both). In contrast, because it takes between 2 and 4 years for an individual to complete a basic nursing education program after they have decided to become an RN and are admitted into an education program, the *long-run* supply of RNs refers to the number of RNs that will be available at some time in the future. Thus, an expansion in the long-run supply of RNs will not address the shortage of RNs that is being experienced today, but it might help resolve the shortage in the future.

This chapter focuses on the short-run supply of RNs in the United States—later, in Chapter 7, we turn our attention to the factors that determine the long-run supply of RNs. We begin by describing the relationships between economic and noneconomic factors that influence the participation and hours of work decisions of existing RNs. After discussing these factors, we review the literature to assess how well these relationships are borne out by empirical studies. Following this, we discuss examples of how RNs' short-run labor supply decisions were influenced when the national economy was booming and when the economy was in a recession. We then conclude the chapter by examining the influence of economic changes on RN employment since 2001 and then look more closely at the characteristics of the RNs who have supplied the hospital RN labor market in the United States over the past few years.

ECONOMIC AND NONECONOMIC FACTORS THAT DETERMINE THE SHORT-RUN SUPPLY OF RNs

The value an RN attaches to spending her or his time working for money in the labor market and the value of spending that same time in nonmarket activities underpin the decision to participate in the labor market and the number of hours spent working. All of us, not just RNs, face the same decision about how we use our time. An individual can go to work and earn money and thereby increase their economic wealth. The increase in wealth allows the individual to purchase essential goods and services and other items that bring satisfaction. In addition to the money earned, spending time working offers social contact and opportunities to learn and improve skills that can lead to gains in overall personal satisfaction. On the other hand, an individual might attach a high value to spending time in nonwork activities (e.g., gardening, playing sports, shopping, doing housework, raising children, being with friends, etc.) such that they spend very little time in the labor market working for pay. From this perspective, the number of RNs employed in the nurse labor market at any given point in time reflects the cumulative total of RNs who have decided that they derive enough value from working that they spend some of their available time working for pay. In the short run, this number of RNs is fixed and cannot be expanded because it takes time to educate additional RNs. The only way that the amount of labor supplied by RNs can be changed in the short run involves influencing the decisions of existing RNs to participate in the labor market and the number of hours they are willing to spend working. What then are the economic and noneconomic factors that influence existing RNs' choices to participate in the labor market and the number of hours spent working?

Economic Factors Impacting RNs' Decisions to Participate in the Nurse Labor Market and Number of Hours Worked

Based largely on the idea of a "labor-leisure tradeoff," economists have developed a fairly precise theory to explain labor supply decisions (Killingsworth, 1983). In their formulation, a combination of economic and noneconomic factors determine the decision of individuals to participate in the labor market and hours worked. Typically, these factors include wages, other sources of income, and demographic characteristics such as the individual's age, gender, marital status, presence of dependents in the household, and other characteristics. Although economists emphasize the role of economic variables over other factors, it is readily acknowledged that noneconomic factors are often more important in determining labor supply decisions than economic factors. However, economists point out that compared to economic determinants, noneconomic factors are slow to change and might not be manipulated easily or at all to bring about short-run labor supply decisions. For this reason, the subsequent discussion and the analysis of RN employment that follow emphasize the effects of economic factors on RNs' short-run labor supply decisions.

Wages and Fringe Benefits

Labor economists break apart the relationship between changes in wages and short-run labor supply (participation and hours worked) into two effects, the *substitution* and *income* effects (Ehrenberg & Smith, 2000). Both effects arise whenever individuals experience a change in their wages. Not only are the substitution and income effects elicited whenever wages change, but they exert an opposite impact on labor supply decisions. We will describe the substitution effect first and then follow with an explanation of the income effect.

Substitution Effect

The compensation an RN receives from an employer in the form of hourly earnings (or a salary) plus fringe benefits (health insurance, vacation time, child care, etc.) exerts an important influence on RNs' decisions to participate in the labor market and on the number of hours spent working. Offering compensation to RNs involves an economic exchange in which the employer gives up financial resources for a certain amount of an RN's time that he or she provides nursing services. Ignoring for a moment all the other factors an RN takes into account when deciding whether to work, and considering only the influence of compensation, when an employer raises wages, the economic value of the RN's time spent working increases. That is, by spending more time working, an RN can increase his or her wealth. Another way to think of the effect of an increase in wages is that it makes the time an RN spends *not* working more costly—by deciding not to work, the RN foregoes the higher wages and the resultant increase in his or her economic wealth. Hence, the effect of a wage increase is to induce an RN to *substitute* some of his or her "leisure," or nonworking, time and spend that time working in the labor market earning additional money. For RNs who are not currently working, a wage increase will stimulate some (but not all) RNs to substitute some of their leisure time so they can participate in the labor market, whereas for RNs who are already working, the wage increase will provide an incentive to work additional hours. *The substitution effect exerts a positive impact on short-run labor supply decisions in response to a wage increase.*

What happens if wages fall, or more realistically, if wage increases fail to keep up with annual increases in the cost of living? From the RN's perspective, and again ignoring all other factors that affect the decision to work and number of hours worked, a *decrease* in wages means that the time spent working becomes *less* valuable because that time will now contribute less toward increasing the RN's wealth. Stated differently, the decrease in wages makes the time an RN spends *not working* less costly. Thus, the effect of a wage decrease tends to result in RNs substituting some of their time working toward spending that time in nonmarket or leisure activities. For RNs who are not currently working, the wage decrease stimulates them to remain nonparticipants, whereas for RNs who are already working, the wage decrease provides an incentive to work fewer hours, shop around for a higher paying job, or even withdraw from the workforce altogether. From the discussion thus far, it is clear that the substitution effect exerts a positive influence on labor supply decisions when wages increase and a negative influence when wages decrease.

Income Effect

In addition to the substitution effect, the income effect also occurs whenever wages change. The income effect, however, exerts the opposite influence from the substitution effect on RNs' short-run labor supply decisions. In the logic of economics, a wage hike increases an RN's wealth, and the increase in wealth means that an RN can purchase more goods and services. One of the goods an RN can purchase with the additional income is more leisure time—that is, less time working. In response to a *wage increase*, therefore, the income effect exerts a *negative* influence on participation and hours worked. However, when *wages decrease* or fail to keep up with inflation, the opposite occurs because the income effect induces some (but not all) RNs to *increase* the amount of their time spent working. This is because the decrease in the RN's wage reduces the ability to purchase more leisure time.

To summarize, whenever wages increase, two opposing forces, the positive substitution and the negative income effects interact and jointly influence RNs' decisions to participate in the nurse labor market, and if they are already participating, the number of additional hours to work. Which effect is stronger than the other for an RN at any given time, holding all else constant, determines the net impact of the wage increase on participation and hours worked. If the substitution effect dominates, the RN will decide to participate, or if working, allocate additional hours to the labor market. If the income effect dominates, the RN will not participate and will not work additional hours. In the case of a wage decrease, the substitution effect now becomes negative and the income effect becomes positive, both interact simultaneously, and the stronger of the two effects determines the net impact on participation and hours worked. Unfortunately, it is impossible to know in advance which effect will dominate in response to a change in wages. Again, the choice of whether to work and the number of hours to work involves decisions about how to spend one's available time. The decision is an explicit tradeoff between the value of the additional wealth that could be acquired by working versus the value of spending that same amount of time doing nonwork activities. **Table 6-1** summarizes the predicted impact of the substitution and income effects on short-run labor supply decisions.

Findings of RN Labor Supply Studies

Given the importance and size of the RN workforce, it is surprising that so few studies have been conducted on the short-run labor supply of RNs in the United States. Moreover, most studies were done years ago using data from previous decades, and they report mixed findings. For example, some studies have

Table 6-1   Predicted Impact on Short-Run Labor Supply (Participation in the Nurse Labor Market and Number of Hours Worked) Elicited by the Substitution, Income, and Pure Income Effects Associated with Changes in RNs' Real Wages and Nonwage Income

Economic Effects	Predicted Impact on Short-Run Labor Supply Following a Change in Wages	
	Wage Increase	Wage Decrease
Substitution Effect	*Positive*	*Negative*
Income Effect	*Negative*	*Positive*
	Predicted Impact on Short-Run Labor Supply Following a Change in Nonwage Income	
	Nonwage Increase	Nonwage Decrease
Pure Income Effect	*Negative*	*Positive*

found a strong, positive, and statistically significant relationship between wages and RN *hours worked*, which would indicate that the positive substitution effect dominates the negative income effect (Sloan & Richupan, 1975; Link & Settle, 1985; Brewer, 1996; Lehrer, Santero, & Mohan-Neill, 1991). Other studies report a weak or statistically insignificant relationship between wage and hours worked, which would indicate that the substitution and income effects essentially offset each other (Askildsen, Baltagi, & Holmas, 2003; Ault & Rutman, 1994; Buerhaus, 1991; Bognanno, Hixson, & Jeffers, 1974; Link, 1992; Link & Settle, 1979; Link & Settle, 1980; Phillips, 1995; Staiger, Spetz, & Phibbs, 1999). Still, others have reported either an inconsistent or no relationship between wages and RN hours worked (Ault & Rutman, 1994; Laing & Rademaker, 1990; Link, 1992; Chiha & Link, 2003). One study (Brewer, 1996) examined the influence of gender and found that the hours worked by RNs who are men are less responsive to the effects of wages than the hours worked by RNs who are women. Overall, the study findings suggest that the relationship between wage changes and number of hours worked is not very sensitive (inelastic), holding all else constant.

With respect to the relationship between wages and *participation*, the evidence is clearer and indicates a stronger relationship than that found for hours worked. Several studies (Benham, 1971; Sloan & Richupan, 1975; Link & Settle, 1981a; Dusansky, Ingber, Leiken, & Walsh, 1986; Link, 1992; Phillips, 1995; Ahlburg & Brown Mahoney, 1996) report a positive relationship between RN wages and participation. In contrast to these results, other investigators (Bognanno, et al., 1974; Ault & Rutman, 1994; Chiha & Link, 2003; Laing & Rademaker, 1990; Link, 1992; and Link & Settle, 1980) find no statistically significant relationship between wages and participation rates, probably because a high percentage of RNs are already employed (Antonazzo, Scott, Skatun, & Elliott, 2003).

The conclusions drawn by Shields and colleagues (2004), after reviewing 16 studies conducted from 1970 to 2003, are helpful in summarizing the evidence on the effect of wages and RNs' labor supply decisions. According to these authors, "With respect to the likely impact of increasing the RN wage rate, although there are considerable differences and inconsistencies across the studies reviewed, the main conclusion is that the wage elasticity is unresponsive (or inelastic) and that very large increases in wages would be needed to induce even moderate increases in nurse labor supply" (p. F493). They go on to indicate that the average of the wage elasticities found across the U.S. studies is around 0.3, suggesting that a 10% increase in the RN real wage rate in the United States would increase the labor supply by only 3%. This estimate is very similar in magnitude to the general consensus elasticity of 0.2 found in studies of the wider female labor market reported by Borjas (2000). Shields and colleagues conclude by noting that the evidence from labor supply studies suggests that wage increases will have a greater impact on increasing RN *participation rates* than on inducing existing RNs to increase their hours of work.[1]

Before moving on to consider other economic and noneconomic determinants of the short-run labor supply of RNs, we pause to consider a phenomenon referred to as a backward bending labor supply curve. As we saw earlier in Chapter 3, the relationship between wages and hours worked is usually depicted graphically by the labor supply curve drawn as a straight line sloping upward and to the right, meaning that, as wages increase, more hours of work will be supplied. Some studies (Bognanno, et al., 1974; Link & Settle, 1980, 1981a; Buerhaus, 1991; Sloan & Richupan, 1975) find evidence that when wages increase and exceed a certain threshold point along the labor supply curve, additional wage increases *reduce* the number of hours worked. Apparently, some RNs determine that despite the greater earnings that could be obtained by working additional hours, they are unwilling to give up so much of their time that is engaged in non-market activities. In this case, the labor supply curve bends backward and to the left when the wage increase exceeds the threshold. Another way to envision this relationship is that at points on the RN's labor supply curve below the threshold point, the positive substitution effect dominates the negative income effect as wages are increasing. When the wage increase exceeds the threshold point, however, the negative income effect dominates the positive substitution effect, resulting in a decrease in hours worked.

To sum up, weighing the available evidence suggests that raising RN wages is likely to result in an increase in the short-run labor supplied by some RNs, but the increase in hours worked is unlikely to be highly responsive; in contrast, the effect on raising participation is likely to be stronger. Thus, facing a shortage of RNs, and having tried other noneconomic ways to resolve the shortage, an employer might decide to raise wages to increase the short-run supply of current RNs in its market or to attract nurses to enter the local market. The resulting increase in participation and hours worked will depend on how much wages increase and on the effect of other factors that an RN takes into consideration when deciding how to use her or his time. Later, in Chapter 11, we discuss shortages of RNs in considerable detail including, in Appendix 11-1, a discusson on why it takes time for some employers to decide to raise RN wages in the presence of a nursing shortage.

Now that we have described the relationship between wage changes and existing RNs' labor supply decisions, we examine another economic variable: RN's nonwage income. As we will see, evidence from labor supply studies indicates

---

[1] These results suggest that the short-run labor supply curve shown in Figure 3-3 would have a relatively steep slope, indicating that any given wage increase would result in a relatively modest increase in employment.

that the influence of this economic factor exerts a more consistent effect on RNs' labor supply decisions.

Nonwage Income and RNs' Labor Market Decisions

Working provides income that is used to acquire essential goods and services that an RN needs in addition to purchasing nonessential items that bring personal satisfaction. Beyond the income received from her or his job working as a nurse, an RN's total income is derived from nonwage sources, including money from investments, alimony payments, a trust fund or inheritance, or other sources. Because the majority of full-time equivalent (FTE) RNs are married (66% in 2004), the income derived from an RN's spouse is a particularly important component of the total nonwage income of married RNs. The more money earned by the RN's spouse, more consumer goods and services can be purchased or, alternatively, more money can be saved or invested. In fact, one of the goods an RN can purchase with this extra income is more of their *own time* spent not working in the labor market.

From the perspective of the RN's *household*, each hour of time the RN spends in the labor market means that hour is no longer available to accomplish activities that benefit the household. Because an RN derives a certain value from time spent on household activities (e.g., raising a child), when the income of an RN's spouse rises, the value of the time the RN spends working falls. In other words, the increase in the spouse's earnings means that more goods and services can be purchased with the added income that would have formerly required a portion of the RN's time to earn. One of the goods that can be purchased by the increase in spouse income is more of the RN's *time* spent on household activities (rather than in the labor market). The effect of changes in the RN's nonwage income is referred to as a *pure income effect* on the labor supply decision of RNs. Because this effect is independent of the RN's own wage, the substitution effect is not elicited. Table 6-1 shows the predicted impact of the pure income effect when RNs' nonwage income changes.

Perhaps a clearer way to understand the pure income effect associated with changes in the RN's nonwage income is to imagine what would happen if an RN receives a large amount of money—say the RN won a lottery. In this event, the economic wealth of the household would increase substantially, and one would not be surprised if the RN decided to quit working or reduce the amount of time working. The added income, which had nothing to do with the RN's own wage rate, makes it possible for the RN to purchase more time out of the labor market. The increase in nonwage income stimulates some, but not all, married RNs to *reduce* not only the number of hours worked but might even encourage some married RNs to withdraw from the labor market altogether.

What happens to RN's labor supply when the income of the spouse of an RN falls, perhaps because he or she has not received a wage increase, lost his or her job, or is worried about losing employment? In this case the nonwage income and the real or perceived economic security of the RN's household are decreased. Consequently, the loss in nonwage income induces some married RNs to decide to reenter the labor market if they are not currently working, while others who are already employed might decide to increase the number of hours worked by working overtime, shifting from part- to full-time status, or even deciding to work a second job. Thus, in the case of a decrease in nonwage income, the pure income effect would exert a *positive* impact on participation and hours worked.

Study Findings

The vast majority of economic studies conducted on the short-run labor supply of RNs referenced above have found that an increase in RN spouse wages exerts the expected negative impact on RNs' labor supply decisions. Moreover, according to the above mentioned review by Shields (2004) of RN labor supply studies conducted from 1970 to 2003, increases in an RN's spouse's wages reduced the RN's participation in the labor market more than it reduced the number of hours worked by RNs who were already participating. One study by Link and Settle (1981a) reported that older RNs were the most responsive to changes in their nonwage income, and a study by Brewer (1996) reported that male RNs are less sensitive to the effects of nonwage income than are female RNs.

Considering the important role of RNs' nonwage income not only expands our understanding of the short-run labor supply decisions of RNs, but it draws attention to the performance of the nation's economy and its effect on spouses' incomes and hence participation and hours worked in the nurse labor market by married RNs. One of the ways economists track changes in the economy's health is by collecting data on levels of employment and unemployment. When the economy experiences a recession, some firms go out of business, and others find that to survive they must lay off some of their employees. If an RN's spouse loses her or his job, or fears that such a loss is likely, then the RN is likely to increase her or his time working in the labor market. That is, because the RN is now (or soon might become) the primary wage earner in the household, the RN's time in the labor market is far more valuable than the time spent in the household, particularly because some of the household activities can be performed by the unemployed spouse or by other family members. As we will see later in this chapter, changes in the performance of the national economy have exerted very large effects on RN employment.

Impact of Noneconomic Factors on the Short-Run Labor Supply of RNs

As noted earlier, the labor supply decisions of most individuals, including RNs, are not driven exclusively by economic factors. Other considerations might in fact drive the decision, particularly when an RN has decided to spend some of her or his time working in the labor market. Labor supply studies have included a variety of noneconomic factors that attempt to explain the variation in participation and hours worked beyond that accounted for by changes in RN wages and nonwage income. These factors include the presence of children and other dependents in the RN's household, RN education, age, race, gender, marital status, and whether the RN is a graduate of a nursing education program outside the United States. As pointed out earlier, because these factors cannot be changed or are not easily manipulated in short periods of time by employers or policy makers, we will generally not discuss the impact of these factors in the same detail as the economic factors previously described.

Dependents in the RN's Household

Whether an RN responds to a wage increase depends on how much earnings are increased, the amount of available nonwage income, and factors that place demands on his or her time. Because the vast majority of RNs are women (91% of those working in 2006), and day-to-day child rearing responsibilities fall more heavily on women than men, the presence of children places additional demands on the RN's time. In particular, young children, who are more dependent on their mothers, offer employers strong competition for an RN's time. The RN must choose whether to spend time with her children or spend that same time working for pay. Again, each person is unique and places a different value on the time spent with children versus time spent working for pay. Nevertheless, as children grow older and become more independent, they demand less time from their parents and, consequently, the RN has more time available to spend doing other things beyond child rearing, including working in the labor market.

Controlling for the effect of wages and nonwage income, nearly all of the studies previously referenced found that the presence of young children exerted the expected negative effect on RNs' participation in the workforce, but older children have little effect on their RN mother's decision to participate. With regard to the annual number of hours worked, there is widespread agreement among study results that young children also reduce hours worked substantially for married RNs. As children become older, studies indicate that the negative relationship between RN hours worked and older children largely disappears. Some studies (Sloan & Richupan, 1975; Brewer, 1996) suggest that older children have a positive effect on RN hours worked, presumably because older children substitute for their mothers in performing some child rearing activities of younger children in the household.

In addition to the presence of children in the RN's household, adults living in the RN's household might exert additional demands on the RN's available time, for example, the RN's parents or perhaps his or her spouse's parent(s). These adults, not unlike an RN's younger children, might exert an important effect on RNs' labor supply decisions. If the older adult is in good health and living arrangements are conducive, he or she can help the RN accomplish household activities and thereby exert a positive effect on the amount of time the RN spends in the labor market. On the other hand, if the older adult(s) is not in good health and requires assistance performing activities of daily living, then the RN is likely to spend less time in the labor market and more time at home. Unfortunately, very few studies of the short-run labor supply of nurses have included a measure of adult dependents in the RN's household. An early study by Sloan (1975) included a variable to measure the number of dependents in the RN's household other than children, but the results were not statistically significant.

The influence of dependents (children and adults) on an RN's participation in the nurse labor market and hours worked is shown in **Figures 6-1** and **6-2**, which are derived from data on RNs aged 36 to 40 obtained from the 2004 National Sample Survey of Registered Nurses (described in Chapter 1). As clearly shown, both participation and hours worked among RNs aged 36 to 40 is lowest among those who report children less than 6 years of age or a combination of both younger and older children at home. As children become older (over the age of 6), participation rates and hours worked increase considerably. The highest participation rates and hours worked by RNs in this age group occur among RNs who report either no children or adult dependents in the household (and by RNs who report that there are adult dependents in the household, regardless of whether there are children of any age). The influence of older adults in the RN's household appears to have a positive influence on short-run labor supply, at least among RNs aged 36-40. These data suggest that older dependents are substituting for the RN's time spent on accomplishing household activities, which makes it possible for these RNs to allocate more of their time in the labor market.

Given the projected rapid expansion in the size and proportion of seniors in the United States population (described in Chapter 4), it is important to develop a better understanding of the potential effects of older adults in the RN's household, particularly among RNs who are older and in their 50s when their children might no longer live at home. In fact, it is well known that older parents are significantly more likely to live with a daughter rather than with a son. As seniors live longer during the years and decades ahead, it is likely that many parents of RNs will live in the RN's household rather than living with their sons or in

Figure 6-1   Percentage of RNs Aged 36 to 40 Employed in Nursing by Status of Children and Adult Dependents at Home, 2004

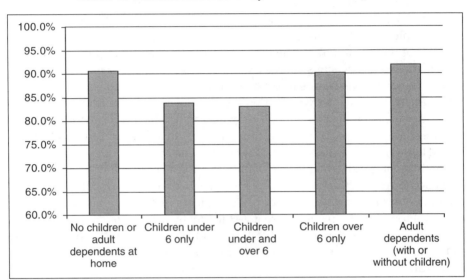

Source: National Sample Survey of Registered Nurses, 2004.

assisted living centers or long-term care facilities. Should many of the elderly who require assistance performing activities of daily living reside with their RN daughters, this might result in an important negative effect on the labor supply decisions and could lead to a potentially large decline in RN participation and hours supplied to the labor market. Already, 16% of all RNs in the 2004 National Sample Survey of Registered Nurses (NSSRN) reported caring for other adults in their home, and 16% also were caring for other adults living elsewhere. The potential reduction in short-run supply is most likely to impact older RNs as the number and proportion over age 50 are increasing faster than any other age group of RNs. The implications of RNs' providing care to adults living in their homes is made clear by a recent study by Johnson and Lo Sasso (2006) that used a sample of women aged 55 to 67 who have elderly parents to estimate annual hours of paid work, controlling for the effects of time needed to assist parents. The study reported that providing informal care to elderly parents substantially reduced the daughters' labor supply. Women in their midlife who helped their parents over a 2-year period reduced their work hours by an average of 41%, or 367 hours per year.

Figure 6-2   Average Hours Worked Last Week by RNs Aged 36 to 40, by Status of Children and Adult Dependents at Home, 2004

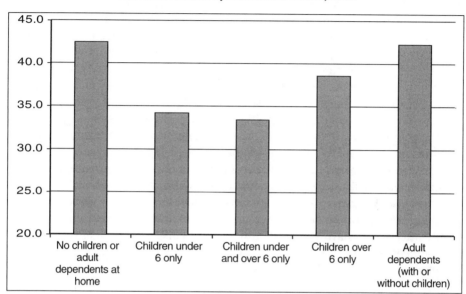

Source: National Sample Survey of Registered Nurses, 2004.

RN Education

The type of nursing education an RN received (associate, diploma, bachelor's, or graduate degree) has been included in short-run labor supply studies. Economists have offered various explanations for why the type of education could account for differences in participation and hours worked. For example, Sloan (1975) suggests that the type of nursing education might affect an RN's attitude toward work as well as his or her tolerance for unfavorable workplace environments. He reasons that more highly educated RNs have higher skills and might therefore derive greater enjoyment from work, and they also might be able to delegate less interesting tasks to others. Thus, RNs with a baccalaureate degree might be more likely to work more hours than RNs who have an associate's degree or diploma in nursing. Altman (1971) offers a different reason for why those with bachelor's degrees might work more hours: He observes that RNs with a baccalaureate degree have greater choices and flexibility in their jobs and occupational choices and that some baccalaureates might be employed in occupations other than nursing to a greater degree. These predictions, however, are not born out by the preponderance of study results, though there is some evidence that RNs with graduate degrees have higher participation rates than RNs with undergraduate degrees or a diploma. In a review of over one dozen RN labor supply studies done in North America during the 1970s and 1980s, Antonazzo and colleagues conclude that, overall, the type of nursing education of participating RNs is not significantly linked to labor supply decisions.[2]

Another way that education has been included in short-run labor supply studies is by accounting for whether participating RNs are enrolled in a nursing education program. To be competitive with other organizations, employers (particularly hospitals) frequently offer tuition assistance to RNs as part of their fringe benefit package. Enrollment in a nursing education program places another demand on the RN's time and is therefore likely to affect labor supply decisions. Over the years that the federal government has been conducting the NSSRN, it has consistently reported that many working RNs are enrolled in nursing education programs. For example, in the 2004 NSSRN, 7.6% of RNs (220,412) were enrolled in formal education programs leading to an academic degree or certificate (U.S. Department of Health and Human Services, Health Resources and Services Administration, 2006). Most of the RN students (172,150) who were enrolled in these programs were in nursing or were in programs that would enhance their nursing careers, and a little more than half (54%) were part-time students employed full-time in nursing. Of the estimated 166,768 RNs pursuing academic degrees in nursing or related to nursing, an estimated 49% were pursuing baccalaureate degrees, 46% were pursuing master's degrees, and 5% were pursuing doctoral degrees (pp. 31–31). Only a few labor supply studies accounted for enrollment into nursing education programs and, not surprisingly, the findings indicate a negative affect on the number of annual hours worked. For example, studies have found that full-time enrollment significantly reduced the hours spent working per year, ranging from a decrease of nearly 450 hours (Buerhaus, 1991) to 285 hours (Brewer, 1996), whereas part-time enrollment decreased hours worked by 65 per year (Buerhaus, 1991).

---

[2] Note that when HRSA (2004) applied FTE workforce participation rates in constructing its projections of the long-run supply of RNs, which is discussed in Chapter 7, it assigned the highest participation rates to RNs with a master's degree, lower rates to both associate's degree and diploma graduates, and the lowest rates to RNs with a bachelor's degree.

RNs' Ages and Other Characteristics

The RN's age is another noneconomic factor influencing the labor supply decisions of existing RNs. Some studies have found a U-shaped pattern in the relationship between an RN's age and amount of time spent working. Young and recently graduated RNs tend to have higher rates of participation in the nurse labor market and spend more hours working, while participation and hours worked decrease during the child rearing years (between age 25 and 40), pick up until the RNs reach their early 50s when children are older, and then decline as RNs approach retirement (see **Table 6-2**). However, other studies find little evidence of a relationship between an RN's age and labor supply decisions.

Some labor supply studies have also included the RN's race, gender, marital status, and whether the RN received his or her nursing education in a country other than the United States (often referred to in the past as a foreign nurse graduate, or "FNG," now more commonly known as an international nursing graduate). Studies generally find that nonwhite RNs, men, unmarried RNs, and international nursing graduates all have a higher rate of participation and work more hours compared to white, female, married and U.S. educated RNs. In an analysis of the 1984 and 1988 NSSRNs, Brewer (1996) found that, in general, ethnic status, children, and continuing education had a smaller affect on RN annual hours for men compared to RNs who were women.

Job Satisfaction

Although seldom included in studies of RN labor supply, job satisfaction might also help explain the variation in participation and hours worked that is not accounted for by wages and nonwage income. Job satisfaction is tied to characteristics of the job (promotion and continuing education opportunities; flexibility of working hours; job security; control over shifts and hours; autonomy; relationships with coworkers, managers, and physicians; etc.) that influence the degree to which RNs derive satisfaction from their workplace and hence influence how much they value time spent in the labor market. Economists have typically considered work satisfaction as captured in the RN's wage rate, reasoning that an employer who provides a poor workplace climate that results in low job satisfaction will have to pay higher wages to attract and retain RNs relative to an employer who provides a positive workplace climate, all other things being equal.

When economic studies have included measures of job satisfaction, they have mostly sought to explain turnover, absenteeism, and intentions of RNs to quit or leave their positions as opposed to explain variations in participation and hours worked. However, Buerhaus (1990) included measures of RNs' work satisfaction in a study of Michigan RN labor supply and found a positive but statistically insignificant relationship with annual hours worked. More recently, Brewer and colleagues (2006) found that job satisfaction was positively related to participation but only for married RNs and not for single RNs. Brewer also reported that decreased job satisfaction compared with a year ago had a small negative effect on the probability that a married RN works on a full-time basis. Finally, we note that the 2000 and 2004 NSSRNs began collecting data on RN job satisfaction in all employment settings. The inclusion of job satisfaction to this large sample longitudinal source of data should enable future studies using these data to assess the effects of the impact of job satisfaction on participation and hours worked.

Because RNs and professional nursing organizations often assert that the main cause of nursing shortages is due to poor working conditions that lead to job dissatisfaction and withdrawal from the workforce, and because from an economic perspective, improving the workplace environment can be accomplished in a relatively short period of time, we devote an entire chapter (Chapter 13) to examining the workplace environment from the perspective of RNs themselves. For now, we continue our examination of the short-run labor supply of RNs by reviewing instances when changes in RNs' wages and nonwage income help explain large changes in hospital RN employment.

CHANGES IN HOSPITAL RN EMPLOYMENT ASSOCIATED WITH RN WAGES AND NONWAGE INCOME

In this section, we examine how changes in hospital and total RN employment levels can be explained by changes in RNs' wages and nonwage income. As discussed earlier, an RN's wage and nonwage income influence the decision to participate in the labor market and number of hours spent working. Both the substitution and income effects are elicited whenever wages change, and the pure income effect occurs with changes in an RN's nonwage income. There have been times when changes in both wage and nonwage income have occurred simultaneously in the nurse labor market, and when these changes were large, they resulted in large and sudden swings in RN participation and employment.

RN Employment Changes in "Bust" versus "Boom" Years

Table 6-3 illustrates how changes in RNs' wage and nonwage income can explain increases (and decreases) in both hospital and total RN FTE employment

Table 6-2   Percentage of RNs Employed and Hours Worked Last Week by Age, 2004*

Age	Percent Employed as an RN	Average Hours Worked Per Week
Less than 25	96.5%	41.8
25–30	92.6%	40.1
31–35	90.8%	38.1
36–40	88.3%	38.8
41–45	88.1%	39.8
46–50	88.5%	41.4
51–55	86.8%	41.2
55–60	78.1%	40.2
61–65	61.9%	36.8
Over 65	40.7%	29.6

*Hours include paid on-call hours.
Source: National Sample Survey of Registered Nurses, 2004.

that have occurred in the nurse labor market over a long period of time. In the bottom two rows of the table, the years between 1979 and 2006 are grouped into "bust" and "boom" periods. During bust periods, the national economy experienced a slowdown in growth (even a recession during some years) as marked by lower average real growth of 1.4% in the gross domestic product (GDP) and higher average unemployment rates of 6.6% compared to boom years when the economy was growing faster. In the boom years, the average real GDP growth was more than twice as high, increasing by 3.8% annually, and average unemployment rates also were lower (5.8%) than in bust periods.

Notice that during the bust periods, average annual real RN wages increased *faster* (1.7%) than during more rapidly growing boom periods (0.9%). The higher wages received by RNs during bust periods would stimulate some RNs to increase their participation and hours worked (a positive substitution effect). At the same time, the slow income growth during the same bust years would stimulate participation and hours worked because many RNs' spouses had undoubtedly lost their jobs (a positive pure income effect). Not surprisingly, during the bust periods, the average annual percent growth in hospital FTE RN employment grew faster (4.6%), as did the total number of FTE RNs (3.5%), than during the average of the boom years (1.0% and 2.4%, respectively).

Although the data shown in Table 6-3 help demonstrate how changes in RN employment are linked to periods of boom and bust in the national economy, by combining several years and summarizing changes as average effects, it is difficult to appreciate how quickly and substantially economic factors that affect RN employment change from year to year. To better understand the swiftness and magnitude of these effects, we examine recent year-to-year changes in hospital and total FTE RN employment that have occurred since 2001.

Table 6-3   Hospital Employment of RNs During Boom and Bust Periods in the National Economy, 1979–2006

Boom and Bust Periods	Real GDP* Growth	Average Unemployment	Average Annual % Growth in RN Wages	Average Annual % Growth in RN Hospital Employment	Average Annual % Growth in Total FTE RNs
1979–1983	1.2%	7.9%	1.8%	3.9%	2.6%
1983–1990	4.0%	6.6%	2.7%	2.4%	3.0%
1990–1992	1.6%	6.5%	0.9%	5.0%	3.3%
1992–2000	3.7%	5.4%	−0.4%	0.5%	2.4%
2000–2003	1.6%	5.1%	2.5%	5.0%	4.9%
2003–2006	3.6%	5.3%	0.0%	−0.9%	0.8%
Bust periods	1.4%	6.6%	1.7%	4.6%	3.5%
Boom periods	3.8%	5.8%	0.9%	1.0%	2.4%

*GDP: Gross domestic product is a measure of the market value of all final goods and services produced within a country in a given period of time
Source: Current Population Survey; Bureau of Labor Statistics.

Recent Changes in RN Employment

As discussed in Chapter 2, total FTE RN employment in the nurse labor market in the United States has been growing steadily for several decades. Recently, total FTE RN employment levels grew at a particularly rapid rate (see **Table 6-4**). From 2001 to 2003, the number of FTE RNs increased by nearly 205,000 FTE RNs. During the next 2 years (2004-2005), however, total RN employment decreased by almost 28,000, and in 2006, total RN employment rebounded, growing by nearly 76,000.

Table 6-4 shows that up until 2006 most of the changes in FTE RN employment occurred in hospitals. In 2002, FTE RN employment increased sharply, rising by nearly 85,000, and in 2003 it grew by an even greater amount, almost 99,000. Our analysis of CPS data shows that this 2-year surge in hospital RN employment growth is the largest increase in over 3 decades. Proving that the hospital RN labor market is dynamic, the growth in hospital RN employment was short-lived because FTE RN employment in hospitals fell by more than 6000 in 2004 and decreased by a much larger number, 51,000, in 2005. In the

Table 6-4   Changes in National Unemployment Rates, Inflation-Adjusted Wages, and Full-Time Equivalent (FTE) RN Employment in the United States, 2001–2006

Year	National Unemployment Rate	Inflation-Adjusted RN Wage Growth		FTE RN Employment and Change from Prior Year	
		Total	**Hospitals**	**Total**	**Hospitals**
2001	4.7%			1,987,389	1,201,003
2002	5.8%	4.3%	5.0%	2,073,283 (85,894)	1,285,718 (84,715)
2003	6.0%	1.7%	1.8%	2,191,981 (118,698)	1,384,482 (98,764)
2004	5.5%	−0.4%	−0.5%	2,191,432 (−549)	1,378,116 (−6,366)
2005	5.1%	−0.3	0.1%	2,164,183 (−27,249)	1,326,914 (−51,202)
2006	4.6%	0.0	0.3%	2,239,873 (75,690)	1,345,711 (18,797)

Source: Current Population Survey.

following year, hospital RN employment rebounded, accounting for 40% of the total growth in RN employment in 2006. Can changes in RN wages and nonwage income once again explain these recent swings in total and hospital RN employment growth?

As shown in Table 6-4, real RN hospital wages increased dramatically, by 5%, from 2001 to 2002. During this same time, other important economic changes were affecting many RNs. In the middle of 2001, the growth rate of the national economy had begun to stall even before the terrorist attacks on 9/11. Thereafter, the stock market declined abruptly, and national unemployment rates began increasing, reaching 6% by the end of 2002. Consumer confidence dropped, and fears of an impending war with Iraq resulted in a general sense of uncertainty about the future. These changes more than likely affected the real or perceived nonwage income and overall economic security of many RN households and, in turn, induced many married RNs to increase their participation and hours worked (a positive pure income effect). In fact, analysis of the CPS data shows that RN employment increased by more than 10% from 2001 to 2002 in the 18 states where unemployment rose by more than the national average between 2000 and 2002. Thus, in addition to increasing wages in 2002, the general slowdown in the economy and rising unemployment reinforced the decision of many RNs to increase their employment activity.

In 2003, both real RN wages and national unemployment rates increased once again (see Table 6-4). Not surprisingly, FTE RN employment in hospitals increased substantially, by nearly 100,000. Over this 2-year period, hospital employment increased by approximately 185,000 FTE RNs, which, according to our analysis of CPS data, is the largest yearly back-to-back employment growth of RNs in over 3 decades. The dramatic effect of the combination of increasing wages and increasing national unemployment rates is further reflected by the increase in the participation rate of RNs nationally, which increased by 1.5% from 2000 (81.7%) to 2004 (83.2%). The 2004 participation rate is the highest RN employment rate ever reported since the NSSRNs have been conducted.

Notice that in 2004 and 2005, these two economic forces quickly reversed direction as both national unemployment rates and RN wages *decreased* at the same time (Table 6-4). Not surprisingly, in 2004 RN hospital employment dropped, falling by a little more than 6000 RNs nationwide. This decrease in employment continued in 2005, as both national unemployment rates and hospital RN wages fell for a second year in a row, resulting in hospital RN employment decreasing impressively, by a little more than 51,000 FTE RNs. However, in 2006, changes in real wages and changes in national unemployment rates moved in opposite directions as RN wages paid by hospitals increased (0.3%), but national unemployment decreased (from 5.1% in 2005 to 4.6% in 2006). The increase in real wages would be expected to positively impact employment, while the decrease in unemployment rates implies that the nonwage income of many RNs was increasing as more spouses were returning to work in 2006, resulting in a negative effect on RN employment. The two economic forces were opposing each other rather than reinforcing each other as they did in the preceding 4 years. But as Table 6-4 shows, the net result was an increase in both total and hospital FTE RN employment.

What might explain why total and hospital RN employment increased in 2006? Three explanations are plausible. First, it is possible that the effect of the increase in real RN wages paid by hospitals (eliciting the positive substitution effect) simply overpowered the negative impact of the rise in household income implied by the falling unemployment rate (the pure income effect). As noted earlier when explaining the impact of economic factors on short-run labor supply, it is impossible to know in advance whether the positive substitution or negative income effect will dominate in response to changes in economic factors. Second, recall that the housing sector of the national economy collapsed during 2006. Conceivably, as the price of houses dropped across regions of the country, many RNs who placed their homes for sale found that their overall household wealth declined because their homes were worth less than they had been the year before. Thus, it is likely that the overall wealth of a good number of RN households fell as the housing market collapsed, resulting in some RNs increasing their employment activity. A third explanation involves changes in the composition of the RN workforce, namely the rapid expansion in the number of foreign-born and foreign-educated RNs who entered the United States in 2006 (see **Table 6-5** in the next section).

In sum, even though economic forces might be of little significance in determining the short-run labor decisions of many RNs, for some RNs economic forces are important. When their decisions are summed over the entire workforce (approximately 2.3 million RNs in 2006), changes in their own wages and in their nonwage income appear to have exerted a substantial impact on both the gains and declines in RN employment that have occurred since 2001 as well as in earlier bust and boom periods in the national economy.

CHANGING COMPOSITION OF THE RN WORKFORCE IN THE UNITED STATES

The above analysis focused on how the large swings in the employment of RNs in earlier decades and during recent years are consistent with changes in both RN wages and changes in RNs' nonwage income (implied by changes in unemployment rates in the national economy). The exceptionally large employment increases that occurred in 2001 and 2002 are intriguing, and they raise the question of who are the RNs who apparently reentered the workplace during this period. We conclude this chapter by taking a closer look underneath these changes in employment and examine the characteristics of the RNs who accounted for this sudden growth in employment.

Increasing Proportion of Foreign-Born RNs

As shown in Table 6-5, the composition of the RN workforce in the United States has become increasingly foreign born and foreign educated.[3] Between 1994 and 2001, the growth of foreign-born RNs averaged 6.0% per year compared to 1.5% among all RNs. However, in 2002 the growth of foreign-born RNs doubled to 12.5%, an increase of nearly 42,000 FTE RNs (Buerhaus, Staiger, & Auerbach, 2003). In fact, this increased employment in the number of foreign-born RNs was just shy of the increased employment growth of RNs born in the United States during 2002. A year later, employment of foreign-born RNs increased by 24,000 for a total growth of roughly 66,000 during this 2-year period. In 2004, when hospital RN employment began to decline (Table 6-4), employment of foreign-born RNs continued to grow, increasing by more than 9000, while the number of United States–born RNs decreased in the same year. In 2005, however, the number of foreign-born RNs in the United States dropped sharply, by more than 21,000, probably as a result of the expiration of visas used to gain entry into the United States in earlier years. Furthermore, of the total decrease (a little more than 51,000) in FTE RN hospital employment in 2005 shown in Table 6-4, foreign-born RNs accounted for 13,000 of this decline. Finally, notice that a year later, in 2006, the number of foreign-born RNs shot up by just over 39,000, once again outstripping the growth in employment among RNs born in the United States. Overall, the rapid growth in employment of foreign-born RNs accounts for more than one-third (37%) of the total growth of total RN employment in the United States since 2002.

An Aging RN Workforce

As shown in **Table 6-6**, a very large proportion of the recent employment growth of RNs came from RNs over the age of 50 years. In fact, employment

---

[3]Because the CPS data used to conduct this analysis do not allow us to identify among foreign-born RNs, the subset of RNs who received their nursing education outside of the United States, employment growth in this group does not solely reflect growth in the number of foreign nurse graduates working in the United States.

Table 6-5   **Total Employment Growth of Full-Time RNs by United States– and Foreign-Born Status, 2002–2006**

Year	United States–Born	Foreign-Born
2002	44,045	41,849
2003	94,503	24,190
2004	–9,824	9,275
2005	–5,897	–21,353
2006	36,616	39,075
2002–2006	159,443	93,036

Source: Current Population Survey.

growth of older RNs increased in every year since 2000 for an astounding net gain of a little more than 257,000 FTE RNs. In stark contrast, the total net employment growth of younger RNs (aged 21-34 years) of roughly 36,000 was effectively washed out by the net decrease (roughly 40,000 FTE RNs) in employment among middle-aged RNs (aged 35-49 years).

As we shall see in subsequent chapters dealing with the supply of RNs, these trends in the increasing number and proportion of both foreign-born and older RNs are not unexpected. Rather, the changes in RN employment and earnings that we have discussed have occurred in the backdrop of more deep-seated trends that are transforming the RN workforce. In other words, while changing economic forces might impact year-to-year RN employment levels and convey visible and important information to those concerned with the performance of the nurse labor market, they are but momentary movements in the current short-run supply of RNs that is occurring on top of longer term forces that are steadily reshaping the composition of the RN workforce. We examine why the RN workforce is becoming older in Chapters 8 and 9 and the long-run implication for the future supply of RNs in Chapter 10. But next, in Chapter 7, we turn our attention to examining the factors that determine the long-run supply of RNs.

Table 6-6   Total Employment Growth of Full-Time Equivalent (FTE) RNs in the United States by Age, 2002–2006

	Employment Growth by Age of FTE RNs		
Year	21–34 years	35–49 years	50–64 years
2002	−21,170	43,152	63,911
2003	87,131	−32,271	65,839
2004	−45,034	21,294	23,212
2005	−31,277	−87,284	91,312
2006	46,172	16,970	12,888
2002–2006	35,822	−40,139	257,161

Source: Current Population Survey.

CHAPTER SUMMARY

The decision of existing RNs to participate in the workforce and the number of hours worked are a function of the RN's wage and fringe benefits, nonwage income (primarily the income of the RN's spouse), presence of children and older adults in the household, enrollment in education programs, demographic characteristics, and job satisfaction. Because it is difficult to change the noneconomic factors that affect RNs' decisions to work, and because improvements in working conditions take time to accomplish, employers rely on changing wages and fringe benefits to influence the short-run labor supply decisions of existing RNs. The substitution and income effects are elicited when RNs' wages are changed, and whichever effect dominates determines employment decisions. Changes in nonwage income also result in a pure income effect that also impacts the short-run labor decisions of RNs substantially.

Studies show that, on average, increases in wages tend to exert a positive but relatively small impact on the number of hours worked by RNs and a greater impact on the decision of nonparticipants to rejoin the workforce, while increases in nonwage income exert a negative impact on these decisions, holding all other factors constant. The combination of changes in real RN wages and RNs' nonwage income implied by movements in national unemployment rates indicate that these economic forces exert a powerful impact on the decisions of many RNs. These changes have led to dramatic swings in national FTE RN employment levels during boom and bust periods in the national economy and were particularly evident in recent years. Underneath these changes in employment, the RN workforce in the United States is becoming older and more foreign born, a sign of what we can expect in the future.

REFERENCES

Ahlburg, D., & Brown Mahoney, C. (1996). The effect of wages on the retention of nurses. *Canadian Economic Journal, 29*, S126–S129.

Altman, S. (1971). *Present and future supply of registered nurses* (DHEW Publication No. 2[NIH] 72–134). Washington, DC: U.S. Government Printing Office.

Antonazzo, E., Scott, A., Skatun, D., & Elliott, R. (2003). The labour market for nursing: A review of the labour supply literature. *Health Economics, 12*, 465–478.

Askildsen, J., Baltagi, B., & Holmas, T. (2003). Will increased wages reduce shortages of nurses? A panel data analysis of nurses' labour supply. *Health Economics, 12*, 705–719.

Ault, D., & Rutman, G. (1994). On selecting a measure of labour activity: Evidence from registered nurses: 1981 and 1989. *Applied Economics, 26*, 851–863.

Benham, L. (1971). The labor market for registered nurses: A three-equation model. *Review of Economics and Statistics, 53*, 246–252.

Bognanno, M., Hixson, J., & Jeffers J. (1974). The short-run supply of nurse's time. *The Journal of Human Resources, 9*, 81–94.

Borjas, G. (2000). *Labor economics.* Boston: Irwin/McGraw-Hill.

Brewer, C. (1996). The roller coaster supply of registered nurses: Lessons from the eighties. *Research in Nursing & Health, 19*, 345–357.

Brewer, C., Kovner, C., Wu, Y.W., Greene, W., Liu, Y., & Reimers, C. (2006). Factors influencing female registered nurses' work behavior. *Health Services Research, 41*(3), 860–866.

Buerhaus, P. (1990). *Economic and work satisfaction determinants of the annual number of hours worked by registered nurses.* Unpublished doctoral dissertation, Wayne State University.

Buerhaus, P. (1991). Economic determinants of the annual number of hours worked by registered nurses. *Medical Care, 29*(12), 1181–1195.

Buerhaus, P., Staiger, D., & Auerbach, D. (2003). Is the current shortage of hospital nurses ending? Emerging trends in employment and earnings of registered nurses. *Health Affairs, 22*(6), 191–198.

Chiha, Y., & Link, C. (2003). The shortage of registered nurses and some new estimates of the effects of wages on registered nurses labour supply: A look at the past and a preview of the 21st century. *Health Policy, 64*, 349–375.

Dusansky, R., Ingber, M., Leiken, A., & Walsh, J. (1986). On increasing the supply of nurses: An interstate analysis. *Atlantic Economic Journal, 24*, 34–44.

Ehrenberg, R., & Smith, R. (2000). *Modern labor economics* (7th ed.). Reading, MA: Addison Wesley Longman.

Johnson, R., & Lo Sasso, A. (2006). The impact of elder care on women's labor supply. *The Journal of Health Care Organization, Provision, and Financing, 43*(3), 195–210.

Killingsworth, M. (1983). *Labor supply.* Cambridge, MA: Cambridge University Press.

Laing, G., & Rademaker, A. (1990). Married registered nurses' labour force participation. *The Canadian Journal of Nursing Research, 22*(1), 21–38.

Lehrer, E., Santero, T., & Mohan-Neill, S. (1991). The impact of employer-sponsored child care on female labour supply behaviour: Evidence from the nursing profession. *Population Research Policy Review, 10*, 197–212.

Lehrer, E., White, W., & Young, W. (1991). The three avenues to a registered nurse license: A comparative analysis. *The Journal of Human Resources, 26*, 362–379.

Link, C., & Settle, R. (1980). Financial incentive and labor supply of married professional nurses: An economic analysis. *Nursing Research, 29*(4), 238–243.

Link, C. (1992). Labor supply behavior of registered nurses: Female labor supply in the future? *Research Labor Economics, 13*, 287–320.

Link, C., & Settle, R. (1979). Labour supply responses of married professional nurses: New evidence. *Southern Economic Journal, 41*, 649–656.

Link, C., & Settle, R. (1981a). Wage incentives and married professional nurses: A case of backward bending supply? *Economic Inquiry, 19*, 145–156.

Link, C., & Settle, R. (1981b). A simultaneous-equation model of labor supply, fertility and earnings of married women: The case of registered nurses. *Southern Economic Journal, 47*, 977–988.

Link, C., & Settle, R. (1985). Labor supply responses of licensed practical nurses: A partial solution to a nurse shortage? *Journal of Economics & Business, 37*, 49–57.

Phillips, J. (1995). Nurses labor supply: Participation, hours of work, and discontinuities in the supply function. *Journal of Health Economics, 13*(5), 567–582.

Shields, M. (2004). Addressing nurse shortages: What can policy makers learn from the econometric evidence on nurse labour supply? *The Economic Journal, 114*, F464–F498.

Sloan, F. (1975). *The geographic distribution of nurses and public policy* (DHEW Publication No. 75–53). Washington DC: U.S. Government Printing Office.

Sloan, F., & Richupan, S. (1975). Short-run supply responses of professional nurses: A microanalysis. *Journal of Human Resources, 10*, 242–257.

Staiger, D., Spetz, J., & Phibbs, C. (1999). Is there monopsony in the labor market? Evidence from a natural experiment. *National Bureau of Economic Research Working Paper Series* No. 7258.

U.S. Department of Health and Human Services, Health Resources and Services Administration. (2006). *The registered nurse population: Findings from the March 2004 national sample survey of registered nurses.* Retrieved November 19, 2007, from http://bhpr.hrsa.gov/healthwork force/rnsurvey04/

CHAPTER 7

The Long-Run Supply
of Registered Nurses

As discussed in Chapter 6, the short-run supply of RNs pertains to the number of *hours* supplied to the nurse labor market by *existing* RNs. In the short run, the total amount of labor that can be supplied to hospitals and other employers is constrained by the number of RNs who are currently licensed and available to participate in the workforce. When thinking about the long-run supply of RNs, however, we are referring to the total *number of RNs* who will be available at some time in the *future*. Because it takes between 2 and 4 years for an individual to complete basic nursing education and then pass a state nurse licensing examination to obtain a license to practice nursing, the long-run supply of RNs adjusts to external forces, such as wage increases, more slowly than does the short-run supply of RNs.

In this chapter we discuss the factors that determine the long-run supply of RNs. Understanding these factors will be particularly helpful in appreciating the topics discussed in ensuing chapters. We begin by providing a brief overview of the major educational options for becoming an RN, including information on the growth of nursing education programs and the number of graduates over time. Following this, we discuss the influence of changes in the size of the population between the ages of 20 and 40 from which nursing education programs have typically drawn. Next, we summarize results of research that address the reasons why people are motivated to become nurses and the importance of societal changes that have shaped the propensity of individuals to become an RN. We then discuss other factors that influence the long-run supply of RNs, including RNs' ages, the availability of alternative sources of RNs, influence of economic factors on people's decisions to become an RN, and factors that appear to be limiting the current capacity of education programs to produce RNs required for the future. We conclude the chapter by summarizing two forecasting models and their estimates of the future number of RNs in the workforce to illustrate how several of the factors described in this chapter have been used to forecast the long-run supply of RNs.

OVERVIEW OF TRENDS IN NURSING EDUCATION

Because nursing education programs are the gateway to becoming an RN, trends in nursing education can have important effects on the long-run supply of RNs. An individual can choose from among three traditional educational options to become an RN: a 4-year baccalaureate degree; a 2-year associate's degree program; or a 3-year diploma program. Baccalaureate programs are based in universities and colleges and generally take 4 years to complete. These programs provide a college education in addition to a professional practice degree with students taking courses in the social sciences and liberal arts in addition to clinical coursework and skill development. The number of baccalaureate degree programs grew slowly after World War II but began increasing in the 1960s and 1970s due to efforts by leaders of national nursing associations to transform nursing from an occupation to a profession, in part by moving nursing education into university and college settings. An increasingly popular option to obtain a baccalaureate degree is what are called "accelerated nursing degree programs" that began in the early 1990s. These programs are offered at both the baccalaureate and master's degree levels and build on the student's previous learning experiences. Over a 12- to 18-month period, students with undergraduate degrees in other disciplines are transitioned through a nursing curriculum emphasizing clinical courses and developing nursing practice skills. In 1990, there were 31 accelerated baccalaureate programs and 12 master's programs; in 2005, the number of these programs had grown to 168 and 50, respectively (American Association of Colleges of Nursing, 2003).

As shown in **Table 7-1,** the number of baccalaureate programs has not grown as fast nor have they been able to catch up to the number of associate's degree programs, which are a second option to become an RN. Associate's degree programs are most frequently based in community and technical colleges and generally take two years to complete. Compared to baccalaureate degree programs, the curriculum is focused more on obtaining clinical knowledge and skill development and less on exposing students to the social sciences and liberal arts.

Diploma nursing programs are the oldest of the three traditional educational options for becoming an RN. Prior to the 1960s, nearly all nursing education took place in these hospital-based programs (see Table 7-1). Nursing students typically received a stipend from the hospital, and graduates received a certificate of completion but not a university or college degree. By subsidizing the costs of nursing education, hospitals virtually guaranteed a steady supply of RNs who were familiar with their particular organizational routines and procedures. After World War II, RNs became more mobile and were not as likely to remain working in the hospital where they received their nursing educations. Eventually, the number of diploma programs began to decrease, particularly as baccalaureate

Table 7-1 Number of Nursing Education Programs Leading to Licensure as an RN, Selected Academic Years, 1950–1951 to 2004–2005

Academic Year	Total	Registered Nursing Baccalaureate Degree	Associate Degree	Diploma
1950–1951	1170	—	—	—
1960–1961	1137	172	57	908
1970–1971	1340	267	437	636
1980–1981	1385	377	697	311
1981–1982	1401	383	715	303
1982–1983	1432	402	742	288
1983–1984	1466	421	764	281
1984–1985	1477	427	777	273
1985–1986	1473	441	776	256
1986–1987	1469	455	776	238
1987–1988	1465	467	789	209
1988–1989	1442	479	792	171
1989–1990	1457	488	812	157
1990–1991	1470	489	829	152
1991–1992	1484	501	838	145
1992–1993	1484	501	848	135
1993–1994	1493	507	857	129
1994–1995	1501	509	868	124
1995–1996	1516	521	876	119
1996–1997	1508	523	876	109
1997–1998	—	—	—	—
1998–1999†	1540	548	899	93
1999–2000†	1513	550	885	78
2000–2001	—	—	—	—
2001–2002‡	1459	526	857	76
2002–2003§	1444	529	846	69
2003–2004§	1504	553	880	71
2004–2005§	1544	573	909	62

†Data are unofficial and unpublished from the National League for Nursing.
‡Data are from the U.S. Statistical Abstract (2007). *Table 152. Health Professions Practitioners and Schools: 1990 to 2004.* Retrieved from http://www.census.gov/compendia/statab/tables/07s0152.xls
§Data are from *Nursing Data Review Academic Year 2004–2005, Baccalaureate, Associate Degree, and Diploma Programs National League for Nursing.*
Source: US Department of Health and Human Services. (n.d.) *National Center for Health Workforce Analysis: U.S. Health Workforce Personnel Factbook, Table 110. Number of nursing students, graduates and schools for selected academic years: 1950–51 to 1999–2000.* Retrieved November 16, 2007, from http://bhpr.hrsa.gov/healthworkforce/reports/factbook.htm

and associate's degree programs started to flourish in the 1960s and 1970s. By 2005, there were only 62 diploma programs in the United States, compared to 909 associate and 573 baccalaureate degree programs. **Table 7-2** shows the number of graduates from each of these three nursing education programs. Since 1969-1970, associate's degree programs have annually produced the largest number of graduates.

According to the National League for Nursing (NLN; 2006), there is a substantial difference in the average cohort size by type of nursing education program. For the most recent academic year in which data are available (2004-2005), the NLN reports that the average cohort size of graduates from associate's degree programs was 71 compared to 58 for baccalaureate programs. This means that while associate's degree programs comprised 59% of all basic RN programs in 2004-2005, they produced 63% of all graduates of RN programs. Baccalaureate programs, which comprised 37% of the programs, produced only one-third (33%) of all RN graduates in that year.

Compared to all 2-year and 4-year colleges and universities, the NLN (2006) reports that nursing programs have relatively high first-year retention rates. One year following initial enrollment, 87% of baccalaureate, 80% of associate, and 75% of diploma students were still enrolled compared to only 72% of students in non-nursing programs in 4-year colleges and 64% of students in 2-year programs.

When examining Tables 7-1 and 7-2, it is apparent that the number of baccalaureate and associate's degree programs and the number of graduates from these programs were generally increasing in most years with the exception of the mid-1980s and again in the latter part of the 1990s. Although the total number of graduates has increased since 2001, the number of baccalaureate degree graduates has not grown as strongly as associate's degree programs. More importantly, when we discuss projections of the long-run supply of RNs later in this chapter, we will see that the federal government's projection model assumes that the future number of graduates is based largely on recent trends. Moreover, these projections use data on graduates during the last half of the 1990s when the number of graduations were decreasing sharply, and they assume that these numbers will reflect future trends, missing the increases in graduations that took place during the current decade.

FACTORS THAT DETERMINE THE LONG-RUN SUPPLY OF RNs

With this overview of trends in the number of nursing education programs and graduates produced during the past several decades, we now focus on examining the factors that determine the long-run supply of RNs. These factors

Table 7-2 **Number of Graduates of Nursing Education Programs Leading to Licensure as an RN, Selected Academic Years, 1950–1951 to 2004–2005**

Academic Year	Total	Registered Nursing Baccalaureate Degree	Associate Degree	Diploma
1950–1951	28,794	—	—	—
1959–1960	30,113	4,136	789	25,188
1969–1970	43,103	9,069	11,483	22,551
1979–1980	75,523	24,994	36,034	14,495
1980–1981	73,985	24,370	36,712	12,903
1981–1982	74,052	24,081	38,289	11,682
1982–1983	77,408	23,855	41,849	11,704
1983–1984	80,312	23,718	44,394	12,200
1984–1985	82,075	24,975	45,208	11,892
1985–1986	77,027	25,170	41,333	10,524
1986–1987	70,561	23,761	38,528	8,272
1987–1988	64,839	21,504	37,397	5,938
1988–1989	61,660	18,997	37,837	4,826
1989–1990	66,088	18,571	42,318	5,199
1990–1991	72,230	19,264	46,794	6,172
1991–1992	80,839	21,415	52,896	6,528
1992–1993	88,149	24,442	56,770	6,937
1993–1994	94,870	28,912	58,839	7,119
1994–1995	97,052	31,254	58,749	7,049
1995–1996	94,757	32,413	56,641	5,703
1996–1997†	91,421	32,813	53,928	4,680
1997–1998†	84,847	31,010	50,394	3,443
1998–1999†	67,189	23,942	40,828	2,399
1999–2000	—	—	—	—
2000–2001	—	—	—	—
2001–2002‡	72,882	30,552	40,073	2,287
2002–2003‡	76,659	31,187	42,922	2,550
2003–2004‡	78,476	26,293	48,980	3,203
2004–2005‡	84,878	28,373	53,118	3,387

†Data are unofficial and unpublished from the National League for Nursing.
‡Data are from *Nursing Data Review Academic Year 2004–2005, Baccalaureate, Associate Degree, and Diploma Programs National League for Nursing.*
Source: US Department of Health and Human Services. (n.d.) *National Center for Health Workforce Analysis: U.S. Health Workforce Personnel Factbook, Table 110. Number of nursing students, graduates and schools for selected academic years: 1950–51 to 1999–2000.* Retrieved November 16, 2007, from http://bhpr.hrsa.gov/healthworkforce/reports/factbook.htm

include the size of the U.S. population from which prospective nursing students are drawn into nursing education programs, changing social preferences for a nursing career, the influence of age on RNs' movement in and out of the RN workforce, the availability of alternative sources of RNs, economic factors that affect individuals' decisions to pursue a career in nursing, and factors affecting the current capacity of nursing education programs. With reference to our model that was discussed in Chapter 3, conceptually, these factors affect whether the long-run supply curve for RNs shown in Figure 3-4, in Chapter 3, shifts out from S_1 to S_2 (an expansion in the long-run supply) or shifts to the left from S_2 to S_1 (a decrease in the long-run supply of RNs).

Changes in the Population

The long-run supply of RNs is determined, in part, by the size of the population of women each year who are between the ages of 18 and 40. Members of this age group make up the pool from which applicants to nursing education programs are typically drawn. Traditionally, most people who have become RNs are women who entered nursing education programs after finishing high school or soon thereafter during their 20s (in 2006 only 9% of the RN workforce were men). Of course, some become RNs when they are in their 30s, a trend that developed in the late 1980s and is discussed in detail in Chapter 9.

The number of women in the applicant pool for nursing has changed due to forces that have affected the overall population. A major change that affected the size of applicant pools for nursing began when a large number of soldiers returned after the end of World War II. The resultant baby boom generation produced the largest ever expansion of the U.S. population, with 76 million children born between 1946 and 1964. In 2007, people who are between the ages of 43 and 61—more than one in three American adults—are members of the baby boom generation. Looking back over time, as women born in the baby boom generation entered their 20s, the size of the applicant pool from which nursing education programs typically draw expanded dramatically.

Figure 7-1 shows the actual number of women in the U.S. population between the ages of 20–29 and 30–39 in 5-year increments beginning in 1955 and projected from 2005 through 2020. Notice that the size of the pool of women in the 20–29 age group began to increase in 1965 as the first wave of baby boomers entered their 20s (and there was an increase in 1975 for those aged 30–39). In 1960, a little more than 11 million women were between ages 20 and 29, but by 1980 there were over 20.6 million women in the U.S. population in this age group. Over the next 5 years, the size of the female applicant pool for nursing in this age group increased more slowly as remaining baby boomers entered their 20s, reaching a peak of just under 21.5 million women in 1985. For the next 15 years, as the baby boom generation aged, the size of the applicant pool of women between the ages of 20–29 began to decrease but still remained above the number of women in this age group from 1975. Overall, from 1985 though projections for 2020, the size of the population of women in the 20–29 age group (the population from which the nursing profession typically draws) has and will remain relatively stagnant. Trends for women in the population between the ages of 30-39 mirror this same trend lagged by 10 years.

Even more important than the size of the applicant pool of prospective nursing students each year is whether people in these pools actually decide to become RNs. As we discuss next, these decisions are determined by changing social preferences for a nursing career and economic factors that individuals take into account when considering the nursing profession.

Changes in Societal Preferences for a Career in Nursing (the Cohort Effect)

Aspirations for a particular career or profession are driven by a variety of interests and motivations. With respect to the nursing profession, studies of nursing

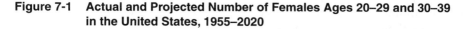

Figure 7-1   Actual and Projected Number of Females Ages 20–29 and 30–39 in the United States, 1955–2020

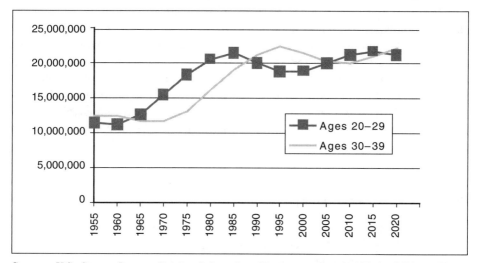

Source: U.S. Census Bureau. Retrieved from http://www.census.gov/cgi-bin/ipc/idbpyrs.pl?cty=US&out=y&ymax=250&submit=Submit+Query

students report that they are motivated to pursue a nursing career due to their desire to help others and serve society (Buerhaus, Donelan, Norman, & Dittus, 2005; May, Austin, & Champion, 1986; Barriball & While, 1996; Kersten, Bakewell, & Meyer, 1991; Boughn & Lentini, 1999; Magnussen, 1998). Other studies point to a long-standing desire to become a nurse that formed in childhood (Boughn, 2001; Okrainec, 1994), a deep interest in science (Kersten, Bakewell, & Meyer, 1991), and the influence of parents, role models, friends, and interactions with nurses (Buerhaus, et al., 2005; Mendez & Louis, 1991). Finally, some authors (Boughn, 2001; Boughn & Lentini, 1999) reported that "practical considerations" defined as salary, benefits, working conditions, and job security were *not* influential in motivating students to become RNs.

Beyond these intrinsic or personal motivations to become a nurse, the overall desirability or attractiveness of the nursing profession is shaped by broader social forces and influences. We use the term "cohort effect" to describe the likelihood, or propensity, of a given person born in a given year to become an RN (this and the other effects described in these sections are defined again more quantitatively, rather than qualitatively, in Chapter 10). In the 1950s, 1960s, and through much of the 1970s, nursing was a popular career choice for women. During subsequent decades, the women's movement resulted in many changes in the role of women in the workforce: participation of women in the workforce increased; the number of career and professional opportunities open to women expanded; and colleges and universities began recruiting women into programs that had traditionally been dominated by men. These changes in society exerted a substantial negative influence on the propensity of individuals born after the baby boom generation to become RNs (the cohort effect). Thus, as we saw above, as the size of the population of women in the United States who might become an RN remains relatively stagnant, the cohort effect becomes extremely critical in determining the long-run supply of RNs. Because changing social forces affecting career choices for women have exerted such an enormous impact on the number of people who have become RNs, we postpone further examination of this trend and instead devote all of Chapter 8 to analyzing these important changes in greater detail, as well as the implications they pose for the long-run supply of RNs.

Influence of RN's Age (Age Effects)

In addition to the population and cohort effects, the long-run supply of RNs is influenced importantly by what we categorize as "age effects." The age effect includes several factors, some of which also impact the short-run labor supply decisions of RNs. First, the age at which the RN enters the workforce will affect the long-run supply of RNs: the older the RN is when he or she enters the work-force, the less time the RN will be in the workforce over his or her work life. Second, at any given age, some RNs might not be employed in the workforce. For example, RNs in their 30s might not be working so that they can be at home for child bearing purposes, or older RNs might be nonparticipants to take care of adult dependents. Third, at different ages, RNs are likely to work a different number of hours in the nurse labor market: Younger RNs are more likely to work a greater number of hours than RNs who are in their mid- to late 50s. And finally, the long-run supply of RNs will be influenced by the age at which RNs retire.

Because the population, cohort, and age effects underpin our model to project the future supply of RNs, we return to discuss these factors in Chapter 10, which describes our updated forecasts of the supply and age of RNs through 2025. For now, we turn our attention to other factors that determine the total long-run supply of RNs.

Alternative Sources of RNs

The number of RNs born or who received their nursing education in other countries and who participate in the U.S. nursing workforce also influences the long-run supply of RNs. Chiefly from the Philippines and Canada, but also from the United Kingdom, Nigeria, Ireland, India, Hong Kong, Jamaica, and Israel, foreign-born and -educated RNs have boosted the supply of RNs in the United States, particularly during times of nursing shortages (Aiken, Buchan, Sochalski, Nichols, & Powell, 2004; Brush, Sochalski, & Berger, 2004; Glaessel-Brown, 1998). For some hospitals, it can be faster to employ already educated RNs from other countries than wait for enrollments and graduations to increase in U.S. nursing education programs (Zachary, 2001). At the behest of hospitals, Congress has enacted legislation specifically intended to make it easier for foreign-educated nurses to receive work visas enabling them to be employed in the United States (e.g., the Immigration Nurse Relief Act of 1989).

As shown in Table 6-5 in Chapter 6, the number of FTE equivalent foreign-born RNs working in the United States increased rapidly in recent years, growing by 93,000 over the period 2002 to 2006.[1] In fact, the increased growth in

---

[1] We note that the CPS data do not allow us to identify among foreign-born RNs the subset who received their nursing education outside the United States. The estimated number of foreign-born RNs derived from the CPS is about three times as large as the estimated number of foreign nurse graduates working in the United States derived from the NSSRNs; therefore, employment growth in this group does not solely reflect growth in the number of foreign nurse graduates (FNGs) working in the United States.

foreign-born RNs had begun in the previous decade. Based on CPS employment data, foreign-born RNs comprised 9% of the FTE RN workforce in the United States in 1994 and grew to 15% of the FTE workforce by 2006 (approximately 350,000 FTEs). More foreign-born FTE RNs work in hospitals than in nonhospital settings, and data from the 2004 NSSRN indicate that about 11% of foreign nurse graduates (FNGs) work in nursing home or extended care facilities. To the extent that foreign-born RNs (or foreign-educated RNs as in the NSSRN) remain in the country for extended periods, or eventually become U.S. citizens, these RNs can exert a material influence on the long-run supply of RNs in the United States.

We recognize that using these RNs to satisfy U.S. employers' demand for nursing labor is a contentious issue, evoking opposition and support by groups who raise ethical, economic, and political arguments justifying their particular positions. However, our interest here is to call attention to the fact that absent a sudden expansion in the domestic long-run supply of RNs, or lacking legislation that restricts entry of foreign RNs into the United States, we expect healthcare delivery organizations to increasingly rely on RNs from other countries to increase the number of RNs in the U.S. nursing workforce. Later, in Chapter 15, we consider the implications of the continued growth of this alternative source of RNs.

Economic Factors and the Decision to Become an RN

In addition to the growth in career opportunities for women that offer attractive earnings relative to a career in nursing, other economic factors influence the decisions of individuals in the population aged 20-40 who are considering whether to become a nurse. At any point in time, it is likely that a good number of individuals are on the brink of deciding to become an RN or to pursue a different career. It is at this point in time when economic factors can be important in influencing the decision to become an RN. These factors include the amount of tuition, the length of time involved in becoming an RN, and earnings in the labor market. When summed over the entire number of people who are considering a nursing career at any given time, these economic factors can affect the decisions of many individuals and, in turn, help determine the long-run supply of RNs.

Tuition

Tuition influences both the decision to become an RN and the choice of which nursing education program an individual selects (the latter decision is discussed in greater detail in Appendix 7-1). When individuals are deciding to be-come RNs, one of the things they consider is the amount of tuition they will have to pay to complete their nursing education relative to the amount of tuition associated with the education required of alternative career choices. If the tu-ition of a nursing education is relatively high, then this might lead to some indi-viduals choosing a different career (a movement along the student's demand curve, holding all else constant). Alternatively, if tuition is relatively low, then more students are likely to choose a nursing education than would otherwise be the case.

The NLN (2006) provides data on the average annual tuition and required fees charged for full-time nursing students and full-time nonnursing undergrad-uate students in 2004-2005. Annual in-state tuition and fees charged by public ed-ucation programs that offered a baccalaureate degree in nursing were slightly higher than those charged in 4-year public institutions for nonnursing degrees. Additionally, there was essentially no difference between private baccalaureate degree nursing programs and 4-year private nonnursing education institutions. With regard to associate's degree programs in nursing, the differences are more significant. Tuition and fees charged in both public and private associate's degree programs in nursing were higher than in 2-year public and private nonnursing in-stitutions. Moreover, when compared to 4-year baccalaureate programs, the an-nual tuition and fees charged by 2-year associate's degree programs, whether public or private, were far less. Thus, students pursuing a baccalaureate degree in nursing face essentially the same annual tuition and fees as other students in 4-year institutions, whereas those pursuing a 2-year associate's degree in nurs-ing face annual costs that are higher than students in 2-year nonnursing institu-tions but much lower than those in baccalaureate nursing programs. The influence of tuition in making choices between a nursing and a nonnursing ca-reer, and in choosing between which type of nursing education program, is likely to be greatest for those individuals who are most sensitive to the costs of an ed-ucation and for those who have narrowed their career decision to a few com-peting choices and are having difficulty making their decision.

To lower tuition costs and thereby increase the demand for a nursing edu-cation, federal and state governments and many hospitals, private corporations, and civic groups have offered students a variety of loans, grants, and stipends. These programs are particularly popular when there are nursing shortages, such as the case today. In 1964, Congress passed the Nurse Training Act to increase the number of RNs in the workforce, and in 1988 they again subsidized the cost of a nursing education by enacting the Nurse Shortage Reduction Act. More re-cently, in 2002, Congress passed but did not fund the Nurse Reinvestment Act, which also contained provisions to lower the costs of a nursing education.

Time Costs

The time required to become an RN represents an opportunity cost that reflects the fact that an individual could instead spend the time it takes to complete a nursing education working and earning an income or earning a degree in another field. The lower (or higher) the amount of foregone income an individual gives up by becoming an RN, the less (or more) time will be needed to recoup this lost income. Therefore, as time costs fall, holding all else constant, an individual will be more likely to decide to become an RN. In addition, because it takes only half as much time to complete an associate's degree program versus a baccalaureate program (2 versus 4 years), the time costs of an associate's degree program are lower. For people in the their 30s who are interested in a nursing career, they will have relatively less time to earn an income from nursing, and thus they will have an incentive to choose the shorter 2-year associate's degree program versus the longer baccalaureate program. Thus, the costs associated with time undoubtedly helps explain the rise in associate's degree programs relative to baccalaureate degree programs shown in Table 7-2.

RN Wages in the Labor Market

As we pointed out earlier, many people choose a profession or occupation based on noneconomic reasons having to do with personal interests and what they perceive will bring them satisfaction. However, if wages in the nurse labor market are increasing and the individual is aware of this information, holding all else constant, then the probability of selecting nursing will be increased for some, but not all, people. (The opposite would occur in the case of wage decreases in the nurse labor market.) In particular, for individuals who are undecided on their choice of a career or profession, direct knowledge or perception of the earnings of RNs can exert an important influence on their decision. In Chapter 6 we described the effects of a wage change on the short-run labor supply decisions of *existing* RNs to participate in the nurse labor market and number of hours they are willing to work. We now see that in addition to these important effects, wages paid in the labor market send critical information that might be particularly influential to individuals who are contemplating their career decisions and comparing nursing to other possible careers. However, because it takes at least 2 years to complete nursing education and become an RN, there is a lag in the time between wage increases (or decreases) in the nurse labor market and subsequent enrollment increases (or decreases). Hence, the long-run wage elasticity of supply of RNs (the sensitivity of the relationship between wage increases and increases in the number of people becoming RNs) is larger than the short-run wage elasticity of labor supply. We note that when the Health Resources and Services Administration (HRSA) forecasts the future supply of RNs, they assume that each 1% increase in real RN wages will increase the number of RN graduates by 0.8% and will increase participation in the nurse labor market on a full-time basis among existing RNs by 0.3%.

Economists use wages and earnings to calculate the economic return of different professions and occupations over time. Unfortunately, there is little empirical research that attempts to determine the economic return associated with becoming an RN relative to comparable career choices. Using data from the 1970s to the early 1990s, Schumacher (1997) compared the wages of hospital-employed RNs, nonhospital–employed RNs, and college-educated women in several occupations, including: executive, administrative, and managerial; professional specialty occupations; technicians and related support; sales; administrative support and clerical; service occupations; teaching; and other careers. The results showed that real earnings fell for all groups throughout the 1970s, and although beginning in the early 1980s real wages increased for all groups, the increase was substantially steeper for RNs, particularly those employed in hospitals. Hospital RNs in 1993 earned wages that were about 16.4% higher than RNs with similar characteristics in 1973. However, the comparison group of women who were not nurses in 1993 earned 9.6% *less* than similar workers in 1973. These results suggest that for the period covered in this analysis and relative to the particular comparison group, earnings growth was greater for RNs than for women who had chosen alternative comparable occupations.[2]

Finally, like wages, other nonpecuniary aspects of working as an RN influence decisions to become an RN. For example, opportunities for job satisfaction, opportunities to work flexible shifts, working as a travel nurse in different locations across the country, or other benefits that might typically come with being an RN are important factors. The extent to which these factors might change over time or how they compare with opportunities in other professions can also have an influence on the long-run supply of RNs.

---

[2] Another useful application of information on the economic returns to a profession is that it provides evidence on whether a shortage of that profession exists. When members of a profession/occupation earn a high rate of return relative to those who belong to other professions/occupations with comparable skills and education, the higher rate of return would indicate the presence of a shortage in the profession/occupation; lower rates of return would indicate a surplus. With respect to the finding of Schumacher, we note that hospitals were reporting shortages of RNs in the early 1980s and again in the latter half of the decade through the early 1990s, the same periods when RN earnings were increasing relative to the comparable group of women that were included in this study.

In Appendix 7-1 we provide additional discussion of how tuition, time costs, and wages paid to existing RNs in the workforce influence an individual's choice of the type of basic nursing education program they will enroll in after they have decided to become an RN. We also describe a federal policy initiative aimed at increasing the number of RNs in the workforce, and we examine the evidence on whether the policy goal was met by lowering the cost of a nursing education to increase enrollment or if the goal was met by increases in real wages paid to the existing supply of RNs.

Number and Capacity of Nursing Education Programs

In addition to the size of the population of prospective nursing applicants, changing social preferences, age effects, foreign-born and -educated RNs, and the influence of economic factors, the long-run supply of RNs depends importantly on the number and capacity of nursing education programs. Even if there is a high demand for a nursing degree, an adequate supply of nursing education programs is needed to meet demand. Capacity chiefly reflects the availability of enough faculty and space (classroom and clinical) to accommodate the learning needs of all those qualified students who want to become an RN. Reductions or increases in either the number of programs or in their capacity affects the efficiency of nursing education programs to produce RNs and, therefore, their ability to add to the long-run supply of professional nurses.

Number of Education Programs

Altering the number of nursing education programs has been an obvious instrument used by policy makers to increase the number of RNs in the United States. Congress has enacted legislation to expand the number of nursing education programs (as noted above), and federal agencies, namely the Division of Nursing within HRSA, have awarded millions of dollars to support nursing education programs and provide student loans. Our earlier overview of nursing education programs indicated that the number of programs had increased since the 1950s. The overall growth in the number of education programs, supported by large numbers of tax dollars, has enabled hundreds of thousands of individuals (particularly those born during the baby boom generation) to become RNs. One might believe that policy makers have always favored expanding the number of education programs, but this is not the case.

In the early 1990s, some observers of the nurse labor market perceived that the expected growth of managed care would reduce employers' demand for RNs in the years ahead. Endorsing this view, in 1995 the Pew Health Professions

Commission projected that the growth of managed care would result in the closure of as many as half of the nation's hospitals, a loss of as many as 60,000 hospital beds, and a resultant *surplus* of 200,000 to 300,000 RNs. Therefore, the existing number of RNs was determined to be more than adequate to meet the demand over the remainder of the decade. Consequently, it recommended closure of between 10% and 20% of basic nursing education programs, mostly from associate and diploma degree programs. Looking back, it is fortunate that this recommendation did not actually result in the closing of many education programs as the managed care decade of the 1990s only slowed the annual growth in demand for RNs from 3% to 2%, as we saw in Chapter 5.

Reported Faculty Shortages

Data indicating the prevalence and magnitude of faculty shortages in nursing education programs are sparse and come mostly from nursing association surveys. The American Association of Colleges of Nursing (AACN; 2003) reported that in 2000 the vacancy rate of nurse faculty positions based on a national sample of 200 member baccalaureate education programs was 7.4%. A study by the Southern Regional Education Board (SREB) in 2002 reported a "serious shortage" of nursing faculty (432 slots) in 16 states and the District of Columbia. When combined with the number of newly budgeted positions to accommodate the growth in enrollments, the SREB reported a 12% overall gap in the number of nursing faculty needed. A 2006 AACN survey of member schools showed that vacancy rates had increased to 7.9% and jumped to 8.8% in its 2007 survey.

One reason for the reported nursing faculty shortage is the lower earnings received by nursing faculty relative to the wages of hospital-employed RNs functioning in clinical and management roles. Given this economic discrepancy, fewer RNs are attracted to teaching roles. In addition to identifying low relative earnings, responses from AACN surveys identified other factors perceived to contribute to the shortage of nursing faculty, including: the additional time, tuition, and loan payback incurred by obtaining a graduate degree required for many faculty positions; work dissatisfaction among younger faculty; changing role expectations of faculty and increased teaching loads; increasing demands for scholarship and service; and a diminishing pipeline of enrollees and graduates from baccalaureate nursing education programs who enter graduate programs where future nursing faculty are prepared.

Two current factors behind the reported faculty shortage, that are expected to exert an even more important impact in the future involve the aging of the existing supply of faculty and the impending retirement of large numbers of faculty in the years ahead. A study by Berlin and Sechrest (2002) found that the average age of 4451 educators with doctorates employed in nursing education programs in the United States in 2001 was 53.2 years. The average age was highest for professors (56.2 years), followed by associate professors (50.4 years) and assistant professors (49 years). The study also reported that the average age of retirement was 62.5 years, and it estimated that, from 2004 to 2012, between 200 and 300 nursing faculty per year will become eligible for retirement. **Figure 7-2** shows that the percentage of faculty over the age of 50 began increasing in the early to mid-1990s, and by 2001, 7 in 10 faculty members were estimated to be 50 years of age or older. As the current supply of nursing faculty ages, the data in **Figure 7-3** indicate that all but 5000 of the estimated 32,000 faculty in 2008 are anticipated to have retired by 2023. If faculty shortages continue and worsen over time, it is likely that large numbers of qualified applicants to nursing education programs could be turned away from careers in nursing, thereby decreasing the long-run supply of RNs compared to what it otherwise would have been.

Reported Constraints on Classroom Space and Clinical Education Sites

According to Clifford (1998), the growth in managed care during the 1990s reduced access to clinical sites needed by nursing education programs to provide hands-on clinical education experiences for students. Because of financial

Figure 7-2   Rising Age of Nursing Faculty, 1993–2001

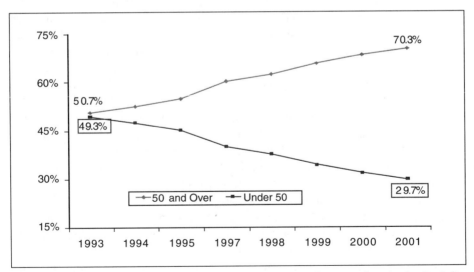

Source: From Berlin, L., & Sechrist, K. (2002). The shortage of doctorally prepared nursing faculty: A dire situation. *Nursing Outlook, 50*(2), 50–56.

Figure 7-3 Anticipated Faculty Retirements in Nursing Education Programs, 2008–2023

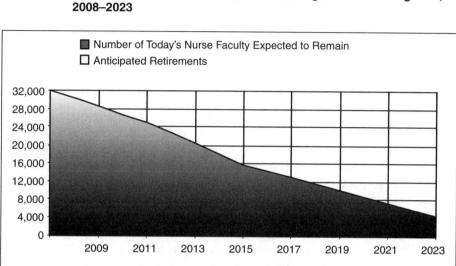

Source: Courtesy of the National League for Nursing. NLN-Carnegie National Survey of Nurse Educators; format adapted from *Charting Nursing's Future*, Robert Wood Johnson Foundation, April 2007.

pressure on healthcare organizations, it was becoming very difficult for many organizations to provide clinical education opportunities that nursing education programs had traditionally relied on to conduct clinical education. The loss of clinical arrangements began to constrain the capacity of nurse education programs during the latter half of the 1990s, and recent AACN surveys (2003 and 2006) indicate that this constraint has continued into the current decade.

With respect to the lack of classroom space, we note that respondents to AACN surveys consistently report that insufficient classroom space is a major reason for turning away qualified applicants. However, we are unaware of any empirical analysis that quantifies the impact of reported reductions in classroom space on enrollments or graduations. Nevertheless, it is possible that these reports were associated with the decrease of nearly 100 nursing education programs between academic years 1998–1999 and 2002–2003 (see Table 7-1).[3] In addition to the possible influence of the Pew Health Professions Commission's recommendations described earlier, reports of insufficient classroom space might also be attributed to falling state budgets caused by the economic

---

[3]Note that over the ensuing 2 years, the number of programs increased, climbing back to essentially the same number as 1998–1999.

recession that began in 2002. Faced with falling revenue, it is likely that some state government allocations to university and colleges, including nursing education programs, fell during this time and hence negatively affected the capacity of some schools, particularly those planning to expand or construct additional space.

Consequences of Faculty Shortages and Insufficient Capacity

Beginning in the early 2000s, a growing number of reports issued by nursing education associations indicated that there was insufficient capacity in nursing education programs. Several surveys (2003, 2006, and 2007) of member baccalaureate programs conducted by the AACN reported that not only had enrollments begun to increase in 2001, but baccalaureate programs were turning away thousands of qualified applicants. **Figure 7-4** shows that over the next several years the number of qualified applicants who could not secure a space in baccalaureate programs grew rapidly, reaching an estimated 37,514 individuals in 2005 and 32,323 in 2006. These survey findings reported by the AACN are supported by a 2004 NLN survey of all basic nursing education programs, which estimated that 125,000 qualified applicants were turned away in 2004 (36,615 from baccalaureate, 86,680 from associate, and 1742 from diploma programs). A year later, the NLN reported the number of qualified applicants estimated to have been turned away increased again, reaching 147,000 nationwide (33,279 from baccalaureate, 110,576 from associate, and 3614 from diploma programs). Both AACN and NLN surveys reported that the reasons cited by survey respondents for why so many qualified students were turned away were due to shortages of faculty, clinical placement sites, and classroom space.

Now that we have discussed the factors that collectively determine the long-run supply of RNs, we conclude this chapter by briefly reviewing different projections of the number of future RNs. As we shall see, in one way or another, the projections we discuss attempt to measure and analyze many of the determinants that we have described.

PREVIOUS PROJECTIONS OF THE LONG-RUN SUPPLY OF RNs: 2000 TO 2020

The first forecast we discuss was made by the authors in 2000, and the second was made 2 years later by the federal government's Health Resources and Services Administration (US DHHS, 2002). These projection models are similar to the extent that they use a 20-year forecast period (2000 to 2020) and rely on data on the size of the population from the U.S. Census Bureau. In

Figure 7-4   Number of Qualified Applicants Turned Away from Entry-Level Baccalaureate Nursing Programs, 2002–2006

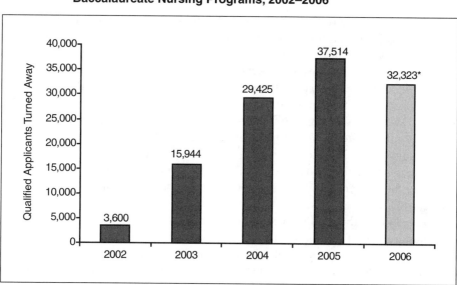

*Preliminary data.

Source: American Association of Colleges of Nursing, Research and Data Center, 2002–2006. Retrieved from http://www.aacn.nche.edu/Media/ppt/02-06TurnedAway.ppt

constructing their forecasts, both models assumed that recent patterns reflecting the number of individuals becoming an RN will continue into the future and that the capacity of nursing education programs is not constrained. The models differ in the source of data on RNs, factors that are measured and included in the models, and analytic methods. The authors' model used 26 years of data and incorporated population, cohort, and age effects in making forecasts, while the HRSA's model used a single year of data but attempted to capture more of the long-run factors discussed in this section in forecasting the RN workforce both for individual states and for the nation as a whole.

Both forecasts projected that the future supply of RNs would grow slowly over the next several years before reaching a plateau near the end of the current decade. Both projections turned out to be more pessimistic than the number of FTE RNs actually observed as of 2006 (though the authors' forecasts were closer to the observed number of FTE RNs). We briefly examine these different methods and projections below, saving for Chapter 10 a more detailed discussion of the authors' updated forecast model, which is similar to the model discussed below that was published in 2000 (Buerhaus, Staiger, & Auerbach, 2000).

Overview of Authors' 2000 Projection Model and Estimates of the Long-Run Supply of RNs Through 2020

Our analysis relied on data from 60,386 RNs obtained from the CPS from 1973 to 1998 (see Chapter 1 for a discussion of the CPS data), data on the U.S. population by age, and forecasts of the U.S. population through 2020 by age from the U.S. Census Bureau. A straightforward statistical model was developed to decompose observed changes in the number and age of RNs over time into the product of the population, cohort, and age effects. Our forecasting model assumed that future cohorts that have not yet been observed would enter nursing at the rate of the five most recently observed cohorts, on average, and that future cohorts would follow the same life cycle pattern of RN FTE production as they age, as had been observed for all previous cohorts. The RN FTE forecasts were summed by year and age to produce aggregate forecasts over the period 2001 to 2020.

The results of the model are shown in **Table 7-3**, and they suggested that the total number of FTE RNs would grow slowly from 2001, reaching 2.1 million FTE RNs by 2006 and peaking at 2.2 million by 2012 before declining to just over 2 million by 2020, a 6% growth over the roughly 1.9 million FTE RNs that was estimated for 2001.[4]

Overview of HRSA's 2002 Projection Model and Estimates of the Long-Run Supply of RNs Through 2020

In 2002, HRSA released a report containing its forecasts of the number of FTE RNs through 2020. This report updated its previous estimates made earlier in 1996. HRSA's projection model tracks RNs by age, state, and highest education level attained (i.e., diploma, associate, baccalaureate degree, or graduate degree) to produce annual, state-level projections of the number of RNs from 2000 to 2020. Starting with the number of individuals who report that they hold a license to practice as an RN (derived from the most recent NSSRN), the supply model adds the estimated number of newly licensed RNs (based on the number of graduates during the latter half of the 1990s), subtracts the estimated number of separations from nursing (due to retirement, mortality, disability, and other factors), and adjusts for changes in level of education attained by

---

[4] In Chapter 10 we provide updated estimates of the long-run supply of RNs extended through 2025. We apply the same forecasting model but update it by including more current RN employment data through 2005, including new population projections, and relaxing some of the key assumptions underpinning our model.

Table 7-3   Projections of the Long-Run Supply of RNs, 2001–2020

Sources of Projections	2001	2005	2010	2015	2020	Change from 2000–2020
B/S/A[1] JAMA (2000)	1,946,000	2,072,000	2,160,000	2,151,000	2,063,000	6.0%
HRSA[2] (2002)	1,990,000	2,012,000	2,069,000	2,055,000	2,002,000	0.6%

Source:
[1] Buerhaus, P., Staiger, D., & Auerbach, D. (2000). Implications of a rapidly aging registered nurse workforce. *The Journal of the American Medical Association, 283*(22), 2948–2954.
[2] U.S. Department of Health and Human Services, Health Resources and Services Administration, Bureau of Health Professions, National Center for Health Workforce Analysis. (2002). *Projected Supply, Demand, and Shortages of Registered Nurses: 2000–2020, July 2002.*

RNs and cross-state migration patterns (to account for the fact that some states are net importers and others are exporters of RNs) to calculate an end of the year estimate of the number of licensed RNs by state. HRSA then applies national rates of workforce participation that vary according to RN age and education level to the projected licensed RN population in each state to produce its estimates of the supply of full time equivalent RNs in each state. The end of year estimate for each state becomes the starting value upon which to make the following year's projections. This iterative process continues with each successive year over the length of the projection period. HRSA produces estimates for each state and also reports estimates for the United States as a whole based on aggregating the state data. Results for the model, when all the state-level estimates are summed to provide a national forecast, are shown in Table 7-3. HRSA's forecasts were roughly 100,000 FTE RNs below those of the authors, which were, in turn, roughly 100,000 below what was observed (at least for 2006).[5] By the end of the forecast period, the difference between the two forecasts had narrowed to 61,000 in 2020, with the authors projecting slightly more RNs than HRSA.

CHAPTER SUMMARY

The long-run supply of RNs refers to the number of individuals holding a license to practice as an RN at any given time in the future. To become an RN, one must complete one of the three basic nursing education programs. Beginning in the 1960s, the number of diploma programs began to decrease as nursing education shifted into associate and baccalaureate degree programs, whose numbers have increased rapidly over time. In most years, the number of RN graduates has increased.

A key factor affecting the long-run supply of RNs is the number of women in the U.S. population between the ages of 20 and 40 that make up the pool of individuals from which nursing education programs typically draw applicants. As large numbers of women born during the baby boom generation entered their 20s, the size of the pool of women increased in the late 1960s and continued expanding for the next 20 years. Since 1985, the size of the pool has remained relatively stagnant and is projected to change very little over the next 10-15 years.

Studies of RN nursing students find that they are drawn into nursing for a variety of personal interests and motivations, yet the growth in new career options for women in the 1980s and 1990s led to a declining propensity of women choosing a nursing career. However, recent increases in the number of enrollments suggest that interest in becoming an RN has increased. Foreign-born (and foreign-educated) RNs who join the U.S. nursing workforce also help expand the long-run supply of RNs; since the mid-1990s, these RNs have been increasing both in number and as a proportion of the nursing workforce in the United States.

Economic factors also determine the long-run supply of RNs by influencing individuals' decisions to become a nurse. For some people, the tuition charged for nursing education programs relative to the tuition required for other careers that the individual is considering is an important factor in their decision to become an RN. The less time it takes for individuals to recoup their investments in a nursing education, given their particular skills and education, the more likely they will become an RN. For individuals who are on the brink of deciding

---

[5] One reason HRSA's forecasts of RN supply is lower than the authors' forecast is that the HRSA model does not capture the effect of RNs who might be out of the labor force in their 30s, perhaps caring for children or elders, and who might return in their 40s, an important component of the age effect previously described. In the 1990s there were many such RNs from the large baby boomer cohorts who would return to the labor force in the 2000s. The authors' model also underpredicted supply over the current period—reasons for this are discussed in Chapter 10 and resulted in an update to the forecast methodology. The HRSA model is also more prone to random error in that by only using a single year of data on which the model is based, the model is only able to "observe" the strength of a given cohort (for example, those born in 1950) one time. The model projects forward the number of RNs observed from that cohort to all future years. If the single year of observation happened to provide an inaccurate picture of the strength of that cohort, the inaccuracy would be present in every year of the forecast. The authors' model uses many years (up to 34 in the current version) of observations over which to gauge the strength of a given cohort. On the other hand, the ability to forecast supply at the state level is a particular strength (and focus) of HRSA's supply model that the authors' model does not share.

to choose nursing or some other career, RN wages in the nurse labor market can influence their decisions, especially if wages are increasing and the individual is aware of the improving economic prospects in nursing.

The number of nursing education programs, in addition to factors that influence their capacity to enroll all those interested and qualified to become an RN, is the final factor that determines the long-run supply of RNs. Shortages of faculty have been reported since the beginning of the current decade, and data suggest that faculty shortages are likely to increase in the future as large numbers of the current supply of faculty retire over the next 15 years. It has been reported that the capacity of nursing education programs has also been negatively affected by shortages of classroom space and clinical placement sites for students. The shortage of faculty and capacity constraints have been cited as reasons for thousands of qualified applicants to be turned away from nursing education programs since 2002.

Recent projections of the long-run supply of RNs made by the authors in 2000 and by HRSA in 2002 suggest that the number of RNs will grow slowly through the current decade, level off for several years, and then decline as RNs retire from the workforce.

Appendix 7-1

The Influence of Economic Factors in Determining the Choice of Nursing Education Programs and Expanding the RN Workforce

As discussed earlier in this chapter, economic and noneconomic factors combine to determine the long-run supply of RNs by influencing individuals' decisions to choose a career in nursing. This appendix provides more background on how, in particular, tuition influences individuals' selection of a nursing education program and the potential for public policies targeting the costs of a nursing education to increase the number of RNs in the workforce.

Because there are three basic nursing education options from which an individual can select to become an RN (diploma, associate, and baccalaureate degree programs), the amount of tuition charged by each type of program will influence the individual's selection. The total tuition at university-based 4-year nursing education programs is higher than 2-year programs based in community colleges or 3-year hospital programs. Individuals who are sensitive to the cost of obtaining a nursing education, as reflected by tuition rates, will be more inclined to select the lowest price program, holding all else constant. Additionally, the effect of tuition on program selection (and on total enrollments) is influenced by the time costs faced by prospective students. For example, a relatively expensive nursing education program (with respect to the tuition) might be located near where an individual who has decided to become a nurse resides. Because it will take less travel time to attend classes, the individual might be less sensitive to the higher tuition price and enroll in the higher priced program versus spend more of their time commuting to a lower priced program located farther away. The large growth in the number of community and technical colleges typically located in smaller cities and towns undoubtedly lowers the time costs for many prospective nursing students. Not only is their tuition cheaper than in many universities, but time costs associated with traveling to classes are lower. The combination of lower tuition and time costs more than likely explains the higher demand for a nursing education in an associate's degree program as seen by the growth in the number of these program and in student enrollments compared to baccalaureate degree programs (see Table 7-1).

An additional reason why many people have selected the 2-year associate's degree program over the 4-year baccalaureate degree option is that the former reduces the total amount of tuition required to become an RN and reduces the foregone income incurred by being a nursing student rather than working. For other individuals who have different preferences for a nursing education and place a different value on the time it will take them to recoup their financial investment in nursing education, the longer baccalaureate degree option is preferred. Many choose this option because they believe a baccalaureate education will expand their future career opportunities, give them an advantage in obtaining positions with increasing responsibility and higher earnings, and make it easier to obtain advanced clinical certifications, earn a master's degree, or complete doctoral education.

Studies have sought to determine whether, over an RN's working lifetime, any wage differential makes up for the higher tuition and lost income given up by spending additional years pursing a nursing education. Studies report that the greater economic return that accrues to an individual who obtained a 4-year baccalaureate degree is very small compared to those who graduated from a 2-year associate's degree or 3-year diploma program. Although many (not all) RNs with baccalaureate degrees in nursing earn higher wages compared to their non-baccalaureate counterparts, the difference in earnings is so small that over time it does not compensate for the foregone earnings and higher tuition costs associated with the additional years of education (Booton & Lane, 1985; Link, 1988, 1992; Mennemeyer & Gaumer, 1983; Spetz, 2002). Investigators have compared the wages of diploma and associate's degree graduates but report mixed findings: Some studies (Booton & Lane, 1985) show that diploma RNs have a wage advantage over associate's degree graduates; others (Mennemeyer & Gaumer, 1983) show the opposite, and one study (Link, 1988) found no difference between the two. Moreover, studies (Mennemeyer & Gaumer, 1983; Leher, White, & Young,

1991) report that the diploma certificate is the least economically attractive option for becoming an RN, whereas the associate's degree is superior to the baccalaureate pathway with respect to providing the individual with a higher level of lifetime earnings (Mennemeyer & Gaumer, 1983; Link, 1988; Leher, White, & Young, 1991; Spetz, 2002). When comparing basic nursing education to graduate nursing education, Mennemeyer and Gaumer (1983) find that employers pay a more substantial wage premium to RNs who hold a master's degree.

EXPANDING THE LONG-RUN SUPPLY OF RNs

Finally, studies have cast doubt over the influence of lowering nursing education tuition as a means to expand enrollments and increase the number of RNs in the workforce. For example, under the Nurse Training Act of 1964 (NTA), Congress allocated $300 million over a 5-year period to increase the number of RN graduates to meet a projected goal of 680,000 RNs available for the workforce in 1970. Most of these dollars were allocated to programs to lower the cost of a nursing education through scholarships and loans, which were distributed by nursing education programs, and to grants to nursing programs for construction, planning, or initiating programs of nursing education and for general financial support. The goal of 680,000 RNs by 1970 was surpassed and was even achieved a year earlier than expected, leading one to believe the NTA had achieved its goal (Feldstein, 1983). However, the number of graduates being produced by schools of nursing in 1969 was roughly 10,000 fewer than the 53,000 targeted by the NTA. Studies (Yett, 1975; Edgren, 1977; Sloan & Richupan, 1975) suggest that increases in real RN wages, which grew rapidly in the latter half of the 1960s, had a far greater impact in stimulating an increase in the RN workforce (increasing the *short-run* participation and hours worked by existing RNs). Furthermore, Sloan and Richupan (1975) found that expanding enrollments into nursing education programs was at least twice as expensive as increasing the wage when attempting to increase the number of working RNs by 10,000. For a further discussion of the role of economic factors with respect to the NTA of 1964, see Feldstein (1983) and Deane and Yett (1979).

REFERENCES

Aiken, L., Buchan, J., Sochalski, J., Nichols, B., & Powell, M. (2004). Trends in international nurse migration. *Health Affairs, 23*(3), 69–77.

American Association of Colleges of Nursing. (2002). *Accelerated programs: The fast-track to careers in nursing.* Washington, DC: Author.

American Association of Colleges of Nursing. (2003). *Faculty shortages in baccalaureate and graduate nursing programs: Scope of the problem and strategies for expanding the supply.* Washington, DC: Author.

American Association of Colleges of Nursing. (2006). *Student enrollment rises in U.S. nursing colleges and universities for the 6th consecutive year.* Retrieved July 19, 2007, from http://www.aacn.nche.edu/06Survey.htm

Barriball, L., & While, A. (1996). The similarities and differences between nurses with different career choice profiles: Findings of an interview survey. *Journal of Advanced Nursing, 23*(2), 380–388.

Berlin, L., & Sechrist, K. (2002). The shortage of doctorally prepared nursing faculty: A dire situation. *Nursing Outlook, 50*(2), 50–56.

Booton, L., & Lane, J. (1985). Hospital market structure and the return to nursing education. *The Journal of Human Resources, 20,* 184–195.

Boughn, S. (2001). Why women and men choose nursing. *Nursing and Health Care Perspectives, 22*(10), 14–19.

Boughn, S., & Lentini, A. (1999). Why do women choose nursing? *Journal of Nursing Education, 38*(4), 156–161.

Brush, B., Sochalski, J., & Berger, A. (2004). Imported care: Recruiting foreign nurses to U.S. health care facilities. *Health Affairs, 23*(3), 78–87.

Buerhaus, P., Staiger, D. & Auerbach, D. (2000). Implications of a rapidly aging registered nurse workforce. *Journal of the American Medical Association, 283*(22), 2948–2954.

Buerhaus, P., Donelan, K., Norman, L., & Dittus, R. (2005). Nursing students' perceptions of a career in nursing and impact of a national campaign designed to attract people into the nursing profession. *Journal of Professional Nursing, 21*(2), 75–83.

Clifford, J. (1998). *Restructuring: The impact of hospital organization on nursing leadership.* Chicago: AHA Press.

Deane, R., & Yett, D. (1979). Nurse market policy simulations using an econometric model. In R. Scheffler (Ed.), *Research in health economics.* Greenwich, CT: JSI Press.

Edgren, J. (1977). *The federal nurse training acts.* Health Manpower Policy Studies Group Discussion Paper Series, School of Public Health, The University of Michigan.

Feldstein, P. (1983). *Health Care Economics* (2nd ed.). New York: John Wiley & Sons.

Glaessel-Brown, E. (1998). Use of immigration policy to manage nursing shortages. *Image: Journal of Nursing Scholarship, 30*(4), 323–327.

Kersten, J., Bakewell, K., & Meyer, D. (1991). Motivating factors in a student's choice of nursing as a career. *Journal of Nursing Education, 30*(1), 30–33.

Leher, E., White, W., & Young, W. (1991). The three avenues to a registered nurse license: A comparative analysis. *The Journal of Human Resources, 26,* 362–379.

Link, C. (1988). Returns to nursing education 1970-84. *The Journal of Human Resources, 23,* 373–387.

Link, C. (1992). Labor supply behavior of registered nurses: Female labor supply in the future? In R. Ehrenberg (Ed.), *Research in labor economics* (Vol. 13; pp. 287–320). Greenwich, CT: JAI Press.

Magnussen, L. (1998). Women's choices: An historical perspective of nursing as a career choice. *Journal of Professional Nursing, 14*(3), 175–183.

May, F., Austin, M., & Champion, V. (1986). *Attitudes, values, and beliefs of the public in Indiana towards nursing as a career.* Bloomington, IN: Indiana University School of Nursing, Sigma Theta Tau International.

Mendez, D., & Louis, M. (1991). College students' image of nursing as a career choice. *Journal of Nursing Education, 30*(7), 311–319.

Mennemeyer, S., & Gaumer, G. (1983). Nursing wages and the value of educational credentials. *The Journal of Human Resources, 18,* 32–48.

National League for Nursing. (2004). *Startling data from the NLN's comprehensive survey of all nursing programs evokes wake-up call.* Retrieved July 19, 2007, from http://www.nln.org/news releases/datarelease05.pdf

National League for Nursing. (2005). *Despite encouraging trends suggested by the NLN's comprehensive survey of all nursing programs, large number of qualified applications continue to be turned down.* Retrieved July 19, 2007, from http://www.nln.org/newsreleases/nedsdec05.pdf

National League for Nursing. (2006). *Nursing data review academic year 2004–2005. Baccalaureate, associate degree, and diploma programs.* New York: Author.

Okrainec, G. (1994). Perceptions of nursing education held by male nursing students. *Western Journal of Nursing Research, 16*(1), 94–107.

Pew Health Professions Commission. (1995). *Critical challenges: Revitalizing the health professions for the twenty-first century.* San Francisco: University of California San Francisco, Center for the Health Professions.

Schumacher, E. (1997). Relative wages and the returns to education in the labor market for registered nurses. *Research in Labor Economics, 16,* 149–76.

Sloan, F., & Richupan, S. (1975). Short-run supply responses of professional nurses: A microanalysis. *Journal of Human Resources, 10,* 242–257.

Southern Regional Education Board. (2002). *SREB study indicates serious shortage of nursing faculty.* Retrieved November 19, 2007, from http://www.sreb.org/programs/nursing/publications/02N03-Nursing_Faculty.pdf

Spetz, J. (2002). The value of education in a licensed profession: The choice of associate or baccalaureate degrees in nursing. *Economics of Education Review, 21,* 73–85.

U.S. Department of Health and Human Services. (2002). *Projected supply, demand, and shortages of registered nurses: 2000-2020.* Health Resources and Services Administration, Bureau of Health Professions, National Center for Health Workforce Analysis.

Yett, D. (1975). *An economic analysis of the nurse shortage.* Lexington, MA: D.C. Health Co.

Zachary, G., (2001, May 24). Labor movement. Shortage of nurses hits hardest where they are needed the most. *The Wall Street Journal,* pp. A1, A12.

CHAPTER 8

Changing Preferences for a Career in Nursing

In the previous two chapters, we discussed the economic and noneconomic factors that determine both the short-run and long-run supply of RNs in the United States. Because it takes time for people to complete their nursing education after they have decided to become an RN, the short-run supply is primarily driven by the decisions of *existing* RNs to participate in the nurse labor market and the number of hours they are willing to work. The long-run supply is concerned with the number of RNs who will be available at some point in the future, and it therefore is primarily driven by the decisions of people to *become* RNs in the first place. As discussed in Chapter 7 and as we will see later in this chapter, the number of people choosing a career in nursing has declined substantially over time. In this chapter we focus on understanding the sources and magnitude of the changes over time in people's interest in nursing as a career.[1]

The most likely explanation for the declining interest in nursing is linked to the women's movement, which began in the 1960s. Social norms and institutions changed dramatically in the 1960s and 1970s in ways that gave married women greater opportunities to work outside the home and resulted in a dramatic rise in the proportion of women participating in the labor force (Goldin & Katz, 2002). This movement spread throughout society and led to an expansion in the number of professional opportunities and careers open to women. By the 1980s, barriers that had kept women disproportionately out of managerial and professional positions had substantially disappeared. As these new opportunities became available, they drew women away from traditional occupations such as nurse, teacher, and homemaker. As we shall see in this chapter, and as has been documented in a number of previous studies (Astin, Parrott, Korn, & Sax, 1997; Greene, 1987; Staiger, et al., 2000), these changing career preferences

---

[1] This chapter is based on Staiger, D., Buerhaus, P., & Auerbach, D. (2000). Expanding career opportunities for women and the declining interest in nursing as a career. *Nursing Economic$, 18*(5), 230–236. The data reported in this chapter are updated through 2006.

of young women have had important and long-lasting implications for the labor supply in traditionally female-dominated occupations, and nursing in particular.

As will be discussed in greater detail in succeeding chapters, the declining propensity of younger women to become RNs has ominous implications for the future, namely, that the RN workforce will become much older in the near term, and the number of RNs in the workforce will eventually fall well below projected requirements in the decades to come. What will happen to the supply of RNs in the long term will critically depend on whether the trend away from nursing as a career continues or reverses. Thus, to forecast what will happen to the supply in the future, this chapter first focuses on understanding the key driving forces behind the declining propensity.

DATA ON CAREER CHOICES OF YOUNG PEOPLE

To track recent trends in the interests of young people in nursing and other careers, we use data from a large survey that asks incoming college freshmen about their probable career choices, with nursing being one option. Of course, many students' actual career choices will differ from their intentions when they started college. Nevertheless, data on the career interests of first-year college students are likely to capture broad trends toward growing and waning interest in nursing, while having the advantage of capturing these trends at an early stage, rather than waiting 2–4 years (at least) before these people are observed entering the labor market.

Our data on the probable career choices of college freshmen come from the Cooperative Institutional Research Program (CIRP) surveys, which have been conducted each fall since 1966 by the Higher Education Research Institute at the University of California, Los Angeles. Each year the CIRP surveys between 250,000 and 350,000 first-year students attending a nationally representative sample of between 300 and 700 2-year and 4-year colleges and universities. The survey provides annual data on background characteristics, attitudes, education, and future goals of new students entering college in the United States. Data were acquired from 1966 to 2006, the most recent year the CIRP survey was conducted at the time our analysis was completed.

Data from the CIRP freshman surveys were obtained on respondents' age, gender, career plans, and average grades in high school. The question on age asks a student's age on December 31 of that year, which makes it possible to accurately determine birth year (i.e., year of the survey minus age). The question on career plans asks students to choose their "probable career occupation" from a list of 48 options including "nurse." The list of options was the same in all years, except for 1973–1975 when a larger list of options was used. As a result, estimates of career plans for 1973–1975 might not be directly comparable to other years. Finally, in all years of the survey, students were asked, "What was your average grade in high school?" and could choose from A, A–, etc. To ensure that estimates are nationally representative, all analyses were weighted by sampling weights provided by the CIRP survey.

In our analysis of these data, the sample was limited to first-year students age 20 and under. Less than 5% of the sample is over age 20 in any given year, while the majority of respondents are age 18. For some years (1966–1970, 1973–1975) data were not available on career plans for the sample that was under age 20. Because data for the sample that was age 20 or under followed similar time patterns to the data for the entire sample, data from the entire sample were used to impute the missing years. In particular, available data from the 1970s were used to calculate the average ratio of estimates from the 20 and under sample to corresponding estimates from the full sample. Estimates from the full sample were then multiplied by this ratio to impute estimates for the 20 and under sample for the years in which data were not available.

While the CIRP survey provides an accurate barometer of the interest of college freshmen in nursing, it does not tell the whole story. College enrollment has increased since 1980, contributing to a larger potential pool of freshmen (Snyder, Dillow, & Hoffman, 2007). More importantly, not all first-year college students who express an interest in nursing will eventually go on to complete their degrees, obtain licenses, and then work as RNs. Therefore, as a more direct method of tracking recent trends in the propensity of young people to become an RN, we use data from the U.S. Census Bureau Current Population Survey (the CPS, which was described in Chapter 1) to generate annual estimates of the percent of individuals actually working as an RN at the age of 25 years. We used age 25 because a substantial proportion of the people who will eventually become an RN are working by age 25. While waiting until age 30 or even 35 would provide an even more accurate measure of how many people are eventually becoming RNs, this would limit our ability to observe the recent entry patterns of young people (e.g., we would have to wait another 5–10 years to learn whether people who are currently 25 are likely to become RNs). Thus, the main advantage of using the CPS data over the college freshman (CIRP) data is that it is a more accurate measure of the actual (as opposed to probable) career choices that were made by young people over time, but at a cost of trading off delay for accuracy. While we use age 25 in this chapter as a reasonable compromise between accuracy and delay, in Chapter 10 we use a more sophisticated method that incorporates data from older ages when available.

DECLINING INTEREST IN NURSING

The declining propensity to become an RN is apparent in **Figure 8-1**. This figure shows the percentage of college freshmen each year that indicated interest in a nursing career (measured on the left hand axis) and the percentage of individuals from the same cohort who actually became RNs by the age of 25 (measured on the right hand axis). To estimate the percentage of a given freshman class that were RNs at age 25, we use 3 years of CPS data from 6–8 years later, which corresponds to the years that these 17-, 18-, and 19-year-old freshmen would turn 25. Because the CPS data run through 2006, the estimates of the percentage who actually became an RN end with the freshman class that was surveyed in the fall of 1998 (who were age 25 in 2004–2006). Because the freshman surveys continue another 8 years through 2006, data from the CIRP freshman survey might provide a more up-to-date indication of what to expect from cohorts who will enter the labor market over the next decade.

As seen in Figure 8-1, there has been a striking decline since 1974 in the proportion of college freshmen who indicate nursing as a probable career and in the percentage of these cohorts who were working as RNs at age 25. The two estimates track each other reasonably well during the 1960s, 1970s, and 1980s, with both showing that interest in nursing roughly doubled from the mid-1960s to the mid-1970s, peaked with the cohort who were freshmen in 1974, and then

---

Figure 8-1   Percentage of College Freshmen Expressing Interest in Nursing Versus the Percentage of the Same Cohort Who Are Working as an RN at Age 25, 1962–2006

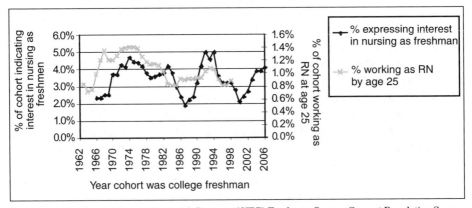

Source: Cooperative Institutional Research Program (CIRP) Freshman Survey; Current Population Survey.

fell roughly 40% by the mid-1980s. However, estimates from the freshman survey show more volatility in students' interest in nursing among the cohorts that graduated from high school in the late 1980s and early 1990s, perhaps reflecting transitory factors and "fads" affecting freshman interest in careers. In particular, there was a large surge of interest in nursing in the freshman survey around 1993 that resulted in only a modest increase in the percentage of this cohort who became RNs by age 25. It might be that such a temporary increase in interest was driven by transitory factors, and many of those who expressed interest in nursing as freshmen later chose other careers as these transitory factors changed.

Data from the freshman survey (but not as clearly from the CPS estimates) also indicate a temporary increase in students' interest in nursing during certain periods, namely the early 1980s and early 1990s, and since 2000. During each of these periods, the nation experienced an economic recession, hospitals were reporting a shortage of RNs, RN wages were increasing, and publicity surrounding the nursing profession was relatively positive (especially after September 11, 2001). These factors more than likely explain the temporary increase in interest in a nursing career among college freshmen.

Explanations for the Decline in Interest in Nursing

Why are young people less likely to enter nursing in recent years as compared to 30 years ago? The most likely explanation is the expansion of career opportunities for women in traditionally male-dominated fields over the last 3 decades. Three trends observed in the freshman survey data support this explanation.

The first trend is that women, but not men, were less likely to have entered a wide range of traditionally female-dominated occupations over the last 30 years. As shown in **Figure 8-2**, the decline in interest in nursing as a career occurred exclusively among women, while men's interest in nursing has increased but still remains quite low. Also, interest in nursing as a career rose in both the early 1990s and since 2000 for both men and women. Economic factors during these periods were increasing the attractiveness of nursing as a career for both men and women; as the national economy was slipping into a recession, unemployment rates were increasing, and RN wages were increasing substantially in response to shortages of RNs. This pattern clearly suggests that while there has been a long-run decline in women interested in nursing as a career since the 1970s, interest in nursing among both men and women freshman college students responds to changing conditions both within the nurse labor market and the larger economy.

Figure 8-2   Percentage of Freshmen Indicating Probable Career in Nursing, 1966–2006

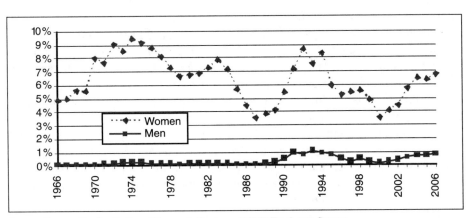

Source: Cooperative Institutional Research Program (CIRP) Freshman Survey.

A similar decline in interest among women has occurred in other traditionally female-dominated careers. For example, **Figure 8-3** shows that interest among women and men in primary school teaching has followed a similar pattern as nursing, with women's interest declining noticeably over this period while interest among men increased slightly but has remained low. Interest among all college freshmen in secondary school teaching, as shown in **Figure 8-4**, has declined

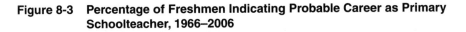

Figure 8-3   Percentage of Freshmen Indicating Probable Career as Primary Schoolteacher, 1966–2006

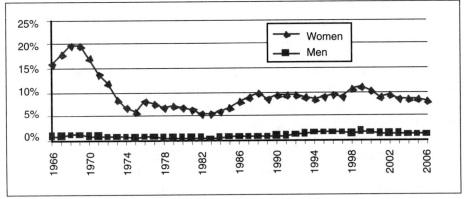

Source: Cooperative Institutional Research Program (CIRP) Freshman Survey.

Figure 8-4   Percentage of Freshmen Indicating Probable Career as Secondary Schoolteacher, 1966–2006

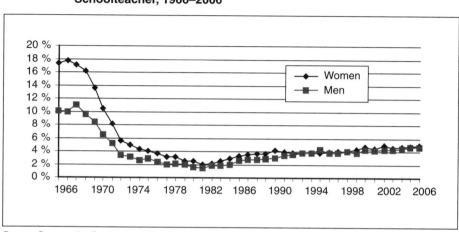

Source: Cooperative Institutional Research Program (CIRP) Freshman Survey.

but more so among women, so that now men and women are equally likely to list this as a probable career.

The second trend reveals a corresponding increase in interest among women in careers that were traditionally dominated by men, particularly in professional and managerial occupations. For example, as shown in **Figure 8-5**, interest among women in business has risen substantially and has narrowed the gap relative to freshmen men. Interest among women in law (**Figure 8-6**) has grown even faster among women and is now at the point where women and men are about equally likely to list this profession as probable a career. With respect to medicine (**Figure 8-7**), however, interest among women has outpaced that of men such that today freshman women are more likely to select a career as a doctor or dentist than their male counterparts. These trends show that many women who in the past might have felt constrained to become RNs and teachers have more recently moved into managerial and professional occupations with higher earnings and perceived prestige.

The final trend is the decline in the average high school grades of women who are interested in nursing relative to all other freshman women. As shown in **Figure 8-8**, the proportion of entering freshman women interested in nonnursing careers who received As in high school increased from 26% to 53% between 1976 and 2006 (reflecting, in part, a trend in general grade inflation, particularly during the 1990s). In contrast, among women interested in nursing, the proportion receiving As in high school increased from 21% to 43% over this time period, lagging behind their freshman counterparts who were interested in nonnursing

Figure 8-5   Percentage of Freshmen Indicating Probable Career in Business, 1966–2006

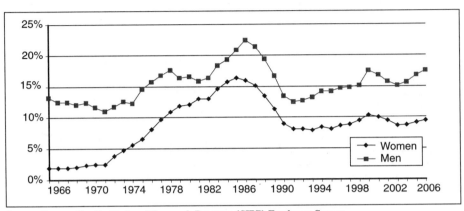

Source: Cooperative Institutional Research Program (CIRP) Freshman Survey.

Figure 8-6   Percentage of Freshmen Indicating Probable Career as a Lawyer, 1966–2006

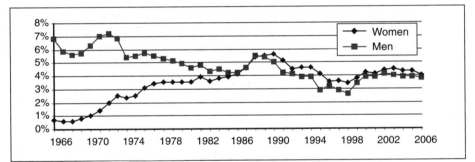

Source: Cooperative Institutional Research Program (CIRP) Freshman Survey.

careers. Moreover, the academic ability of women who were interested in nursing reached its lowest point in 1989, around the same time that interest in nursing was at an all time low, with only 13% receiving As in high school as compared to 28% among all other freshman women at the time. Thus, it appears that the expanding career opportunities in business, law, and medicine have drawn away some of the most promising candidates for a nursing career.

Taken together, these data suggest that two countervailing forces have influenced the decisions of young people to enter nursing over the last 4 decades. First, the social changes that expanded the careers open to women drew many women away from traditional occupations such as nursing, leading

Figure 8-7　Percentage of Freshmen Indicating Probable Career as a Doctor or Dentist, 1966–2006

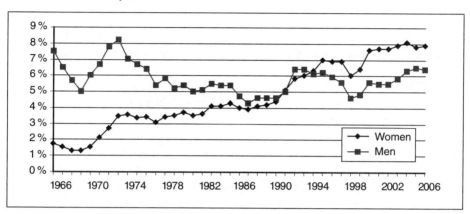

Source: Cooperative Institutional Research Program (CIRP) Freshman Survey.

Figure 8-8　Percentage of College Freshmen Women Interested in Nursing Who had A– or Better in High School, Compared to All Other Women

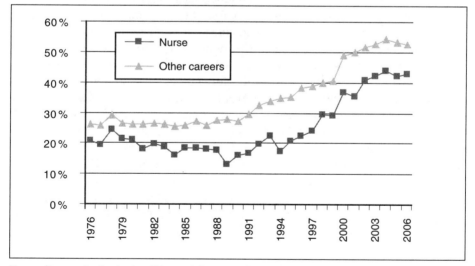

Source: Cooperative Institutional Research Program (CIRP) Freshman Survey.

to a long-term decline in the number of women becoming professional nurses. But second, rising wages of RNs combined with high national unemployment rates have contributed to brief periods of rekindled interest in nursing as a career for both men and women. An interesting question is whether the most recent rise in interest in nursing seen among college freshmen beginning in 2000 will be more permanent and lead to a more sustained increase in the number of women entering nursing.

WHAT IS BEHIND THE RECENT RISE IN INTEREST IN NURSING?

Since 2000, there has been a steady rise in the percentage of college freshmen expressing an interest in nursing. It might be that the rising interest in nursing among freshmen is an early indicator of renewed interest in nursing as a career, perhaps in response to rising wages and growing awareness (through press coverage and publicity campaigns) among the public that the looming shortage will increase the attractiveness of nursing as a career in the coming decades. If so, this would suggest that market forces are already working to increase the long-run supply of nurses and thereby reduce the magnitude of future shortages. But, as we saw in the early 1990s, career preferences of freshmen can be volatile and are far from perfect predictors of actual career choices.

Other data, however, appear to confirm that growing numbers of young people see nursing as an attractive and respected career. A 2001 survey of high school students in the United States, conducted by the National Research Center for College & University Admissions, found that nursing was ranked ninth among career paths that students would consider. In 2002, the survey found that nursing had moved up to fourth place. Annual surveys conducted by the American Association of Colleges of Nursing of its member baccalaureate degree institutions (which attract proportionately more younger age students) reveal that annual enrollments, which had fallen from 1995 through 2000, have increased over the past 6 consecutive years—3.7% in 2001, 8.1% in 2002, 15.6% in 2003, 14.1% in 2004, 9.6% in 2005, and 5.0% in 2006 (AACN, 2006). Similarly, the AACN reports turning away thousands of qualified applicants from baccalaureate degree programs—3600 in 2002, 15,944 in 2003, 29,425 in 2004, 37,514 in 2005, and 32,323 in 2006. And finally, a 2007 national survey of the American public found that 92% of Americans would likely advise a qualified high school or college student to pursue a career in nursing—63% definitely would advise, and 29% probably would advise (Donelan, Buerhaus, DeRoches, & Dittus, 2007).

CHAPTER SUMMARY

The evidence presented in this chapter supports the view that the primary reason for the declining interest in the nursing profession has been the expansion of career opportunities for women in traditionally male-dominated occupations over the last 4 decades. The number of young women entering the RN workforce has declined because many women who would have entered nursing in the past, particularly those with high academic abilities, are now entering managerial and professional occupations that used to be traditionally male. Thus, the declining interest in nursing is driven by fundamental, permanent shifts in the broader, nonnursing labor market that are unlikely to reverse anytime in the immediate future. As a result, while interest in nursing might yet revive, it is doubtful that women will again enter nursing careers at the rate that occurred during the boom years of the 1970s when the peak of the baby boom generation was graduating from high school and nursing was still one of the major career opportunities available for women. While there has been a recent increase in the proportion of freshmen who indicate an interest in nursing, it remains to be seen whether this upturn will be temporary, as occurred in earlier decades during times of RN shortages, economic recession, and RN wage increases, or if this upturn represents a renewed interest in nursing as a career. Overall, however, the evidence suggests that there might be a modest increase in the number of young RNs entering the labor market in the near future.

While the analysis presented in this chapter has established the sources of the declining interest in nursing as a career and presented key trends in the expansion of career opportunities for women, we have not yet discussed the implications for the long-run supply of RNs. As we will see in Chapter 10, these implications will profoundly alter the future of the RN workforce for years to come.

REFERENCES

American Association of Colleges of Nursing. (2006). *Student enrollment rises in U.S. nursing colleges and universities for the 6th consecutive year.* Retrieved July 19, 2007, from http://www.aacn.nche.edu/06Survey.htm

Astin, A., Parrott, S., Korn, W., & Sax, L. (1997). *The American freshman: Thirty year trends.* Los Angeles: Higher Education Research Institute, UCLA.

Donelan, K., Buerhaus, P., DeRoches, C., & Dittus, R. (2007). Unpublished preliminary results of a 2007 national public opinion survey of the nursing profession.

Goldin, C., & Katz, L.F. (2002). The power of the pill: Contraceptives and women's career and marriage decisions. *Journal of Political Economy, 110*(4), 730–770.

Green, K. (1987). What the freshmen tell us. Nurses for the future: A provocative debate on economics, enrollment and essentials. *American Journal of Nursing,* 1593–1648.

Snyder, T.D., Dillow, S.A., & Hoffman, C.M. (2007). *Digest of education statistics 2006* (NCES 2007-017). National Center for Education Statistics, Institute of Education Sciences, U.S. Department of Education. Washington, DC: U.S. Government Printing Office.

Staiger, D., Buerhaus, P., & Auerbach, D. (2000). Expanding career opportunities for women and the declining interest in nursing as a career. *Nursing Economic$, 18*(5), 230–236.

CHAPTER 9

Associate Degree Graduates and the Rapidly Aging Registered Nurse Workforce

It has been suggested that the increase in associate degree programs over the past several decades is a major cause of the rising average age of the RN workforce. This chapter, while brief, addresses this question and also provides new data on trends and changes in the age of individuals seeking to become RNs over recent decades and in the type of programs from which RNs received their basic nursing education. Examining these trends builds upon the information provided in Chapter 8 and enhances our understanding of the factors that are driving the changing age composition of the current RN workforce. Additionally, by sorting through these trends in some detail, we will obtain a greater appreciation of the forces that we consider in making our projections of the future age and supply of the RN workforce, which are discussed next in Chapter 10.

Using data from the National Sample Survey of Registered Nurses (NSSRN, discussed in Chapter 1), we begin this chapter by describing patterns in the age of individuals who have become RNs and the type of education programs from which RNs have obtained their basic nursing education. Next, we examine the large increase in the percentage of new RNs that graduated from associate degree programs in the 1990s and the older age of those graduates. Following this, we focus on how these patterns are explained by changes in the underlying propensity of people from different birth eras in the United States (cohorts) to become RNs. Finally, the chapter documents an emerging trend that is also discussed in Chapter 10: the increase in the average age of new entrants to nursing education programs compared to students who entered nursing programs in previous decades.

RISE IN ASSOCIATE DEGREE GRADUATES

As discussed earlier, the average age of the RN workforce has increased dramatically since the 1980s, from just under 38 to over 45 between 1980 and 2004 according to the NSSRN. The rapid aging of the RN workforce has been attrib-uted, among other things, to the older age of graduates of 2-year associate de-gree nursing programs, a trend believed to have begun with the swift increase in the number of these programs (see **Table 9-1**). Associate degree programs seem to have attracted older individuals, relative to traditional nursing students interested in a career in nursing, who did not want to enroll in longer, 4-year bac-calaureate degree nursing education programs (McBride, 1996). [1]

As discussed in Chapter 7, **Figure 9-1** shows that the percentage of new RNs who graduated from associate degree programs has grown steadily since the mid-1970s, from 37% among graduates from 1973 to 1977 to more than 60% of graduates from 1992 to 1996 (the percentage dipped back under 60% from 1996 to 2004). Most of this growth appears to have come at the expense of diploma ed-ucation programs, because the percentage of graduates from baccalaureate pro-grams has remained between 30% and 40% of graduates over most of this time period. What might explain this enormous growth in associate degree graduates?

Table 9-1   **Growth of Associate Degree Programs, 1960–2005**

Year	Number of Programs
1960–1961	57
1970–1971	437
1980–1981	697
1990–1991	829
1999–2000	885
2004–2005	909

Source: National League for Nursing. (2006). *Nursing data review academic year 2004–2005. Baccalaureate, associate degree, and diploma programs.* New York: Author.

---

[1] See Appendix 7-1 for a further discussion of the factors that individuals consider in making this decision

Figure 9-1   Program in Which RN Received Basic Nursing Education, by Year of Graduation, 1973–2004

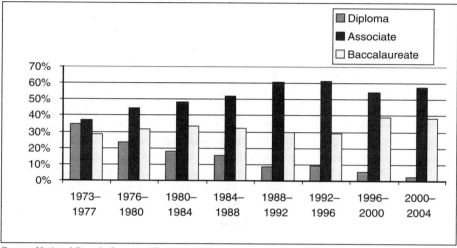

Source: National Sample Survey of Registered Nurses

Explaining the Increase in the Percentage of Associate Degree RN Graduates

One explanation for the increase in the percentage of associate degree RN graduates is simply that associate degree programs have become increasingly available (Table 9-1), which, in turn, could have drawn students into these programs relative to other nursing education options. This explanation can be assessed by examining whether the proportion of graduates *of any given age* who entered the workforce via associate degree programs has been increasing over time. For example, if in the past, 30-year-old nursing students tended to graduate from baccalaureate programs or diploma programs but now tend to graduate from associate degree programs, this would indicate that there has been a shift toward these programs or that these programs were drawing more 30-year-old graduates into nursing.

A second explanation for the increase in associate degree programs and in the age of graduates could be that older students are entering nursing programs in large numbers. If this is the case, then within a given age range (e.g., 26 to 30), we should observe no increase over time in the proportion of graduates from associate degree programs. In other words, if people in their 20s tended to enter baccalaureate programs while people in their 30s tended to enter associate degree programs, and if there were a sudden burst of people in their 30s who were interested in becoming RNs, then one would expect to observe an increase in the number of people entering associate degree programs. This would have nothing to do with whether these programs were attempting to attract students.

To evaluate these two explanations, we first examine the trend in the percentage of graduates obtaining associate degrees over time, separating graduates into different age categories. As shown in **Figure 9-2**, there has been remarkably little change in these percentages, by age category, over the years 1980 through 2004. Among graduates between the ages of 20 and 25 years, about one-third have always graduated from associate degree programs Among graduates aged 26 to 30, roughly two-thirds graduate from associate degree programs, a proportion that has also not changed appreciably over time. With regard to older graduates (those over age 30), the proportion graduating from associate degree programs has generally hovered around 75% to 80%. Thus, the data in Figure 9-2 establish that there has been no increased tendency over the last few decades to seek out associate degree programs by those who have decided to become an RN. Younger people who are interested in becoming RNs have always favored baccalaureate programs while older people have always favored associate degree programs. Based on this examination, our first explanation for why there has been an increasing percentage of RNs graduating from associate degree programs does not seem likely. We next turn to evidence that would

Figure 9-2   Percentage of Recent Graduations Coming from Associate Degree Programs, by Age at Graduation, 1980–2004

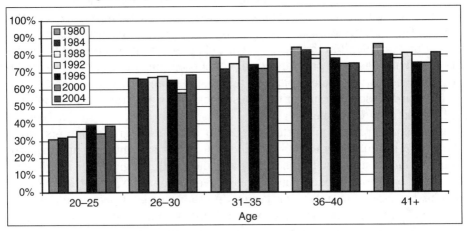

Source: National Sample Survey of Registered Nurses

support our second explanation, which involves tracking cohorts of individuals over time and observing their choices of nursing program type as the cohorts age.

Changing Patterns of Ages of Graduates

Figure 9-3 shows the ages at which RNs have graduated over time. Among graduates in the late 1970s, nearly half finished their education by age 22, indicating that these individuals entered nursing programs directly or soon after graduating from high school. This proportion had fallen to less than 20% by 1990, with a corresponding increase in graduates of all older ages. Generally, between 1976 and 1996, there was a large decline in the percentage of graduates from the 20 to 25 age group and a rise in the percentage of graduates from the older age groups, particularly among graduates over the age of 30. This pattern suggests that because older graduates are more likely to obtain associate degrees, *whatever is causing the older mix of RN graduates has indirectly led to an increase in the percentage of graduates obtaining associate degrees over time.* A close examination of Figure 9-3 shows that after 1996, the trend of an older age of graduates subsided slightly because there was a small resurgence of graduates aged 23 to 25 and a small decline in graduates older than 30 years. This change matches the slight decrease in the proportion of new RN graduates from associate degree programs since the mid-1990s.

Figure 9-3   Percentage of RN Graduates at Various Ages, 1976-2004

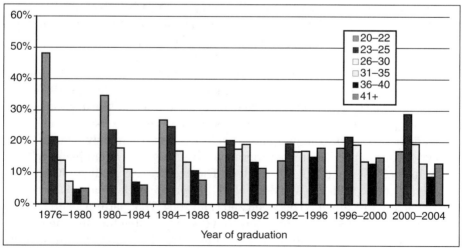

Source: National Sample Survey of Registered Nurses

The data presented in Figure 9-2 and Figure 9-3 suggest that the changing age distribution of graduates appears to drive the pattern observed for the percentage of graduates by degree program. What then is behind the changing age pattern of RN graduates?

Cohort Effects as an Explanation for Patterns and Trends Observed for Associate Degree Graduates

The changing age pattern of RN graduates over time appears to be explained by the large baby boom cohorts (the term *cohort* refers to all the individuals born in any given year) who enrolled in nursing programs and became RNs in record numbers. The baby boomers who entered nursing education programs in their 20s (during the 1970s and 1980s) were more likely to enter baccalaureate programs, as were RNs from earlier and later eras. Subsequently, the baby boomers who entered nursing at later ages were more likely to enter associate degree programs. The cohort effect is discussed in more detail in Chapter 10 because this effect is the key to understanding not only observed changes in the age composition of the current RN workforce but in forecasting the age and supply of the RN workforce for years to come. For now, there is more to learn by analyzing graduation patterns from a cohort perspective.

Figure 9-4 shows the decade in which graduates from all nursing education programs were born. For example, in the bars depicting graduates from 1973 to 1977, 73% were born in the 1950s, 17% were born in the 1940s, and 10% were born earlier (not shown). Those born in the 1950s accounted for most of the graduates of the late 1970s as well, comprising nearly 78% of all RN graduates. *Never again would a single decade of birth account for much more than 50% of graduates*; in fact, people born in the 1950s comprised a significant portion (nearly 30%) of RN graduates even into the mid-1990s when these individuals had aged into their late 30s and 40s. When the 1950s cohorts finally stopped entering nursing education programs in large numbers by the late 1990s, the proportion of associate degree graduates began to fall and, the average age of all nursing graduates began to decrease as shown in **Figure 9-5**.

While associate degree graduates tend to be approximately 5 years older than graduates of baccalaureate programs, the average age of graduates of both programs has risen and fallen in tandem. The average age of all graduates was roughly 25 in the mid-1970s and grew to 31.8 years by the mid-1990s, before falling back to just under 30 between 2000 and 2004. That pattern again reflects the dominance of the 1950s cohorts who were responsible for inflating the age of RN graduates as they continued to enter nursing education programs in large

Figure 9-4 **Percentage of RN Graduates by Decade of Birth, 1973–2004**

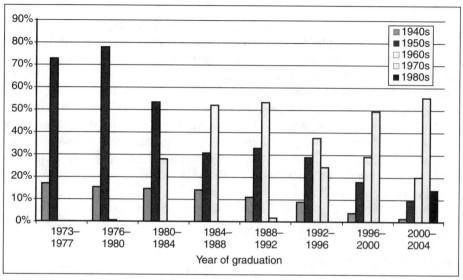

Source: National Sample Survey of Registered Nurses

Figure 9-5 **Average Age of RNs Who Graduated from Different Programs, 1976–2004**

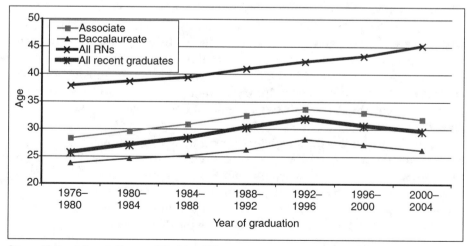

Source: National Sample Survey of Registered Nurses

numbers well into their 30s and 40s. As the number of students born in the 1950s continues to diminish, we can expect the trends in the age of graduates as shown in Figure 9-5 to stabilize.

Note also that while the age of RN graduates rose and fell with the entrance and exit of the 1950s cohorts, the average age of working RNs continued to rise after 1996. Our earlier research (Buerhaus, Staiger, & Auerbach, 2000), which is updated and described in greater detail in Chapter 10, found that the cohort-based explanation has driven both trends. Not only were the 1950s cohorts larger in number than the cohorts that came before and after them, but there has been a dramatic decline in the propensity of younger birth cohorts (those born after the 1950s) to choose nursing as a career because opportunities for women outside of nursing have expanded. This declining propensity of young women to choose a career in nursing is the primary factor behind the aging of the RN workforce, the age trends of graduates of both major types of degree programs, and the proportion of graduates entering associate degree programs.

OLDER AGE OF NEW GRADUATES

Figure 9-6 focuses on one additional nuance to the pattern of age and graduation trends dominated by the 1950s cohorts. As in Figure 9-3, which showed graduation patterns by age over time, Figure 9-6 focuses on the graduation age of the majority of nursing students who graduated by age 30. Among individuals born in the 1930s through the 1950s, the great majority who would eventually become RNs finished their nursing education during their early 20s. Of RNs born in the 1940s who became RNs by age 30, 90% graduated by age 25. In other words, there were roughly 10 RNs who graduated by age 25 for every one who graduated between the ages of 26 and 30. For those born in the 1950s who would become RNs by age 30, 80% had graduated by age 25. Yet for those born in the early 1970s, this ratio fell to nearly 60%, meaning that for every three individuals who became RNs by age 30, two became an RNs by age 25, and one became an RN between the ages of 26 and 30.

Figure 9-6 illustrates the later age of entry into RN education that is explored in more detail in Chapter 10. We have observed this trend in our CPS data, and this seems to reflect an increasing number of people who enter nursing from other careers rather than directly from high school as was the more common route in earlier years. Yet, at the same time, the number of these new entrants does not appear to be large enough to reverse the decline in the average age of nurse graduates (Figure 9-5), resulting from the loss of the aged 40 and older nursing students born in the 1950s who were still enrolling in nursing programs in large numbers in the mid-1990s.

Figure 9-6   Ratio of RN Graduates by Age for Different Cohorts

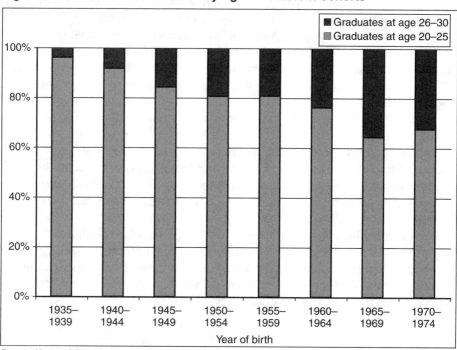

Source: National Sample Survey of Registered Nurses

CHAPTER SUMMARY

It has been suggested that the increase in associate degree programs over the years is a major cause of the rising average age of RNs. Stated differently, the large expansion of these programs over the past several decades made it easier for women in mid or late career to decide to become RNs where, without these programs, they would have been unable to make such choices. The analysis reported here shows that in recent years a growing proportion of new RNs have indeed graduated from associate degree programs. However, rather than the presence of associate degree programs driving the aging of the RN workforce, the exceptional size of the cohorts of women born in the 1950s and early 1960s who would eventually become RNs as they aged into their 30s explains the rising growth in demand for these programs. These large cohorts of women were in their 30s or 40s in the late 1980s and 1990s. Because the shorter-to-complete associate degree programs attract the majority of people who enter nursing in their 30s and 40s, the burst of associate degree graduates in the 1980s and 1990s reflects these underlying large cohort effects.

This result also implies that because cohorts of women born *after* the 1950s are smaller in population size and are also less likely to enter nursing as a profession, the trend toward ever larger numbers of new RN graduates in their 30s and 40s would eventually fade, just as what has been observed beginning in the late 1990s and early 2000s. This decline resulted in a small decrease in the average age of RN nursing students, but it did not impact the overall aging of the RN workforce, which will continue until the large number of baby boomer RNs begin to retire.

Finally, there is an emerging trend toward later entry into nursing programs among newer cohorts of students. That trend, combined with the loss of the 1950s cohorts from nursing education programs, should help stabilize the average age of nursing students in the years ahead and could result in nursing programs needing to adjust their recruitment strategies and curriculum because increasing numbers of new students will not enter nursing education directly from high school.

Now that we have examined the factors that determine the short- and long-run supply of RNs in Chapters 6 and 7, the changing preferences for a career in nursing in Chapter 8, and the importance of the cohort effect in explaining the rising age of the current RN workforce, we move to Chapter 10, which brings many of these factors together, quantitatively, to make our projections of the future age and supply of FTE RNs through 2025.

REFERENCES

Buerhaus, P., Staiger, D., & Auerbach, D. (2000). Implications of an aging registered nurse workforce. *Journal of the American Medical Association, 283*(22), 2948–2954.

McBride, A. (1996). Professional nursing education today and tomorrow. Commissioned paper in G. Wunderlich, F. Sloan, & C. Davis, (Eds.), *Nursing staff in hospitals and nursing homes. Is it adequate?* (pp. 333–360). Washington, DC: National Academies Press.

National League for Nursing. (2006). *Nursing data review academic year 2004–2005. Baccalaureate, associate degree, and diploma programs.* New York: Author.

CHAPTER 10

Forecast of the Supply and Age of Registered Nurses Through 2025

In Chapters 8 and 9, we have seen how two long-run trends have affected entry into the RN workforce. First, we noted the declining interest among young women in becoming RNs that resulted from more career opportunities opening up for women in other fields. Second, we discussed the recent trend toward entering nursing education programs at later ages as more individuals chose to enter the nursing profession, particularly through accelerated baccalaureate and 2-year associate degree programs, after first working in other fields or raising children.

In this chapter, we use data from the Currrent Population Survey (CPS) to incorporate these trends in constructing a model to forecast the supply and age composition of the RN workforce through 2025. We begin by providing an overview of our forecasting model and briefly describing the overall results. Following this, we provide a more comprehensive description of the forecasting model we developed, focusing on how the model captures the population, cohort, and age effects. Next, we describe how observations of the nursing workforce since our initial forecast in 2000 have led to changes in the forecasts and in the model itself. We then describe these new forecasts in detail to the year 2025 and how forecasted shortages would change if future cohorts enter the nursing profession to a greater or lesser extent than expected.

OVERVIEW OF FORECASTING MODEL AND KEY RESULTS

One key trend that is captured by our model is how the number of RNs peaked with the large baby boom cohorts. These cohorts were large in size and supplied many individuals who entered the nursing workforce in years when many other professions were not as open to women as they are today. Those cohorts of RNs were followed by cohorts that were smaller in number and whose members found more abundant career opportunities in the 1980s and beyond. These effects resulted in a large wave of RNs entering the nursing workforce followed by smaller waves, which has resulted in an aging workforce as the large wave grows older, and it will result in structural shortages as this wave of RNs retires from the workforce in numbers that are unlikely to be replaced by new incoming RNs.

A second key trend captured by our model is that relatively large numbers of people have recently entered the profession in their late 20s and early 30s. Though it is unclear why people are becoming RNs at later ages and in higher numbers, there is some evidence that the nursing profession is attracting interest from different segments of the potential workforce than it was in the 1970s and 1980s. The recent entry into nursing of relatively older individuals will contribute to an older workforce in the future, but it also will help to offset some of the large losses when the baby boom cohorts retire.

Both of these trends have important implications for long-run forecasts, which are described in the remainder of this chapter. More specifically, the workforce is projected to plateau in size and in average age by the middle of the next decade at an overall size of roughly 2.55 million FTE RNs and an average age of nearly 45 years. From that point forward, with the demand for RNs likely to steadily increase, an overwhelmingly large shortage of RNs will develop, reaching a projected 500,000 FTE RNs by 2025. This shortage could be lessened based on promising emerging trends wherein many people born in the early 1970s and early 1980s are becoming RNs. However, even a large growth in the RN workforce among these cohorts would not forestall shortages in the latter part of the next decade due to the effect of the retirement of large numbers of baby boom RNs. The implications of those shortages (which have already been experienced in some areas for several years) and of an aging workforce are discussed in subsequent chapters.

COMPONENTS OF OUR FORECAST MODEL

As with the Health Resources and Services Administration (HRSA) forecast model described briefly in Chapter 7, our model first compiles data on key features of the current RN workforce. Then we apply assumptions as to how those key data elements might change in the future to forecast the future age and supply of the RN workforce. Our model, however, differs significantly from the HRSA model in both the specific approach and in the data on which it is based. In the following section, we provide a nontechnical overview of the key features of the model. The model first decomposes data on past and current RN employment into *cohort, population,* and *age* effects, and then uses these three effects to describe trends in the current workforce and make forecasts about the future workforce.[1] For a more complete description of the model, how it was estimated, and how forecasts were constructed, see Appendix 10-1.

Cohort, Population, and Age Effects

The forecast model we used to project the RN workforce is based on *cohort, population,* and *age* effects. A helpful analogy in explaining these terms is to imagine a large conference center in 2000 holding a reunion for everyone who went to a certain high school over a span of many years. Each room in the conference center has a sign that indicates the graduating class that will be holding its reunion in that room. When the reunion convenes, each room counts the number of graduates from its class who are employed as RNs. For example, the class of 1990 might have seven RNs among its attendees while the class of 1980 might have five and the class of 1970 might have 10. All else equal, the class of 1970 would therefore have twice the *cohort effect* of the class of 1980—that is, the class of 1970 produced twice as many RNs as the class of 1980.

However, there are at least two other considerations that make this analysis slightly more complicated. First, the class of 1970 might simply have been larger in size than the class of 1980, and that could have led to the larger number of RNs. That is the *population effect*, which is included in our projection model as well. Second, in the reunion year (2000), members of the class of 1990 were 28 years old (born in 1972) while members of the class of 1970 were 48 years old. The count of working RNs among the class of 1990 might be artificially low because some members might still be matriculating in their nursing education programs at the time of the reunion, while some RNs might be caring for children or dependent adults and thus temporarily working part time or not working at all. Thus, to arrive at a fair comparison between the likelihood of becoming an RN for two different classes, each class should be compared when they are the same

---

[1] Note that RN wages, which are also discussed in Chapter 7 as a determinant of the long-run supply of RNs, are not used in our forecast model. When national average RN wages are used as one factor attempting to describe the observed workforce in multiple regression models, they are found to have an insignificant effect on the observed supply. Other researchers have noted this paradox (that it makes economic sense that wage levels would affect people's decisions to become RNs, but that effect has not been strongly observed in models such as these). Furthermore, there is little basis for estimating what wages in the future might be, so an effect of wages would not add much certainty to the forecast model.

age. The pattern describing the extent to which more FTE RNs might be expected from a cohort when it is age 48 versus age 28, for example, is called the *age effect.*[2]

Cohort effects, therefore, describe the likelihood, or propensity, of a given person who was born in a given year to become an RN. In Chapters 7 and 8, we described some of the reasons why these propensities have varied over time, with expanding opportunities for careers for women being a major factor. As with population effects, cohort effects are defined quantitatively in our forecast model such that one can assess their combined impact with statements such as the following: There were 34% fewer 45-year-olds in 1990 (the 1945 birth cohort) than in 2000 (the 1955 birth cohort), *and* a given person born in 1945 was 38% less likely to be working as an RN by age 45 as was a person born in 1955. Combining these two effects implies that there were roughly 60% fewer 45-year-old RNs in 1990 than in 2000 (i.e., the number of 45-year-old RNs more than doubled between 1990 and 2000).[3]

These percentages for both population and cohort effects, by birth year, are plotted together in **Figure 10-1** for the full range of years of observation that were included in our forecasting model (based on CPS data from 1973 to 2006). As in the preceding example, all of the population and cohort effects are defined in terms of their size relative to the cohort that was born in 1955. The population effects show the number of births attributed to the baby boom peaking around 1960, followed by a decline in births through the mid-1970s, and then a slight rebound in births through the early 1980s. The cohort effects follow a pattern that is quite similar to what we observed in Chapter 8 with the interest of college freshman in nursing, which peaked with the 1955 cohort (who were college freshmen around 1973) and declined thereafter, with a temporary rise seen for cohorts born in the mid-1970s (corresponding to freshmen in the early 1990s).

Taken together, changes in the population and cohort effects describe trends in the number of people who became RNs since the 1940s. Beginning with those born during the 1940s, there was a strong increase in population sizes and propensities to become RNs, the latter peaking for those born in 1955. That increase explains the robust growth in the nursing workforce over the last few decades. For those born after 1955, the explanations behind the trends in Figure 10-1 that show the number of nurse FTEs produced by a given

---

[2] Note that while population effects account for immigration to the United States in that the model uses updated census population figures, which include immigrants and their children, the sudden influx of foreign nurse graduates (FNGs) in a given future year would not be captured by this model. While this is not an insignificant factor, FNGs still make up only about one in eight nurses in the workforce today.

[3] Note that the two effects (cohort and population) are multiplicative, not simply additive.

Figure 10-1 Population and Cohort Effects for Birth Cohorts Relative to 1955 Birth Cohort, 1924–1983

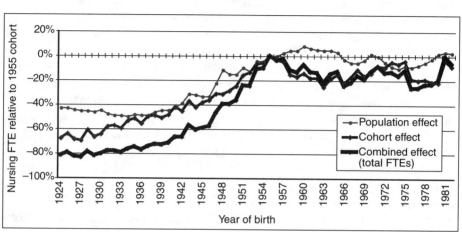

Source: Authors' forecast model based on Current Population Survey

birth year are more complicated. The population of each birth cohort continued to grow until the mid-1960s, while the propensity to become an RN declined. The decline in the propensity to become an RN was much stronger than the population growth, however, so that the number of people becoming RNs began to drop. The low point (after 1955) in total FTE RNs produced is the 1966 cohort, which is projected to produce 25% fewer RNs at age 45 (this will occur in 2011) than did the 1955 cohort.[4] For the next 10 years, births generally remained below the level in 1955 while propensity to become an RN grew. Although those born in 1975 were nearly as likely to become RNs as those born in 1955, a low number of births in that year ensured that the total number of RNs produced by the 1975 cohort would remain about 10% below the 1955 cohort. The population effect began growing again in the late 1970s while the propensity to become an RN dropped in the latter 1970s only to rebound in the early 1980s. Those latter effects are based on only a few years of data and might well change in the future after these recent cohorts have been observed for longer periods of time.

The age effect, as discussed in Chapter 7, describes the output of a cohort of RNs relative to their output at age 45. The age effect combines several factors, including the age of entry into the workforce; the likelihood that an RN is employed

---

[4] This result is technically a projection from the model that has not yet been fully described. It is based on the 18 years of observations of the 1966 cohort (from 1989 to 2006) combined with the full dataset of observations on age effects, which are used to predict FTEs at age 45 compared to FTEs at age 40, for example, for a given cohort, as described in the next section.

in nursing at a given age (compared to working in another field or to not working at all, for example, staying home to care for family members); the number of hours worked at a given age; and the age at which RNs retire.

The age effect, averaged across all RN cohorts observed in the CPS data, is presented in **Figure 10-2**. The overall pattern of the age effect is consistent with expectations of how work effort varies over the life cycle. There is a rise in FTEs through age 45 as many RNs finish nursing education and enter the labor force while others increase labor force activity as they pass out of the child-rearing years. For example, within a given cohort, say people born in 1960, the number of observed RN FTEs among that group at age 30 (which occurred in 1990—there were 51,400 FTE RNs among this group) was about one-third fewer than the number observed among the same group at age 45 (which occurred in 2005—there were 84,570 FTE RNs). Total FTEs are relatively stable from roughly age 45 to age 55, followed by a rapid decline as RNs approach the usual retirement age of 65. Note that the age effect reflects the number of RNs in the labor force at any given age and the average hours worked among those RNs. Thus, while average hours worked *among RNs in the labor force* generally peaks prior to age 40, we find that total FTEs peak somewhat later because of an increased number of RNs who are *in* the labor force at older ages.

With the exception of cohorts born after 1965, which will be discussed shortly, the age effect has been relatively stable over time because each successive cohort has followed the same pattern. Thus, Figure 10-2 shows the age effect using one main line with two small branches with lower the branch representing the age effect for cohorts born after 1965. Consistent with what we

Figure 10-2   Age Effect (FTEs Produced by a Cohort at a Given Age) Relative to Age 45

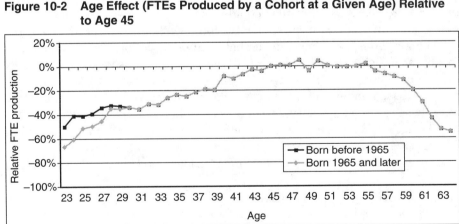

Source: Authors' forecast model based on Current Population Survey

discussed in Chapter 9, these more recent cohorts appear to have begun their nursing careers later, on average, and thus exhibit a slightly different life-cycle pattern.

PRIOR WORKFORCE SUPPLY MODEL AND FORECASTS

As summarized in Chapter 7, our initial modeling efforts were published in 2000 and were based on data through 1998 (Buerhaus, Staiger, & Auerbach, 2000). This study used data on individuals between the ages of 23 and 64 who reported their occupation as an RN between January 1973 and December 1998 and a forecast model based on the previously mentioned population, age, and co-hort effects to describe the current RN workforce (at the time) and to project the future age and supply of FTE RNs. Further details of our methods and fore-casting model are provided in Appendix 10-1.

The key assumptions required to make forecasts based on this model are that: (1) future cohorts that have not yet been observed will enter nursing at the rate of the five most recently observed cohorts, on average; and (2) future cohorts will follow the same life-cycle pattern of RN FTE production as they age (age ef-fects) as has been observed for all previous cohorts. These assumptions, combined with population projections from the U.S. Census Bureau, are all that is required to forecast the nursing workforce many years into the future. To evaluate our model's accuracy at that time, we showed that using data only through 1988, we were able to project the supply and age of the RN workforce over the next 10 years (from 1989 to 1998) quite accurately, including the overall growth in size of the workforce and the dramatic increase in the number of RNs in their 40s along with a dramatic decline in the number of RNs in their 20s during those years.

Our initial projections indicated that the average age of working RNs would increase from 42.0 years in 2000 to 45.4 years in 2010 (when 40% of the RN work-force would be over age 50) and would hold steady at this level over the next decade. Further, our forecasts indicated that the number of FTE RNs would grow slowly until 2012, peaking at 2.2 million, and subsequently decline to 2.05 million FTE RNs by 2020, roughly the size of the RN workforce that existed in 2000. The latest projections of the future *demand* for RNs at the time were re-ported in 1996 by HRSA (U.S. Department of Health and Human Services, 1996).[5] Comparing our supply projections to HRSA's demand projections revealed a

---

[5] For more details about HRSA's demand model, see *"What is Behind HRSA's Supply, Demand and Projected Shortage of Registered Nurses?"* at http://bhpr.hrsa.gov/healthworkforce/ (April 2006).

shortage of RNs developing over the 20-year forecast period, eventually growing to more than 400,000 by 2020.

In 2002 HRSA published new RN workforce projections. These revised forecasts indicated that the demand for RNs would be 20 percent greater than its previous forecast, reaching 2.8 million RNs by 2020. Applying our projections of the future supply of RNs to HRSA's latest demand estimates, the future shortage was then estimated to be twice the in size, reaching roughly 800,000 by 2020.

When we published our RN age and supply forecasts in 2000, the cohorts born in the 1970s were primarily in their early 20s, and the slow rates with which they were becoming RNs were interpreted as a continuing decline in the propensity to become a nurse, leading to pessimistic future labor supply forecasts. Although we observed what appeared to be a trend toward later entry into nursing, we did not have strong corroborating evidence of its impact and thus did not incorporate this trend in our forecasting model.

In subsequent studies of the RN workforce, we observed substantial growth in RN employment (Buerhaus, Staiger, & Auerbach, 2004). This growth, roughly 300,000 from 2000 to 2005, was larger than either we or HRSA had projected,[6] and it suggested the need for a fresh examination of the assumptions underpinning our forecasting model. This growing trend toward later entry into nursing, described in the next section and also in Chapter 9, was incorporated into our new, updated model by allowing for a different life-cycle pattern of FTE production, prior to age 30, for cohorts born after 1965 (as shown in Figure 10-2).

UPDATING OUR FORECAST

Our new forecast reflects two changes observed in the nursing workforce since the initial forecast was published (in 2000). The two changes are related to observations of the propensity of the 1970s cohorts to become RNs. The first is that members of these cohorts are, in fact, becoming RNs to a much greater extent than was previously thought. The second related observation (as mentioned earlier) is that members of these cohorts simply began their nursing careers later. These two effects are illustrated in **Figure 10-3**, which shows the rate at which those born in different time periods became RNs as they aged.

---

[6] According to our initial projections made in 2000, which used data through 1998, the projected total workforce was expected to grow by roughly 220,000 FTE RNs from 2000 to 2005. HRSA's 2002 report, which used data through 2000, projected growth at 120,000 RNs over this same time period. The actual growth from 2000 to 2005, according to the CPS, was 293,000.

Figure 10-3   RN FTEs per 100,000 U.S. Residents in Three 3-Year Birth Cohorts, by Age

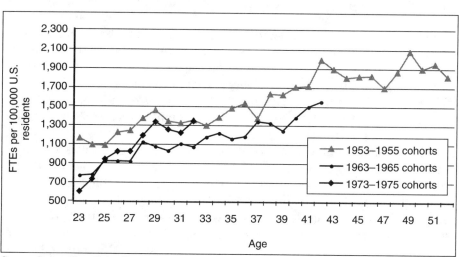

Source: Current Population Survey

Among those born in the mid-1950s, by age 23, roughly 1200 per 100,000 (1.2%) were FTE RNs. The numbers of working RNs grew gradually among these cohorts throughout their 30s and 40s before leveling off at nearly 2000 FTEs per 100,000 by age 50. In contrast, among those born 10 years later (from 1963 to 1965), the number of working RNs was roughly 20% lower at every age. This drop in RN employment reflects that fewer people chose to become RNs due, primarily, to the growth of other professions that were increasingly attracting women who were graduating from high school in the 1980s (Goldin, 2006).

Importantly, a different pattern has emerged among the most recently observed cohorts. For those born in the mid-1970s (1973 to 1975), few had become RNs by their early 20s—fewer than their predecessors born in the 1960s. But over the next 7 years, those born in the mid-1970s entered nursing at an unprecedented rate of increase such that by age 32, there were as many RN FTEs among this cohort (controlling for cohort population size, which was larger for the 1950s cohorts) as there were among the cohorts born in 1953 to 1955, that produced the largest number of RNs in the workforce ever observed in the United States. Thus, the first effect that makes recent forecasts different from earlier ones is that the 1970s cohorts are to be producing more RNs than those that came before them in the 1960s.

The second effect reflecting the shift in the age at which recent cohorts are becoming RNs—from their early 20s to their late 20s and early 30s—is revealed in greater detail in **Figure 10-4**, which plots RN FTEs produced by a given single-year birth cohort at ages 29 to 30 versus at ages 23 to 24. For example, among people born in 1950, the number of working RNs are counted in 1973 to 1974 and then again in 1979 to 1980 and the two points are plotted on the graph. The two lines corresponding to RN production track fairly well for those born before roughly 1965, but then they diverge. That is, in earlier years, the number of FTE RNs observed for a given cohort in their *late* 20s was roughly 20% greater than had been observed for that same cohort in their *early* 20s. For cohorts born after 1965, however, the number of FTE RNs at ages 29 and 30 is roughly double the number observed for the same cohorts at ages 23 and 24. If we did not account for this trend, the model would, for example, observe the 600 FTE RNs per 100,000 population produced by the 1975 cohort at age 23 (in 1998) and assume that this would forever be a small RN cohort, growing to perhaps 800 FTE RNs by age 30, instead of the 1200 that were actually observed. This entry into the nursing profession at later ages is reflected as a structural change to the forecast model, and it is shown by the second line referred to earlier in Figure 10-2, indicating a slightly different life-cycle pattern for cohorts born after 1965.

Figure 10-4   FTEs per 100,000 U.S. Residents at Ages 23 to 24 vs. at Ages 29 to 30 for Birth Cohorts 1950–1976

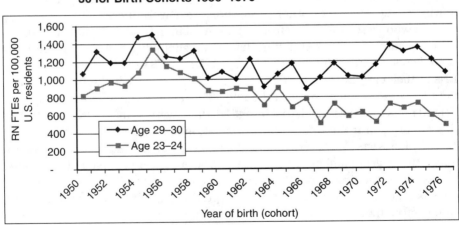

Source: Current Population Survey

AGE AND SUPPLY FORECASTS THROUGH 2025

Using this updated model, we forecast the age and number of FTE RNs to the year 2025. The workforce has grown steadily from 1972 to 2006, adding roughly 50,000 FTEs per year (3.9% annual growth) to reach roughly 2.3 million RNs in 2006. Our initial forecast (Buerhaus, Staiger, & Auerbach, 2000) predicted a slowdown beginning around 2012 and had forecast smaller numbers of RNs in 2006 than were actually observed. As shown in **Figure 10-5**, using our revised projection model, the future number of FTE RNs in the workforce in 2020 is projected to be significantly larger (by about 500,000) than our previous forecast. We estimate that about one-fifth (80,000) of this increase is attributed to using more recent census data that indicates higher projected populations of working-age Americans over the next few decades. The majority (about 400,000) of the increase relative to our earlier forecasts is due to the fact that the cohorts born in the 1970s (and early 1980s) are becoming RNs at faster rates than was earlier projected, which is captured by the model's cohort effects and by the model's re-vision that is better able to account for the later entry of these cohorts into nursing school and, eventually, into the RN workforce.

Figure 10-5   Actual and Forecast FTE RN Workforce Supply and Average Age, 1973–2025

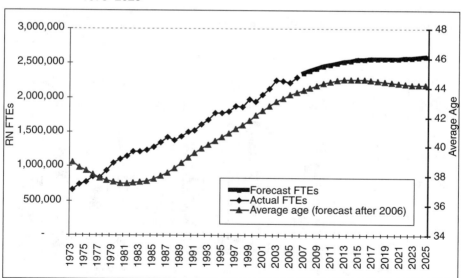

Source: Authors' forecast model based on Current Population Survey

Despite this improvement in the forecast of the long-run size of the RN work-force, the dominant trend facing the workforce is unchanged: the eventual re-tirement of the large 1950s cohorts. Our new forecast indicates that the observed historical growth in total RN supply will begin decelerating by the end of the cur-rent decade, when the first of the 1950s RNs approach their 60s (see Figure 10-5). The growth in the total workforce is projected to pause around 2019 at 2.56 million FTE RNs when RNs born in the 1950s who are retiring in great numbers will offset new entry into the workforce. The workforce is then projected to begin growing slowly again from 2020 to 2025 when the smaller 1960s cohorts are leaving the workforce and the 1970s cohorts will reach their productive years in their late 40s.

In 2006, the average age of the FTE RN workforce was 43.7, and the largest age group was composed of RNs in their 40s (see **Figures** 10-5 and **10-6**). These RNs reflect the large number of people born in the baby boom generation who entered the nursing profession in the 1970s and 1980s (as is evident in the large growth in the bars representing RNs in their 30s and 40s in the 1989 distribu-tion compared to the 1972 distribution). By 2012, with the aging of this group of RNs, the average age of the FTE RN workforce will have increased 0.8 years to 44.5, and RNs in their 50s will be the largest age group. We project the aver-age age of the workforce to peak at 44.6 in 2015, and by 2018 it will drop slightly to 44.5 years. By then, many baby boomer RNs will continue working in their 60s (at 12% of the workforce, matching the numbers of RNs in their 20s), but

Figure 10-6   Past and Projected Age Distribution of RN Workforce, 1972–2025

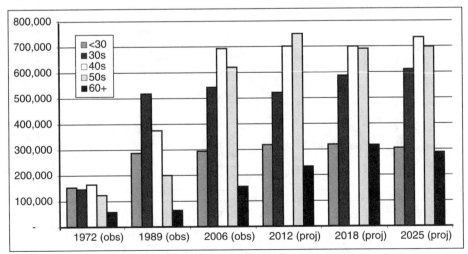

Source: Authors' forecast model based on Current Population Survey

most will have retired. Finally, by 2025, the age distribution of the RN workforce will begin to assume a more "normal" shape because the 1950s cohorts will have mostly retired.

Figure 10-7 shows how different assumptions about the size of future cohorts of RNs not yet observed in our data (i.e., those born after 1983) affect our forecasts. It also compares those forecasts, as well as our baseline forecast, to the RN requirements projected by HRSA in 2002. The baseline forecast indicates a deficit relative to the requirements for RNs beginning in 2015 that grows to 285,000 RNs, or 9.3%, by 2020. Though requirements have not been published for 2025, if they were to grow at the same annual rate as the HRSA projections to 2020 (about 50,000 RNs per year), the requirements for RNs would reach roughly 3.1 million FTE RNs by 2025. This estimate, compared to a projected workforce of 2.6 million, suggests a deficit of roughly 500,000 RNs (or 16%) in 2025.

As shown in Figure 10-7, if future entering cohorts are not the same size as the average of the five most recently observed cohorts (1979 to 1983), but rather are 10% larger (which would make them as large as the 1955 cohort), the RN workforce would still experience a shortfall of 200,000 FTE RNs by 2020 and 370,000 FTE RNs by 2025 (12%). If future cohorts are 10% smaller than the most recent cohorts (e.g., similar to the 1962 cohort), the shortfall would be nearly

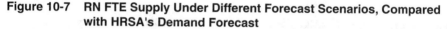

Figure 10-7   RN FTE Supply Under Different Forecast Scenarios, Compared with HRSA's Demand Forecast

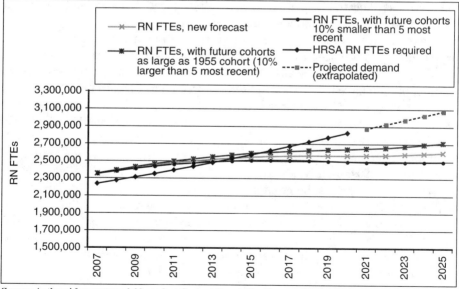

Source: Authors' forecast model based on Current Population Survey; HRSA, US Department of Health and Human Services

600,000 FTE RNs in 2025. Extrapolating from these alternative forecasts suggests that future cohorts would have to be 40% larger (controlling for population size) than those observed over the last 5 years to erase the projected shortfall of RNs by 2025. This is very unlikely because those cohorts would have to be about 30% larger than those of the mid-1950s who, as discussed before, flocked to nursing partly because many other professions had significant barriers to entry for women at the time.

IMPLICATIONS OF THE RESURGENCE OF THE 1970s COHORTS

It is hard to predict which scenario, with respect to the propensity of future cohorts to become RNs, might be closer to the truth. Yet the observed workforce participation of RNs born in the 1970s is striking and suggests that the forces leading individuals to pursue careers in nursing are dynamic enough to lead to significant change. Not only are these individuals entering the workforce later than previous cohorts, but they are entering in greater numbers than the 1960s cohorts, thereby countering predictions of a continued decline in interest in nursing (U.S. Department of Health and Human Services, 2002; Buerhaus, Staiger, & Auerbach, 2000).

The trend toward later entry began with the cohorts born after 1964 who began entering the nursing workforce in the late 1980s and early 1990s. RNs today are less likely to obtain their basic nursing education immediately after high school, as was more common in the past. Instead, two routes of entry into nursing have become increasingly common. First, people are entering the nursing profession by graduating from 2-year associate degree programs after a substantial period in their early 20s spent in other careers or not in the workforce. Second, people have increasingly entered nursing via 12 to 18 month "accelerated" bachelor of science degree programs designed for those with other (and usually unrelated to nursing) bachelor's degrees as was described in Chapter 7. With its relatively attractive entry wage, high job security, and relatively small educational investment, nursing has become a very attractive career option for people in their 20s or early 30s who might have begun careers in other fields.

What, then, explains the greater propensity of the 1970s cohorts to eventually become RNs relative to the 1960s cohorts? Today it appears that the nursing profession is drawing entrants from a different, and potentially larger, pool than in earlier years, particularly undecided "20-somethings" who are looking for a fresh start, as opposed to career-minded late teens in earlier cohorts who aimed for one of the few professions then available to them.

At least three other developments have contributed to the increased production of the 1970s cohorts. First, in response to the current shortage of RNs, a substantial number of foreign-born RNs have entered the United States (foreign-born RNs now account for 14% of the current workforce, up from less than 9% in 1994). Most of these recent entrants were under age 40, thus contributing materially to the size of the 1970s cohorts. Second, the Johnson & Johnson Campaign for Nursing's Future began in early 2002 and thus far has spent $50 million on national strategies aimed at recruiting more people into the nursing profession and increasing the capacity of nursing education programs (Johnson & Johnson Health Care Systems, 2002). Third, the authors have had many conversations with officials in nursing education programs who have indicated that 9/11 was a tipping point in the decision of many people to become a nurse. Taken together, these developments fueled interest in nursing and might have helped boost entry into the profession among the 1970s cohorts. Still, their potential impact on the current number of RNs in the workforce is obscured by the fact that many individuals who might have been encouraged to enter nursing in 2002 and beyond have not yet been observed in the workforce by 2006.

Our latest supply projections are more likely to materialize if additional developments, akin to those mentioned above, do not occur. At the present time, the trend toward later entry into nursing seems fairly stable, and there is no reason to expect that the entry age will increase much beyond the 30s or revert back to the early 20s. There is greater uncertainty in the level of participation in the workforce among the late 1970s and 1980s cohorts, who are just beginning to be observed. Future changes in the economy, in immigration policy, in educational subsidies or incentives, in wages, in the organization and financing of health care, or in society generally could affect the propensities of future cohorts to enter the nursing profession.

However, as the sensitivity analyses (Figure 10-7) show, our updated forecast is not very sensitive to the potential size of future cohorts that have not yet been observed. This insensitivity is due to the fact that even by 2020 these future cohorts (born after 1983) will comprise barely a third of the total workforce. With respect to those who are already participating in the workforce, changes in retirement trends (which have been relatively stable among RNs over the last three decades) or hours worked (for example, if wages were to increase) could substantially affect the size of the future RN workforce. Additionally, our forecasts of future shortages are dependent on the accuracy of HRSA's projected demand for RN FTEs, which is based on projected changes in population demographics, insurance coverage, income, and wages.

CHAPTER SUMMARY

Many of the factors discussed in Chapter 7 that determine the long-run supply of RNs were used to construct a model of the RN workforce. The model includes variables that assess the importance of life-cycle aspects such as child rearing, hours worked, and retirement, as well as effects of population size and the propensity of people born in a given period to eventually become RNs. Changes in these effects over time have had a profound impact on the size and age distribution of the RN workforce. When analyzed quantitatively, these factors enable us to observe important trends, such as the resurgence in the number of individuals in their late 20s and 30s, who were born in the early 1970s, becoming RNs.

Equally important, our forecasting model provides a relatively straightforward approach to forecasting the size and age distribution of the RN workforce far into the future, assuming that future cohorts that have not yet entered the profession in large numbers will behave as have recent cohorts. Those assumptions were varied to generate alternative scenarios to show that the projections did not change appreciably.

Forecasts produced from this model indicate that the growth in the RN workforce that has been observed over the last few decades will decelerate and eventually plateau around 2020 at roughly 2.6 million RNs. Because HRSA projects continued growth in the demand for RNs during the foreseeable future, shortages are expected to develop around 2015 and grow to roughly 300,000 RNs by 2020 and approximately 500,000 by 2025. Of course, forecasts are uncertain, and it is possible that large wage increases, nursing school expansions, continued promotion of nursing as a career, or other events could stimulate new waves of interest in nursing. The cohorts born in the 1980s, only just now entering nursing, show signs of increased entry, though it is still too early to tell if those trends will be sustained.

Appendix 10-1

How the Projection Model was Estimated

The analysis in this chapter relies on a straightforward statistical model that is commonly used by demographers and economists (Deaton, 1997), which decomposes observed changes in the size and age of the RN workforce over time into three distinct components: population, cohort, and age effects. The term *population* refers to the size of the total population in the United States of a given age in a given year. Population effects are expected to play an important role because the overall age distribution in the United States has changed recently with the aging of the baby boom generation. The term *cohort* refers to all the individuals born in any given year. Likewise, the term *cohort effect* refers to the propensity of individuals born in any given year to work as RNs. Cohort effects are expected to be important because women who were born in recent years have had much broader career opportunities and therefore are less likely to choose nursing over other professions. Finally, the term *age* refers to a person's age in a given year. Age effects reflect the relative propensity of RNs to work at any given age and are expected to capture the tendency of RNs to work less during their childbearing years and as they approach retirement age.

More formally, the number of FTE RNs of a given age (a) that were born in a given year (b) can be described by the following equation:

(1) # FTE RN$_{a,b}$ = (POPULATION$_{a,b}$)(π_b)(α_a), for a = 23,...,64 and b = 1909,...,1983

The observed cohorts, born between 1909 and 1983, correspond to the cohorts that were between the ages of 23 and 64 at some point in the CPS sample years (1973 to 2006). The first term on the righthand side of equation (1) captures population effects, with POPULATION$_{a,b}$ referring to the total population in the United States of a given birth cohort (b) at a given age (a). The second term captures cohort effects, with π_b representing the propensity of individuals from a given cohort to work as RNs. The final term captures age effects, with α_a representing the relative propensity of RNs to work at a given age. Thus, the total number of FTE RNs of a given age that are working in a given year is the product of the size of the population, the propensity of that cohort to choose nursing as a career, and the propensity of RNs to be working at that age.

Estimating the Model

Both the cohort effects (π_b) and the age effects (α_a) are parameters that must be estimated. Rearranging equation (1) and taking logs yields the following estimating equation:

(2) ln(# FTE RN$_{a,b}$ / POPULATION$_{a,b}$) = ln(π_b) + ln(α_a), for a = 23,...,64 and b = 1909,...,1983

Analysis of variance (ANOVA) was used to estimate the parameters of this equation. The unit of observation was an age-cohort group (e.g., the 1955 cohort at age 30). The dependent variable was the logged fraction of a given birth cohort at a given age whose members are working as RNs (defined on an FTE basis). The numbers of FTE RNs were estimated from the CPS data, while data on the U.S. population by year and age were obtained from the U.S. Census Bureau. The data cover 42 years of age (23 to 64) and 34 calendar years (1973 to 2006) for a total of 1428 observations. The ANOVA model estimated main effects for cohort (birth year) and for age. These parameter estimates were exponentiated to yield estimates of π_b and α_a. Standard errors for these estimates were calculated by the bootstrap method (Efron & Gong, 1983) in a manner that accounted for the existence of multiple observations in the sample for some individuals and households, and they ranged from 5% to 15% on the age and cohort estimates.

It is important to note that the ANOVA model in equation (2) does not include main effects for the year in which the RNs were working (i.e., year effects). If year effects were included, then age and cohort effects would no longer be uniquely identified because year, cohort (or birth year), and age are linearly related to each other (year = birth year + age). Thus, in the context of our model, a major change to conditions facing the entire RN workforce in a given year might be manifested via the cohort effect for future cohorts, but not via a uniform effect on RNs of all ages working in a given year. For example, a sudden jump in RN wages might make nursing more attractive to new cohorts of RNs entering the labor market, but it would not encourage older cohorts to work more. This assumption is supported by findings from many studies discussed in Chapters 6 and 7, which show that variation in RN wages have small effects on labor supply, suggesting that year effects are likely to be small and can be safely ignored. In our earlier work (Buerhaus, Staiger, & Auerbach, 2000), year effects were not found to be jointly statistically significant when added to the model.

Forecasting Using the Model

Forecasts of the total number of FTE RNs of each age in the years 2007 to 2025 were constructed based on equation (1). The FTE forecasts were summed by year and by age to produce aggregate forecasts. Constructing forecasts for a given age group in a given year required estimates of the population by age in future years, along with estimates of the cohort (π_b) and age (α_a) effects for the age group in that year. Population estimates were obtained from the U.S. Census Bureau's "middle series" projections. The ANOVA model, equation (2), provided estimates of age effects (α_a) for each age (23 to 64). The model also provided estimates of cohort effects (π_b) for cohorts born between 1909 and 1983. However, the model does not provide estimates of cohort effects for cohorts that were born after 1983 (not yet 23 years old by 2006, which is the last year of our data). Therefore, to construct forecasts of the cohort effect (π_b) for cohorts born after 1983, we used the average cohort effect from the five most recent cohorts observed in the estimation period (the cohorts born from 1979 to 1983). If future cohorts behave like recent cohorts, then this will yield accurate forecasts. We also investigated the sensitivity of forecasts to this assumption. Standard errors on the forecasts were estimated by the bootstrap method in a manner that accounted for the existence of multiple observations for some individuals and households, and they were under 5% for most forecasts.

Incorporating Recent Changes in Age Effects

Our original model, which was developed in the late 1990s, assumed that future cohorts would follow the same life-cycle pattern of RN FTE production as they age (age effects) as has been observed for all previous cohorts. To incorporate the recent trend toward later entry into nursing, we updated this model by relaxing this assumption. Specifically, we allow for a different life-cycle pattern of FTE production, prior to age 30, for those cohorts born after 1965. More explicitly, in the ANOVA estimates of equation (2), we added an additional set of age effects only for cohorts born after 1965 and for ages 23 to 29 (a total of three additional parameters: for the age groups 23 to 24, 25 to 26, and 27 to 29). A new age pattern was not forced; if the raw data indicated that recent cohorts had the same age pattern of FTE production as earlier cohorts, this new model would yield similar forecasts to our original model.

REFERENCES

Buerhaus, P., Staiger, D., & Auerbach, D. (2000). Implications of a rapidly aging registered nurse workforce. *Journal of the American Medical Association, 283*(22), 2948–2954.

Buerhaus, P., Staiger, D., & Auerbach, D. (2004). New signs of a strengthening nurse labor market? *Health Affairs*. Web exclusive. W4-526-W4-533.

Deaton, A. (1997). *The analysis of household surveys*. Baltimore, MD: Johns Hopkins University Press.

Efron, B., & Gong, G. (1983). A leisurely look at the bootstrap, the jacknife and cross-validation. *The American Statistician, 37*(1).

Goldin, C. (2006). The quiet revolution that transformed women's employment, education, and family. *The American Economic Review, 96*(2), 1–21.

Johnson & Johnson Health Care Systems. (2002). *Discover nursing*. Retrieved March 14, 2006, from www.discovernursing.com

U.S. Department of Health and Human Services. (1996). *Basic workforce report: National Advisory Council on Nurse Education and Practice.* Rockville, MD: Health Resources and Services Administration, Bureau of Health Professions, Division of Nursing .

U.S. Department of Health and Human Services. (2002). *Projected supply, demand, and shortages of registered nurses: 2000–2002.* Rockville, MD: Health Resources and Services Administration, Bureau of Health Professions, National Center for Health Workforce Analysis.

CHAPTER 11

Shortages of Registered Nurses: Then and Now

Anyone who has been involved with the healthcare system in the United States, either as a patient, a health professional, or a member of the media, is aware that hospitals have experienced recurrent RN shortages. The frequency of hospital RN shortages has led many people to accept nursing shortages as an inevitable part of the way the healthcare system functions in the United States. Yet, because RNs are central to hospitals' and other healthcare delivery organizations' ability to provide healthcare services and ensure access to health care, whenever RN shortages develop, they elicit the attention of federal and state legislators, workforce planners, hospitals, and nursing organizations who are intent on resolving the shortage as rapidly as possible. From the point of view of the nursing profession, no other issue has affected so many nurses so greatly over so many years.

In this chapter, we use an economic perspective to analyze key factors that lead to the development and resolution of hospital RN shortages. We begin by defining an RN shortage with respect to hospital settings, then we explain how shortages develop and are resolved in a competitive and properly functioning labor market, and then we discuss how hospital RN shortages are typically measured. Next, we examine how shortages have developed over the past 25 years, focusing first on instances when RN wages did not adjust quickly, preventing the market from reaching a new equilibrium, thereby prolonging the length of the shortage. We then examine instances when hospital RN shortages resulted from sharp increases in the demand for RNs. Following this, we focus on how supply side factors, namely the changing age composition of the RN workforce that was discussed in Chapter 10, led to the development of the current RN shortage, which began in 1998 and continues to the present.

DEFINING, EXPLAINING, AND MEASURING HOSPITAL SHORTAGES OF RNs

Given the frequency with which hospitals have experienced RN shortages, one might reasonably expect that there would be a clear and universally accepted understanding of how shortages are defined, why and how they develop, how they are measured, and how they are resolved. This is not the case, however, because researchers, nurses, and observers of the nurse labor market have used various theoretical perspectives, along with observations based on personal experiences, to guide their understanding of nursing shortages. However, it is beyond the scope of this chapter to describe or evaluate these different approaches; rather, we adopt an economic perspective to guide our analysis of hospital RN shortages. We use an economic perspective because it provides a clear and widely understood definition of a shortage, data exist over a long period of time to evaluate the presence of shortages, measures exist to assess their magnitude, and an economic perspective allows us to more easily discuss how forces external to hospitals have significantly influenced the development and resolution of hospital RN shortages.

Economic Definition of a Hospital RN Shortage (and Surplus)

A shortage is a market disequilibrium in which labor demanded by hospitals exceeds labor supplied by RNs because the wage lies below the equilibrium wage—the wage level in which demand and supply are in balance.[1] The shortage will not begin to disappear until wages increase to a level that induces an increase in the RN short-run labor supply (an increase in participation, hours worked, or both) that satisfies the hospital's demand. If, however, a hospital's demand for RNs continues to expand at the same time that wages are rising, the shortage might persist. As we will see later in this chapter, how the interaction of wages, demand, and supply unfolds during actual shortages gives texture to what might otherwise appear to be rather straightforward concepts.

It is useful to discuss RN shortages by reintroducing two figures we discussed in Chapter 3 that illustrate how supply and demand interact to determine RNs' wage and employment levels. As shown in **Figure 11-1**, because the labor supply curve is upward sloping while the labor demand curve is downward

---

[1] When we refer to the RN wage, we are also including nonwage benefits that employers provide as part of the compensation package aimed at attracting RNs.

sloping, they will cross at a single point. At the point where demand and supply intersect, the wage level (W_1) is such that the supply of RN labor is exactly equal to the demand for RN labor at employment level, E_1. At any higher wage level, such as W_2, there will be a surplus of workers looking for jobs because the higher wage increases supply while reducing demand. In Figure 11-1 the surplus is reflected in the horizontal distance between the supply and demand curves at wage level W_2. Competition among the surplus workers to obtain the limited number of jobs will place downward pressure on wages, pushing wages back toward W_1 until the supply and demand cross at the equilibrium wage, W_1. Similarly, at any wage level below W_1, such as W_3, there will be a shortage of RNs as the lower wage reduces the supply of RNs and increases employers' demand for RNs. The shortage is shown in Figure 11-1 as the horizontal distance between the demand and supply curves at wage level W_3. During a shortage, competition among employers to obtain the limited number of workers will put upward pressure on wages, pushing wages back to their equilibrium level. Thus, shortages should not exist (or at least they should be short lived) in a competitive labor market as long as there are no restrictions that prevent wages to from increasing.

Figure 11-1   Equilibrium Hours and Employment in a Competitive Labor Market

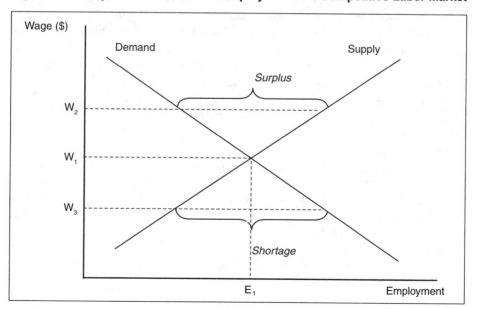

If a hospital's demand for RNs should increase, the hospital might find that there are not enough RNs willing to supply their services at the prevailing wage it is offering, and a shortage will develop. We illustrate the development of the shortage in **Figure 11-2**. Initially, in the long-run equilibrium wage is W_1, at which the short-run and long-run supply of RNs are equal to the demand for RNs. In the short run, the outward shift in RN demand from D_1 to D_2 results in a shortage of RNs. The shortage develops because not enough RNs are willing to supply their time to hospitals at the prevailing wage rate, W_1. However, as soon as RN wages increase and reach a new equilibrium at the point where the new labor demand curve (D_2) crosses the short-run labor supply curve, the shortage will disappear. This movement along the short-run labor supply curve results in much higher wages and somewhat higher employment in the short run (increased participation and hours worked by existing RNs) from E_1 to $E_{2,\ SR}$. Stated differently, the increase in RN wages will first stimulate some existing RNs to respond in the short run by rejoining the workforce, moving from nonhospital settings into hospitals, or by working additional hours (switching from a part- to full-time basis, working overtime, or even working a second job). Eventually, in the long run, new individuals will choose to become RNs (drawn to nursing by the wage increase) thus multiplying the effect of the initial short-run response to the wage increase. Thus, over time, the new equilibrium will move to the point where the new labor demand curve (D_2) crosses the long-run labor supply curve at $W_{2,\ LR}$ in Figure 11-2. Thus, outward shifts in the labor demand curve tend to primarily increase wages in the short run, while having more of an impact on employment (and less on wages) in the longer run.

As noted earlier, shortages of RNs tend to be transitory and are corrected by increases in the wage rate unless hospitals do not increase RN wages or for some reason are blocked from raising them. Unless demand is continuing to expand at the same time, the increased long-run supply of RNs will, in turn, exert downward pressure on wages. As the wage rate decreases, employers will be willing to hire additional RNs until they reach the point depicted by $E_{2,\ LR}$, and the labor market for RNs will once again adjust to a new long-run equilibrium wage and employment level of RNs.

If a hospital's demand for RNs should increase again, the hospital might find that there are not enough RNs willing to supply their services at the prevailing wage it is offering, and consequently a new shortage will develop. The series of short- and long-run adjustments will begin anew, and eventually a new market wage will be reached where the long-run demand and the long-run supply of RNs are in balance and employment levels are higher. The repetition of this cycle of demand, supply, and wage adjustments is often referred to as the "cyclical" shortage of nurses.

Figure 11-2   Impact of Outward Shift in Labor Demand on Short-Run and Long-Run Competitive Equilibrium

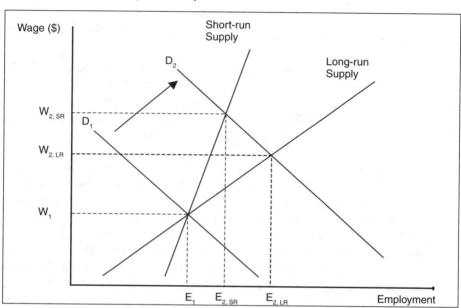

The speed with which shortages are resolved depends on several factors, including how high and how quickly a hospital increases RN wages, how sensitive RNs are to the wage increase,[2] and how sensitive the hospital's demand is for RNs over the range of wage increases it is considering offering to RNs (the employer's wage elasticity of demand for RNs). These factors and others, which help explain why hospitals are often slow to increase RN wages in response to a nursing shortage, are described further in Appendix 11-1. Additionally, as hospital decision makers realize that they will have to increase wages to resolve the shortage, they will have an incentive to substitute lower wage LPNs, or perhaps unlicensed caregivers, for RNs. Although from an RN's perspective, LPNs and nursing assistants do not represent a substitute (or at least a close substitute) for the services that RNs provide, LPNs and nursing assistants might be readily available and willing to work, and some hospitals

---

[2] Recall from Chapter 6 that studies show that RNs are not very sensitive to wage increases in the short run, meaning that a large increase in wages would result in a moderate increase in short-run supply, at best.

that are experiencing an RN shortage might believe that the shortage can be alleviated by employing non-RNs.[3]

Measuring Hospital RN Shortages

While an economic perspective provides a conceptually clear definition of a shortage of RNs, there are no widely agreed upon standards for how to measure shortages of hospital RNs. Shortages have been measured chiefly on the basis of individual or hospital self-reports, by government agencies that define health professional shortage areas throughout the country, and by calculating the ratio of RNs to the population in a state or county and comparing the ratio to other areas. A study by Grumbach, Ash, Seago, Spetz, and Coffman (2001) assessed various definitions of nursing shortages using data from large samples of hospitals in the United States in 1990 and 1992. These researchers examined various ways that shortages have been measured, including the percentage of individual hospitals self-reporting a moderate to severe shortage, the mean hospital RN vacancy rate, mean RN turnover rates, and mean number of RNs per inpatient year. These same measures were aggregated to broader health service areas to determine whether any of the measures would detect a shortage at this level better than other measures. Additionally, these investigators included the average ratio of RNs per 100,000 people in a county. The study reported that at the level of individual hospitals, there were relatively weak but statistically significant correlations among the different shortage measures. When examined at the health system area level, the correlation among most of the measures was considerably stronger. Of the measures analyzed, the strongest statistically significant correlation was found between hospital reports of a moderate or severe shortage and nurse vacancy rates at the individual hospital level (0.43) and at the health system level (0.57).

The study by Grumbach et al. (2001) is useful in providing some support for the use of hospital RN vacancy rates as a measure, though imperfect, of hospital shortages of RNs. Indeed, economists, nurses, and others have often used hospital vacancy rates to measure shortages, and there are data showing hospital RN vacancy rates during many of the years in which shortages have been reported over the past 50 years. Hospital RN vacant positions are defined as the

---

[3] For an excellent and straightforward discussion of labor shortages and wage increases, the reader is urged to see the classic article by Kenneth Arrow and William Capron (1950). Dynamic shortages and price rises: The engineer-scientist case. *Quarterly Journal of Economics, 307,* 292–308.

number of full-time equivalent (FTE) RN positions that hospitals are *actively* trying to fill. (Some hospitals might report vacant positions, but they are not truly attempting to fill them.) The RN vacancy rate is simply the number of vacant RN positions divided by the sum of the number of vacant RN positions plus the number of staffed (filled) RN positions. Although there is no well-recognized level of hospital vacancy rate that indicates the presence or absence of an RN shortage, it is common to hear hospitals report shortages of RNs when their FTE RN vacancy rate exceeds 5%. As we shall see next, there have been a number of years when the national average hospital FTE RN vacancy rate exceeded this level.

THE DEVELOPMENT OF HOSPITAL RN SHORTAGES IN THE UNITED STATES

In this section, we review the development of shortages of hospital RNs since the 1960s in order to illustrate the importance of allowing for flexibility in wages to appreciate the impact of changes in the demand for RNs. As we shall see, all of the shortages were initially driven by increases in the demand for RNs that pushed the hospital RN labor market out of equilibrium. These demand-induced shortages were transitory shortages that resolved when hospitals increased RN wages. The increase in wages led to adjustments initially in the short-run and later in the long-run supply of RNs along the lines discussed earlier. However, in a few cases, hospitals did not increase RN wages with the result that the shortage lingered because the expected adjustments needed to bring the long-run demand and supply of RNs into equilibrium did not take place. In the following section, we examine the current hospital RN shortage that began as a result of changes in the age composition of the RN workforce that, in turn, reduced the supply of RNs in surprising ways.

In discussing hospital RN shortages, we use average national RN vacancy rates reported by hospitals to indicate the presence and magnitude of shortages. Because data on hospital RN vacancy rates are unavailable for the latter half of the 1960s and for much of the 1970s, we rely on sources reported in the literature for average national hospital RN vacancy rates during those years; since the 1980s, more complete data are available on RN vacancy rates.

Inflexible RN Wages and Hospital RN Shortages in the 1960s and 1970s[4]

In the late 1950s and early 1960s, hospitals reported acute shortages of RNs as indicated by very high RN vacancy rates. According to Yett (1975) national RN FTE hospital vacancy rates were 23.2% in 1961 and 23.0% in 1962. In his classic study, *An Economic Analysis of the Nurse Shortage,* Yett found evidence supporting the hypothesis that throughout the 1950s and up until 1966 hospitals might have acted as a cartel, colluding to set RN wages below the wage that would bring the demand and supply of RNs into balance. The reason hospitals would behave as a cartel would be to lower their labor-related costs, particularly the costs associated with higher wage RNs. At the same time, however, keeping RN wages below the equilibrium market wage would mean that shortages would persist. To compensate, hospitals substituted lower wage LPNs and nursing assistants for RNs and employed foreign nurse graduates. In addition, hospitals lobbied Congress to enact legislation to subsidize nursing education to expand the long-run supply of RNs, which would exert downward pressure on wages (see the discussion of the Nurse Training Act of 1964 in Appendix 7-1).

With the enactment of the Medicare and Medicaid programs in 1965, hospitals soon faced a large increase in demand as individuals over the age of 65 had increased access to acute hospital care (Medicare) as did those with low incomes (Medicaid). Given shortages of RNs and the complexities associated with providing care to the elderly, hospitals obtained an extra 2.0% added to the costs they were being reimbursed by the Medicare program. Hospitals used these extra dollars, in part, to increase RN wages. Over the next few years, as RN wages increased toward the market equilibrium level, RN vacancy rates began to fall, decreasing to 18.1% in 1967, 15.0% in 1968, 11.2% in 1969, and 9.3% in 1971 (hospital RN vacancy rates are from Yett, 1975). Although the shortage of RNs was not totally eliminated, at least as indicated by the relatively high vacancy rates, the shortage had eased considerably.

Throughout the 1970s the demand for health care increased substantially due to an increasing population, advances in technology, favorable hospital payment policies, and the growth in insurance coverage. Consequently, the healthcare delivery system expanded as discussed in Chapter 2, and hospitals' demand for RNs grew considerably: The number of FTE RNs employed by hospitals increased 69% between 1972 and 1980 (Aiken, Blendon, & Rodgers, 1981). However, during this period, RN wages did not increase appreciably for two reasons.

---

[4] For a more in-depth discussion of the shortages of RNs during this time period, see: Buerhaus, P. (1987). Not just another nursing shortage. *Nursing Economic$, 5*(6), 267–279.

First, in 1971, the Nixon administration implemented price and wage controls that were left in place in the healthcare industry until 1974, even though they were removed from the rest of the economy in 1972. The second reason RN wage increases were blunted during the 1970s was due to the high rate of inflation in the economy during the Carter administration, which began in 1976. With demand increasing rapidly and RN wages not keeping up with the cost of living, the supply of RNs was unable to catch up to the steadily rising demand even though nursing education programs were expanding the long-run supply of RNs by graduating ever-increasing numbers of RNs (as described in Chapter 7). Throughout the 1970s, hospitals consistently reported a shortage of RNs, and by 1979 national RN vacancy rates had climbed to 14%. The inability of RN wages to rise fast enough prevented the supply and demand for RNs from reaching a new equilibrium level.

Demand-Driven RN Shortages in the 1980s

As shown in **Figure 11-3**, hospitals substantially increased real RN wages in the early 1980s, with the result that the short-run supply of RNs increased as reflected by the notable rise in national RN participation rates (the percentage of licensed RNs who were employed) from 76.6% in 1980 to 78.4% in 1984.[5] Following the increase in real RN wages and RN participation rates, the hospital RN shortage ended quickly as indicated by hospital RN vacancy rates that plummeted to a national average of 4.4% in 1983 to 1984.

In 1983, just as the hospital RN shortage ended, the demand for RNs received a sudden shock as the Medicare program began implementing its new hospital prospective payment system based on Diagnosis Related Groups. Rather than decrease the demand for RNs, as many expected because hospitals would begin to be paid a fixed price for inpatient care, hospitals' demand for RNs *increased* markedly. Unlike the former cost-based retrospective reimbursement system, the new fixed prospective pricing system provided hospitals with an economic incentive to produce patient care more efficiently, to keep patients in the hospital only for as long as necessary, and to increase the throughput of patients. For hospitals to remain profitable or at least maintain their financial positions, they needed to admit only those patients who were acutely ill, shift the care of less acutely ill

---

[5] Real wages represent the change in annual wages after taking into account the effects of inflation, as measured by annual changes in the Consumer Price Indexes. By adjusting for the effects of inflation, real RN wages measure how well the annual growth rate in wages reflects whether RNs are economically better or worse off in relation to changes in the prices of goods and services they purchase.

Figure 11-3   Two-Year National Average Hospital Vacancy Rates and Real Wages for FTE RNs, 1979–2006

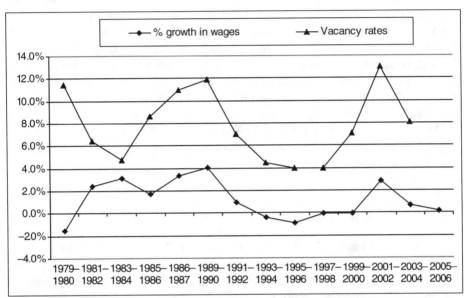

Source: Data on real RN wages are from author calculations of CPS data, 1979 to 2006.
Data on hospital RN vacancy rates for 1979 to 1994 are from Buerhaus, P. (1995). Economic pressures building in the hospital employed RN labor market. *Nursing Economic$*, 123(3), 137–141; vacancy rates for 1995 to 1998 are estimated; vacancy rates for 1999 to 2000 are from J. Walter Thomspon, Inc.; vacancy rates for 2001 are from the First Consulting Group, and vacancy rates for 2002 to 2006 are from the American Hospital Association surveys published in its annual reports, "Trends Affecting Hospitals and Health Systems."

patients into less costly outpatient settings, and reduce the length of time these sicker patients remained in the hospital. To provide inpatient care more efficiently, hospitals needed to use the least costly method of providing nursing care to treat an increasingly ill inpatient population. Because state nurse practice acts allow RNs to provide a greater number and variety of nursing procedures and tasks than LPNs or assistive nursing personnel, RNs are relatively more versatile and productive in producing nursing care. Moreover, because RN wages did not exceed LPN wages by an appreciable amount, RNs were a relatively cheaper input in the production of inpatient care. As a result of their increased productivity and relatively low wage, hospitals' demand for RNs increased substantially throughout the 1980s. Every year between 1983 and the end of the decade, the number of hospital beds decreased; at the same time, the ratio of total nursing personnel per hospital bed increased. The ratio of RNs per bed increased 32% between 1983 and 1990, compared with a decline of 14% and an increase of 1% in the ratio of LPNs and aides per bed, respectively (Buerhaus

& Staiger, 1996). Overall, from 1983 to 1990, we estimate that average growth in hospital RN demand increased roughly 3% per year.

The strong growth in hospitals' demand for RNs resulted in a period of annual real wage growth during the same period, as seen in Figure 11-3. However, despite the growth in real wages, hospital vacancy rates increased steadily, rising from 4.4% in 1983 to just below 12% in 1990. The rise in vacancy rates implies that the supply of RNs was not increasing fast enough to meet the rising demand, and hospitals could not fill all the RN positions they wanted. Thus, from 1983 through the end of the decade, hospitals reported a shortage of RNs.

The RN Labor Market in the 1990s: Another Shock in Demand

In the 1990s, the growth in demand for RNs *decreased* substantially as a result of a slowdown in the demand for health care and hospital care brought about by the surging growth in managed care. As discussed in Chapter 5 (see Figure 5-1), by the late 1980s managed care organizations had emerged as an important option for employers who were anxious to reduce the annual growth of employee health insurance premiums. In 1988, Health Maintenance Organizations (HMOs) and Preferred Provider Organizations (PPOs) accounted for 27% of workers covered by employer-provided health insurance plans. By 1993 this percentage had doubled to 54%, and by 1996 it had reached 73%. At the end of the decade, 92% of workers covered by employer-provided health insurance plans were enrolled in some form of managed care. As shown in Chapter 5, *as impressive as the growth of managed care was, it did not stop the demand for RNs from growing; rather, it merely slowed the rate of growth in demand by about 1% per year. Thus, during the 1990s, we estimate that the annual growth in demand for RNs was roughly 2% per year.*

Compared to the 3% rate of annual growth in demand during the 1980s, the slowdown in the growth of RN demand was important because by 1993 it appears to have allowed the supply of RNs (which had been growing during the 1980s) to finally catch up to the demand for RNs, thereby ending the RN shortage that had begun in the mid-1980s. As shown in Figure 11-3, vacancy rates decreased to 4% by 1993, and by this time the growth in real RN wages had already begun decreasing. In fact, some observers of the nurse labor market declared that the nurse labor market was experiencing a *surplus* of RNs (see the discussion of the report by the Pew Health Professions Commission in Chapter 7).

As shown in Figure 11-1, a surplus of RNs is reflected by the supply of RNs *exceeding* the number of RNs demanded at the prevailing market wage. This market disequilibrium places downward pressure on the wages of RNs, and the pressure will continue until the demand and supply of RNs are again brought into balance. Figure 11-3 shows that, in fact, real RN wages stopped growing and actually decreased from 1993 to 1997, and during this same period vacancy rates remained at or slightly below 4%. The drop in real wages appears to have brought the demand and supply of hospital RNs into equilibrium between 1997 and 1999 (notice that real wages flattened in these years). Thereafter, vacancy rates once again increased as did real RN wages, indicating the development of yet another RN shortage. However, before examining this shortage, we first consider another important change in the nurse labor market that involved the deterioration in RNs' working conditions in hospitals.

Deterioration in Hospital RN Working Conditions

After the shortage of hospital RNs abated in the early 1990s, many RNs believed that conditions in hospitals were beginning to worsen and that the quality of patient care was beginning to decline. Hospitals were adjusting to the rapid growth of managed care organizations, which were demanding and obtaining discounts from hospitals in exchange for agreements to admit patients to hospitals belonging to their network of providers. In addition, hospitals faced the threat of mergers and aquisitions and were having to adjust to the economic discipline brought about by increasing price competition and ever-tightening government cost containment policies. To survive under these pressures, hospitals took deliberate actions to lower their costs, including labor costs, which are the largest component of hospitals' operating expenses. Some hospitals employed consultants to analyze hospital production processes and advise on how to restructure the organization and delivery of nursing care. From the perspective of many hospital RNs, however, these changes resulted in the elimination of certain RN positions (particularly in nursing research and clinical education) and cutbacks in support services and personnel (aides, orderlies, and other assistants). As hospitals continued to face economic pressures to reduce patient length of stay, RNs had shorter periods of time to provide nursing services to an increasingly ill and needy patient population. Newspaper accounts flourished describing stories of overworked RNs and poor quality of care, and national nursing associations spoke out frequently about how the changes occurring in hospitals were affecting the RN workforce negatively.

Complaints became so numerous that in 1995 the secretary of Health and Human Services requested that the Institute of Medicine (IOM) convene a study to investigate these and other concerns extending beyond the hospital workplace (Wunderlich, Sloan, & Davis, 1996). The IOM Committee on the Adequacy of

Nurse Staffing in Hospitals and Nursing Homes examined a wide range of issues involving hospital staffing levels, future supply and demand for nurses, use
of unlicensed assistive personnel, and the potential adverse impact of hospital
restructuring on nurses and patients. With regard to the relationship between
hospital nurse staffing and quality of care, the lack of empirical evidence at the
time prevented the IOM from reaching definitive conclusions on this matter.[6] The
report issued by the IOM committee emphasized how the role of RNs was expected to change in the future as a consequence of managed care and other
forces affecting hospitals, and although it made no recommendations on the
supply and demand for nurses, the report seemed to support the prevailing view
that there would be enough RNs during the foreseeable future.

Only 2 years after the IOM issued this report in 1978, hospitals began to report another shortage of RNs. But this time, unlike hospital RN shortages of
previous decades, the nursing shortage was concentrated in intensive care units
(ICUs), step-down units, operating rooms (ORs) and postanesthesia recovery
units (PARUs; American Organization of Nurse Executives, 1998; Kuhl, 1999;
"Acute Shortages," 1999). Although later in 2001, hospitals reported that the
shortage had spread to general medical and surgical units, during the late 1990s
it was not apparent why this new shortage had begun in these hospital specialty
care units. To understand this trend, we need to examine how the aging of RNs
that we have described in previous chapters was already affecting the age composition of the RN workforce by the late 1990s.

INFLUENCE OF A CHANGING AGE COMPOSITION OF THE RN WORKFORCE ON THE DEVELOPMENT OF THE CURRENT SHORTAGE OF RNs[7]

In this section, we will see that work settings that rely on younger RNs and
older diploma-educated RNs, both of which were decreasing by the late 1990s,
were susceptible to shortages of RNs. To appreciate how substantially the age
and educational composition of the RN workforce was changing, it is useful to
recap the two major factors driving the long-run supply of RNs. First, there have
been smaller numbers of people entering the age 20 to 29 pool of potential

---

[6] As we shall see in Chapter 12, the findings of the IOM report stimulated the development of studies that later provided evidence of the impact of hospital nurse staffing on patient outcomes, including
mortality.

[7] This section and the following section are adapted, in part, from Buerhaus, P., Staiger, D., & Auerbach, D. (2000). Why are shortages of RNs concentrated in hospital specialty care units? *Nursing
Economic$, 18*(3),111–116.

nursing students each year during the 1970s and 1980s compared to the large number of people who were born during the baby boom years (1946 to 1964, discussed in Chapter 7). Second, the women's movement that began in the 1960s had resulted in expanding career options for women in the 1980s and 1990s, leading many to choose nonnursing careers (as described in Chapter 8). The combination of these developments resulted in a much smaller percentage of younger women who were born in the late 1960s and 1970s choosing to become RNs after graduating from high school compared to those born in earlier decades (the 1950s). Consequently, the number of younger RNs who entered the workforce each year in the late 1980s and 1990s was much smaller compared to the number of younger age RNs who were born years earlier during the baby boom generation.

Aging RN Workforce

Over the past 25 years, these changes have been profoundly altering the age composition of the hospital RN workforce. Based on our analysis of CPS data shown in **Figure 11-4**, through about 1995 there was a dramatic growth in the number of middle-aged RNs (those between 35 and 49 years of age) and an equally dramatic decline in the number of younger RNs (those between 21 and 34 years of age). Since 1995, the number of middle-aged and younger RNs has been relatively stable, but the number of older RNs (those over 50 years of age) has increased substantially. A close look at Figure 11-4 shows that in 1983 there were approximately 250,000 middle aged FTE RNs, but by 1998 the number had more than doubled to more than 600,000. The decline in the number of younger RNs in the hospital RN workforce over the same period is equally remarkable, falling from an estimated 500,000 in 1983 (the largest age group in the hospital RN workforce at the time) to roughly 350,000 by 1998. Additionally, as seen in Figure 11-4, in 1983 there were a little more than 100,000 older FTE RNs, but by 1998 the number had doubled, reaching approximately 200,000 (and had quadrupled to nearly 400,000 by 2006).

When these trends in the aging of the RN workforce are projected into the future (as described in Chapter 10), we expect that baby-boomer RNs over the age of 50 will dominate the RN workforce in the near future, and as they begin to retire in large numbers around 2015, a very large shortage of RNs will begin to develop. However, we have already observed a declining number of certain types of RNs, particularly the number of younger RNs and those who received their basic nursing education in diploma programs. Age and education data derived from the National Sample Survey of Registered Nurses in **Figure 11-5** indicate that although the total number of FTE RNs increased steadily from 1977

Figure 11-4   Hospital FTE RNs by Age, 1983–2006

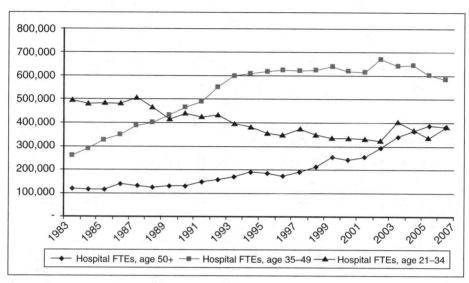

Source: Current Population Survey data

through 2004, the number of diploma-prepared FTE RNs in the workforce has declined since 1988, and the number of RNs under 40 years of age has declined since 1992.

RN Shortages in Intensive Care Units and Operating Rooms

The declining numbers of both younger RNs and older RNs who were educated in diploma nursing programs implies that shortages of RNs will develop first in settings that rely on these types of RNs. **Figure 11-6** shows that more than half of RNs who worked in ICUs in 2000 were under the age of 40. Two reasons likely explain why ICUs attract relatively younger RNs. First, the development of ICUs began to expand in the 1960s, and the number of hospitals with ICUs increased rapidly in the 1970s and 1980s. Nursing students in the 1970s and 1980s, who, by the latter part of the 1990s, would have aged into their late 30s and early 40s, would have been more likely to have had clinical rotations in ICUs during their nursing education compared to those who received their education in the 1960s. After graduation, therefore, these RNs would have been more likely to have taken positions in ICUs compared to RNs who entered nursing during earlier decades when ICUs were far less prevalent. The second

Figure 11-5   Total FTE RNs, RNs Under Age 40, and Diploma-Prepared RNs, 1977–2004

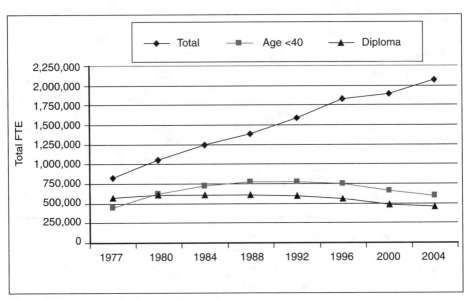

Source: National Sample Survey of Registered Nurses

explanation for why ICUs employ a large percentage of younger RNs is based on numerous conversations with clinicians and administrators who indicate that the greater use of technology combined with the excitement and challenge of the ICU environment attracts younger RNs more than older RNs.

As indicated in Chapter 7, the size of graduating classes of RNs was beginning to shrink beginning with the 1997–1998 academic year compared to the size of graduating classes in the 1970s and 1980s. Additionally, data in Figure 11-4 indicate that there were far fewer younger RNs in the late 1990s than in the 1980s, the very ages in which many RNs tend to be attracted to the ICU setting. The current shortage of hospital RNs, which began in 1998 with reports of a shortage of ICU RNs, developed in part because of the shrinking supply of younger RNs from which ICUs have typically drawn. Stated differently, the propensity of younger RNs to work in ICUs, combined with the decrease in the number of younger RNs in the workforce, resulted in too few younger RNs available to satisfy ICUs' demand by the late 1990s.

With respect to the declining number of older RNs who received their education in diploma programs, data in Figure 11-6 show that the highest percentage (greater than 30%) of diploma-prepared RNs work in ORs, PARUs, and in the

Figure 11-6   RNs Working in Various Inpatient Settings under Age 40 and Percentage with Diploma Education in 2000

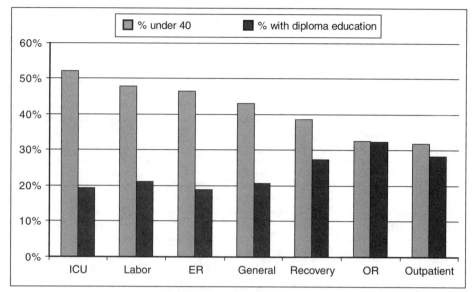

Source: National Sample Survey of Registered Nurses

outpatient setting. We believe the reason diploma-prepared RNs are more likely to work in these settings is explained by examining when these RNs completed their basic nursing education in hospitals. Before the 1970s, more RNs received their basic nursing education in 3-year diploma programs than from associate or baccalaureate degree programs (see Chapter 7, Table 7-4). Because 3-year diploma programs are based in hospitals, students had significantly greater exposure to all hospital clinical units, including the OR, than did 2-year associate and 4-year baccalaureate degree nursing programs that were steadily replacing hospital-based diploma programs in the 1980s. The shift away from diploma programs meant that younger college-educated nursing students in the 1970s and 1980s were less likely to have had the same amount and quality of exposure to the OR than RNs who had been educated principally in hospital-based diploma programs. Therefore, the large numbers of diploma graduates of the 1950s, 1960s, and 1970s would be more likely to have taken positions in the OR and recovery room following graduation compared to graduates of associate and baccalaureate programs.

In addition, the timing of the changeover in nursing education programs accounts for why the average age of diploma graduates is much higher than nondiploma graduates as shown in **Figure 11-7**. In 1996, diploma graduates

Figure 11-7   Average Age of FTE RNs by Degree, 1977–2004

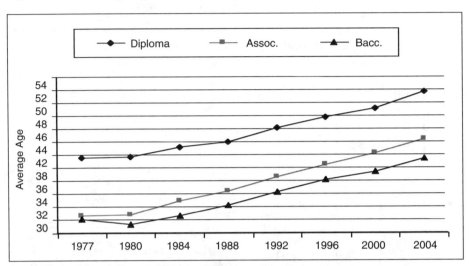

Source: National Sample Survey of Registered Nurses

were, on average, 8 years older than associate degree graduates and 10 years older than RNs with a baccalaureate degree. Also notice that in **Figure 11-8** the proportion of the RN FTE hospital workforce composed of diploma graduates had been shrinking rapidly since 1977 and that the percentage of the workforce with an associate's degree exceeded those with a diploma certificate by 1996.

Taken together, these trends suggest that many older RNs, particularly those who were diploma graduates working in ORs and PARUs, were beginning to reduce the number of hours worked or retire altogether during the late 1990s, with the result that hospitals reported shortages of RNs in these specialty units. Moreover, the shortage of RNs in ORs and PARUs was probably exacerbated by the increasing demand for RNs, as reflected by the increasing number of surgeries that were being performed, particularly in the growing number of lower overhead ambulatory care surgi-centers, which required RNs with operating room experience (Patterson, 1998).

Changes in RN Wages and Reported Hospital Vacancy Rates: 2002 to 2006

The initial development of the current hospital RN shortage started as a result of the changing age and education composition of RNs, which decreased the

Figure 11-8 FTE RN Workforce by Degree and Percentage of Total, 1977–2004

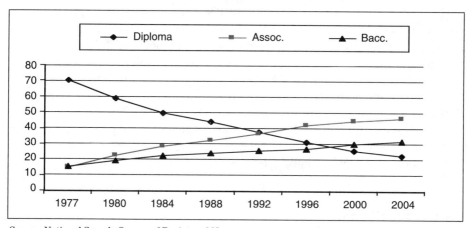

Source: National Sample Survey of Registered Nurses

supply of RNs in specialty care settings. Over the next few years, the shortage spread into other units throughout hospitals as inpatient RN demand began to increase considerably (outpatient demand had been increasing strongly throughout the 1990s) coincident with the decreasing impact of managed care that had begun to occur. In addition, as discussed earlier, hospital-employed RNs had experienced a difficult workplace environment throughout much of the decade, and their real wages had grown very little since 1993. Enrollment into nursing education programs also had been falling rapidly since 1995, and the production of new graduates began to decrease significantly by the late 1990s.

In 1999, hospital RN vacancy rates had increased to 5.6%, and in 2000 they increased again to 8.1% (see Figure 11-3). By the end of 2001, vacancy rates had jumped to 13%, and a survey conducted for the American Hospital Association found that nearly one in five hospitals reported vacancy rates averaging more than 20% (First Consulting Group, 2001). The survey also reported that nationally hospitals were unable to fill 126,000 full-time RN positions. A year later, in 2002, the federal government's Health Resources and Services Administration reported that 30 states were experiencing shortages, and they estimated that total demand for RNs exceeded supply by 110,000 (U.S. Department of Health and Human Services, 2002). Not since the early 1990s had the average national hospital RN vacancy rate exceeded 10%.

As described in Chapter 6, hospitals responded to the shortage of RNs by increasing RN wages substantially (see Table 6-4) in 2002 and 2003, which led to a very large growth in hospital RN employment (nearly 185,000, the largest

2-year increase in RN employment in more than 25 years) and a subsequent decrease in vacancy rates to 8.1% (see Figure 11-3).

In 2004 and 2005, the growth in real RN wages stopped, hospital RN employment subsequently decreased by more than 50,000 FTE RNs, and the RN vacancy rate increased to 8.5%. In 2006, hospitals raised real RN wages slightly
and vacancy rates dropped back to 8.1%, but hospitals still reported that 116,000
RN positions remained unfilled. Unlike the hospital RN shortages of the 1960s,
1970s, 1980s, and early 1990s that were transitory until wage increases brought
the demand and supply of RNs into equilibrium, the current shortage that began
in hospital specialty units in 1998 has lasted 10 years. Based on the analyses reported in this chapter, it appears that further wage increases will be needed to
bring about a new equilibrium in the hospital RN labor market.

CHAPTER SUMMARY

Although hospitals have reported shortages of RNs in every decade since
the 1960s, there is no overall agreement about how to define and measure hospital RN shortages. Adopting an economic perspective in which an RN shortage
is reflected by hospitals' demand for RNs exceeding the existing supply of RNs
at the prevailing wage rate, and measuring RN shortages by vacancy rates reported by hospitals, we have shown that most hospital RN shortages since the
mid-1960s were driven by increases in the demand for RNs and were resolved
after hospitals increased real wages.

The new financial resources provided by the Medicare program in 1966 allowed hospitals to increase RN wages, which subsequently reduced vacancy
rates to below 10% by 1969. During the 1970s, the demand for RNs continued to
grow, but wage controls imposed by the federal government and very high inflation rates combined to restrict the increase in RN wages from rising fast
enough to bring the demand and supply of RNs into equilibrium. Consequently,
shortages of RNs were reported during the decade, and vacancy rates once again
exceeded double digit levels by 1980. After hospitals responded by increasing
real wages in the early 1980s, RN vacancy rates fell, and the shortage ended
quickly. With the beginning of Medicare's prospective payment system in 1983,
hospitals faced new incentives for efficiency and began to employ more RNs
compared to LPNs and aides due to their greater productivity and relatively low
wages. Through the decade, hospitals' demand for RNs increased approximately
3% annually, and despite increases in real wages, the supply of RNs was unable
to catch up to the significant growth in demand, resulting in hospitals once again
reporting RN shortages throughout the 1980s.

During the 1990s, the growth in the demand for RNs slowed to about 2% per year as managed care developed rapidly and slowed the growth in demand for health care overall and hospitals specifically. This lower demand for RNs led to lower wages and to lower vacancy rates, ending the RN shortage. The increased number of RNs graduating from nursing education programs and joining the RN workforce resulted in an apparent surplus of RNs during the mid-1990s, and real earnings and vacancy rates declined. Hospitals reacted to external economic pressures that forced them to become more efficient, but, in the eyes of RNs, their workloads grew more difficult and working conditions deteriorated as support services were scaled back at the same time that increasingly ill patients spent ever shorter amounts of time in the hospitals. By the end of the decade, yet another RN shortage was reported by hospitals, but, in this case, the shortage was concentrated in intensive care units and operating rooms.

When we analyzed data on RNs by age categories, hospital unit, and educational background, we found that the shortage broke out in these units because they were the first to experience the implications of underlying changes in the age and educational composition of the RN workforce that resulted in a decreased supply of certain types of RNs. Shortages reported by ICUs and step-down units resulted from a decrease in the number of younger RNs entering the workforce who have a greater propensity than older RNs to work in these settings. Shortages in ORs are explained by the decline in the number of older diploma-educated graduates, who had a greater propensity to work in this setting, as they left the workforce due to retirement. This analysis demonstrated that unlike the earlier shortages that were driven by increases in demand, the shortage that developed in 1998 was driven by supply-side factors reflected by the changing age composition of the RN workforce.

Finally, in the early 2000s, the hospital RN shortage had spread hospital wide, vacancy rates had increased again to double-digit levels, and despite increases in real RN wages in 4 of the last 5 years, national vacancy rates remained above 8.0% by the end of 2006. As the shortage continued in 2007, it became the longest lasting shortage of hospital RNs in the past 50 years.

Next, in Chapter 12, we peer behind the numbers that indicate the presence of RN shortages and examine how different clinicians and administrators perceive the impact of the current hospital nursing shortage on hospitals, nurses, and patients. Data obtained from national surveys of RNs, physicians, hospital chief executive officers, and chief nursing executives reveal how the current shortage has affected care delivery processes, the capacity of hospitals to provide patient care, the ability of RNs to provide patient care, and the quality and safety of patient care.

Appendix 11-1

Why Hospitals Are Often Slow to Increase RN Wages When Experiencing a Shortage of RNs

Given that increasing wages has a positive impact on increasing employment from the existing supply of RNs (the substitution effect), one might reasonably think that whenever there are shortages, hospitals would automatically raise wages to increase the amount of short-run labor (increased participation and hours worked) by existing RNs. Yet hospitals do not necessarily react in this manner and, in fact, it might take considerable time before they determine that it is in their economic interest to raise RN wages. For a number of reasons, hospitals might be slow to react to a shortage of RNs by increasing RN wages.

Hospitals Might Not Realize a Shortage Exists

It takes time for hospitals to realize that a shortage of RNs exists. Hospitals face constant fluctuations in nurse staffing, and therefore it takes some period of time before enough data are available for hospital decision makers to comprehend that a shortage of RNs actually exists as opposed to staffing fluctuations. For example, hospitals might realize they are experiencing staffing shortfalls, but they might believe the shortfall is due to local, temporary factors arising from, say, a sudden increase in demand due to an outbreak of flu in the community or some other illness that has increased admissions. Alternatively, hospitals might perceive that a shortage is caused by RNs leaving their organizations due to a wave of nurses who take maternity leaves at the same time. Additionally, there might have been some unanticipated development within the local nursing education program that is causing nursing students to unexpectedly withdraw their employment or reduce their hours. In these and similar cases, hospitals might believe that the shortage is temporary and will resolve itself in a matter of weeks or months as these conditions subside, and thus they would be reluctant to increase RN wages. Hospitals also might believe that there are existing nurses in their community who are available to fill these vacant positions and decide to run advertisements to inform nurses that nursing positions are available. In sum, shortages of RNs take time to develop and often originate from temporary and unique local circumstances, and it takes hospitals time to realize that a shortage of RNs is occurring and understand why it has developed.

Hospitals Do Not Know How Much to Raise Wages

When hospital leaders realize the hospital is facing a shortage of nurses that is not explained by temporary changes in local circumstances, they must decide how to react. To be sure, raising RN wages and advertising this information is one strategy. However, when contemplating whether to implement this strategy, hospitals must first decide how much to increase wages. Should they increase RN wages by $0.25 per hour, $0.50 per hour, $1.00 per hour, $1.50 per hour, or $4.00 per hour? Hospitals simply do not know how much wages will have to increase to raise participation and hours worked from the existing supply of RNs. As discussed in detail in Chapter 6, economists have conducted studies aimed at determining the effect a wage increase will have on inducing an increase in participation and hours worked. However, those studies are not particularly helpful because they are not current and were based on national, regional, or state level data. Consequently, hospital decision makers rarely have access to timely analysis of the effects of wage changes on the short-run labor supply decisions of RNs in their local labor market. Because labor costs account for the largest component of hospital expenditures, and nurses account for the largest portion of labor costs, a wage increase will have a direct and significant impact on raising hospital costs. Guessing at what might be the right wage increase is a risky undertaking, and hence hospitals are understandably cautious in making such a decision.

Fear That Raising Wages Might Actually *Decrease* Employment

Labor economists have identified the existence within the nurse labor market of what is termed a "backward bending labor supply curve" (see Chapter 6). As wages rise, holding other things constant, some RNs might decide to reduce their participation, or if they are already working, decrease their time by switching from full- to part-time status. The wage increase raises the total level of income available to the RN, and one of the things a nurse might purchase with this added income is more leisure time (the negative income effect dominates the positive substitution effect in response to the wage increase). Not all nurses are likely to react to a wage increase in this way, but some RNs might, and a hospital has no way of knowing which nurses are likely to react in this manner or at which wage level an increase in wages will result in nurses reducing their employment rather than increasing it.

Less Costly Alternatives

Because increasing wages to combat a shortage of RNs raises a hospital's labor costs substantially and might not result quickly in a sufficient increase in participation and hours worked, hospitals have an economic incentive to pursue other, less costly means to increase the short-run supply of RNs. Although some collective bargaining agreements might limit the options a hospital can pursue, hospitals are likely to offer overtime hours at increased pay per hour, pay a premium for working double shifts, hire RNs from temporary employment agencies, develop in-house supplemental staffing teams, hire nursing students or non-RNs such as licensed practical/vocational nurses, employ "traveler" nurses, or hire RNs who received their nursing education in other countries. Many hospitals believe that such responses are less expensive than granting a wage increase, particularly if they believe the shortage is temporary. Moreover, from a hospital's perspective, if they were to raise wages, the increase would apply to the RNs they already employ as well as any new RNs they seek to hire. In addition, any new hires would receive not only the higher wage, but the hospital would have to pay nonwage fringe benefits to all of the additional nurses it employs, adding further to its total labor costs. Such a decision has enormous economic consequences that understandably cause some hospitals to carefully assess the costs of all available alternatives to raising RN wages, all of which takes time.

Collusion Among Hospitals

In many communities, the hospital is the sole employer of RNs whereas in other communities two or three hospitals dominate the labor market for RNs (monopsonists). In such communities, it is possible that hospitals might explicitly, or more likely tacitly, agree not to increase RN wages even in the presence of a shortage. From the perspective of hospitals who are in such markets, if one hospital raises wages, it is likely that others will feel pressure to increase their wages to avoid losing some of their RN employees to the hospital that raised RN wages. Thus, hospitals experience powerful incentives to work together to control the labor market for RNs; by cooperating, they can avoid a large increase in operating costs associated with raising wages as well as avoid other costs associated with turnover and adding new employees.

Prior to the enactment of the Medicare and Medicaid programs in the mid-1960s, evidence suggests that the hospitals likely colluded to set RN wages below the equilibrium level. However, studies by economists to determine whether widespread hospital collusion to prevent wage increases has continued since the

1960s offer mixed findings. Thus, while it is likely that some hospitals in certain markets behave as monopsonists with respect to controlling nurse wages, it is difficult to ascertain the extent to which hospitals act like cartels and exert their economic power over the nurse labor market. Data discussed throughout this chapter, which shows that hospitals consistently increased real RN wages following the outbreak of shortages in the 1980s, 1990s, and during the 2000s, suggest that at least in these years it is unlikely that the majority of hospitals were behaving as monopsonists.

In sum, the preceding factors represent a formidable set of considerations that can reduce the speed with which hospitals increase wages in response to a shortage of RNs.

REFERENCES

Acute shortages of health-care professionals fester nationwide. (1999, September 14). *The Wall Street Journal*, p. A1.

Aiken, L., Blendon, R., & Rodgers, D. (1981). The shortage of hospital nurses: A new perspective. *Annals of Internal Medicine, 95*, 365–372.

American Organization of Nurse Executives. (1998). *Research on nurse shortages*. Scottsdale, AZ: The HSM Group, Inc.

Arrow, K., & Capron, W. (1950). Dynamic shortages and price rises: The engineer-scientist case. *Quarterly Journal of Economics, 307*, 292–308.

Buerhaus, P. (1987). Not just another nursing shortage. *Nursing Economic$, 5*(6), 267–279.

Buerhaus, P. (1995). Economic pressures building in the hospital employed RN labor market. *Nursing Economic$, 123*(3), 137–141.

Buerhaus, P., & Staiger, D. (1996). Managed care and the nurse workforce. *The Journal of the American Medical Association, 276*(18), 1487–1493.

Buerhaus, P., Staiger, D., & Auerbach, D. (2000). Why are shortages of RNs concentrated in hospital specialty care units? *Nursing Economic$, 18*(3), 111–116.

First Consulting Group. (2001). *The healthcare workforce shortage and its implications for America's hospitals*. American Hospital Association. Retrieved December 10, 2007, from http://www.aha.org/aha/content/2001/pdf/FcgWorkforceReport.pdf

Grumbach, K., Ash, M., Seago, J., Spetz, J., & Coffman, J. (2001). Measuring shortages of hospital nurses: How do you know a hospital with a nursing shortage when you see one? *Medical Care Research and Review, 58*(4), 387–403.

Kuhl, A. (1999). Emerging responses to the specialty nurse shortage: Leveraging critical care training. *Nursing Watch, 2*. Washington, DC: The Advisory Board Company, The Nursing Executive Center.

Patterson, P. (1998). Salary/career survey: Hospitals. *OR Manager, 14*(10), 18, 20.

U.S. Department of Health and Human Services. (2002). *Projected Supply, demand, and shortages of registered nurses: 2000–2020*. Washington, DC: Health Resources and Services Administration, Bureau of Health Professions, National Center for Health Workforce Analysis.

Wunderlich, G., Sloan, F., & Davis, C. (Eds.). (1996). Institute of Medicine, Committee on the Adequacy of Nurse Staffing in Hospitals and Nursing Homes. *Nursing staff in hospitals and nursing homes. Is it adequate?* Washington, DC: National Academies Press.

Yett, D. (1975). *An economic analysis of the nurse shortage.* Lexington, MA: D.C. Heath.

CHAPTER 12

Impact of the Current Shortage of Hospital Registered Nurses

As we discussed in Chapter 11, shortages of hospital RNs have occurred in every decade since the 1960s. When hospitals increased RN wages, most of these shortages eventually resolved, some sooner than others. The current shortage that began in 1998 and entered its 10th year in 2007 has not yet ended. For several reasons the current hospital RN shortage has generated an unusual amount of public policy attention and media coverage. First, unlike previous shortages, it developed at the same time that a global shortage of nurses was unfolding (Buchan & Calman, 2004). Second, shortly after it was first being reported, forecasts were published of a much larger shortage developing in the United States due to the anticipated retirement of large numbers of RNs between 2012 and 2020 (Buerhaus, Staiger, & Auerbach, 2000). Third, the current shortage developed at the very same time that a national interest in the quality and safety of health care was taking root in the United States. Initially thought to be a fad by some, the quality movement has proven to be remarkably persistent. More importantly, quality improvement organizations and prominent health policy leaders and researchers have begun to view the current nursing shortage less as a problem for the nurse labor market and hospitals to sort out but more as a serious threat to the quality and safety of patient care provided in hospitals.

Our purpose in this chapter is to probe inside the current nursing shortage, getting underneath vacancy rates reported by hospitals and changes in RN wages, and to focus on how the shortage has affected the quality and safety of patient care in U.S. hospitals. We begin by providing an overview of the development of the quality and safety improvement environment and how this movement began changing views about the current nursing shortage. Following this, we summarize some of the major studies that have provided evidence that patients who are treated in low staffed hospitals are at increased risk of experiencing complications of care, adverse outcomes, and even death. We conclude the chapter by describing the results of national surveys of RNs, physicians, and hospital chief executive and chief nursing officers that were conducted in the midst of the current shortage of hospital RNs to determine their perceptions of its impact on hospitals, nurses, and patients.

OVERVIEW OF THE QUALITY AND SAFETY IMPROVEMENT ENVIRONMENT

The shortages of hospital RNs between the 1960s and early 1990s that were described in Chapter 11 occurred when there was much less national interest in improving either the quality or safety of patient care. In contrast, when the current shortage of hospital RNs developed, there was a tremendous amount of activity occurring that coalesced into a national focus on improving patient care quality and safety. **Table 12-1** identifies several of the main organizations that have led this improvement and provides a brief description of selected initiatives that are related to the quality and safety of hospital care provided by RNs.

Development of a National Movement to Improve Quality and Safety

In the 1990s, studies began to quantify the incidence of injuries and threats to patient safety (Leape, et al., 1991; Brennan, et al., 1991; Leape, Lawthers, Brennan, & Johson, 1993; Leape, 1994). As the number of avoidable adverse events and their effects on patients began to be broadly recognized, efforts quickly developed that were aimed at motivating healthcare organizations and individual clinicians to change their thinking and behavior to reduce the occurrence of adverse events. Leaders of the nascent quality and patient safety improvement movement embraced a systems perspective that stressed identifying and correcting failures in the organization of healthcare delivery systems rather than blaming individual clinicians for mistakes and injuries caused by accidents (Leape, et al., 1995). Human factors research influenced this perspective by providing insight into how non-healthcare industries have designed quality and safety into the production of goods and services.

In 2000, the concern over patient safety reached a tipping point when the Institute of Medicine (IOM) of the National Academies of Science published *To Err is Human: Building a Safer Health System*. This report indicated that medical errors resulted in as many as 98,000 deaths in hospitals each year. The intense media attention that this report received prompted Congress to allocate millions of dollars to federal agencies to fund research on the quality and safety of care. Subsequently, not only did the volume and breadth of studies that focused on improving safety and quality accelerate dramatically, but over time the Agency for Healthcare Research and Quality (AHRQ), Center for Medicare and Medicaid

Table 12-1   **Selected Quality and Safety Organizations and Sample of Initiatives Affecting RNs in Hospitals**

Organization	Major National Initiatives Since 2000 Related to Nurses
Institute of Medicine	• Published high-profile reports on quality and safety of patient care: *To Err is Human: Building a Safer Health System* (2000) *Crossing the Quality Chasm: A New Health System for the 21st Century* (2001) *Keeping Patients Safe: Transforming the Work Environment of Nurses* (2004) • Advocated six aims to improve the quality of health-care systems (patient centered, safe, effective, equitable, timely, and efficient) (2001)
National Quality Forum	• Endorsed 15 national voluntary consensus standards for nursing sensitive care in hospitals (2004)
Institute for Healthcare Improvement	• Implemented national hospital "100,000 Lives Campaign" (2005) • Implementing national hospital "5 Million Lives Campaign" (2006–2008)
Joint Commission	• Established a national Nursing Advisory Committee (2003) • Endorsed National Quality Forum's 15 national voluntary consensus standards for nursing sensitive care in hospitals (2005) • Included nurse-sensitive measures in hospital accreditation process (2005)
Robert Wood Johnson Foundation	• Developed the Transforming Care at the Bedside initiative (2005) • Partnered with the Institute for Healthcare Improvement and American Organization of Nurse Executives (2007) • Developed Interdisciplinary Nursing Quality Research Initiative (2006)

Services (CMS), and many private organizations began publishing quality and safety indicators for identifying, monitoring, comparing, and publicly reporting the performance of organizations (Romano, 2005).

The IOM produced follow-up reports on the quality and safety of patient care, including two reports that gained particular attention. In 2001, *Crossing the Quality Chasm: A New Health System for the 21st Century* identified a comprehensive agenda for transforming the healthcare system, and it advocated six aims for improving the quality of systems of care in the United States. According to the report, healthcare systems should aim to provide care that is safe, timely, effective, patient centered, equitable, and efficient. These aims were subsequently recognized by the Accreditation Council for Graduate Medical Education, which now mandates graduate medical education and postgraduate training programs to provide education in systems-based thinking and practice-based learning and improvement (Leach, 2002). Moreover, medical specialty boards began to establish requirements for physicians to demonstrate appropriate competency in each of these six aims for acquiring and maintaining clinical licensure (Brennan, et al., 2004). Another IOM report released in 2004, *Keeping Patients Safe: Transforming the Work Environment of Nurses* (Page, 2004), focused on improving patient safety linked to nursing and provided 17 recommendations to improve the work environment of nurses (Chapter 13 examines in detail how the hospital work environment has changed during the current RN shortage).

Another stimulant to the development of the quality and safety movement in the United States was the development of the National Quality Forum (NQF). In the late 1990s, the NQF was established as a private, not-for-profit membership organization to develop and implement a national strategy for healthcare quality measurement and reporting. The NQF also embraces the six aims for improving the quality of healthcare systems advocated by the IOM. The NQF has conducted projects aimed at endorsing and promoting voluntary use of consensus-based national standards for various conditions and healthcare organizations, including mammography centers, ambulatory care, serious reportable events, nursing home and hospital care, cardiac surgery, palliative and hospice care, adult diabetes care, home care, behavioral health care, and others. Through 2006 NQF has endorsed more than 300 measures, indicators, events, practices, and other products to help assess quality across the healthcare continuum.

In 2004, the NQF was funded by a grant from the Robert Wood Johnson Foundation (RWJF) to evaluate the quality of nursing care. After carefully assessing the scientific evidence supporting more than 150 potential measures, the NQF endorsed 15 national voluntary consensus standards for nursing sensitive care—eight patient-, three nursing-, and four systems-centered standards. The patient-centered standards include death among surgical inpatients with treatable serious complications (failure to rescue), pressure ulcer prevalence, falls prevalence, falls with injury, restraint prevalence, urinary catheter-associated urinary tract infection for intensive care unit (ICU) patients, central line catheter-associated bloodstream infection rate for ICU and high-risk nursery patients (HRN), and ventilator-associated pneumonia for ICU and HRN patients. The three nursing-centered standards include smoking cessation counseling for patients with acute myocardial infarction, heart failure, and pneumonia. The four systems-centered standards include skill mix of nurses, nursing care hours per patient day, the practice environment of nurses, and voluntary turnover of nurses. The NQF acknowledged the mixed evidence in the literature on these standards and recommended that additional research be conducted to expand the evidence base on these and other potential standards. Importantly, however, the involvement of the NQF focused attention on the contributions of nurses and the ongoing nursing shortage with respect to the quality and safety of hospital patient care. In 2007, the NQF received funding from the RWJF to establish a tracking system for capturing and reporting adoption and use of the NQF-endorsed consensus standards, identify the successes and challenges experienced by users of the standards, and identify technical and other issues that are barriers to uniform implementation, and communicate these to measure developers and key stakeholders.

The programs and initiatives developed by the Institute for Healthcare Improvement (IHI) are another important development in helping build the national focus on improving the quality and safety of patient care. The IHI has engaged hundreds of hospitals, clinics, and other organizations in dozens of initiatives aimed at educating providers, creating a culture of safety, making and testing change, and monitoring individual and systems level processes and outcomes. Among its most visible initiatives, the IHI and partner organizations launched the "100,000 Lives Campaign," which was a national voluntary effort aimed at reducing preventable deaths in U.S. hospitals. The IHI estimates that 3100 hospitals participated in the campaign and that by adopting six changes in how they provided patient care, these hospitals saved an estimated 122,000 lives during an 18-month period. IHI has followed this initiative with a "5 Million Lives Campaign" that is aimed at enlisting 4000 hospitals to adopt six new changes in providing patient care (in addition to the six used in its earlier campaign) with a goal of preventing 5 million injuries to patients. IHI estimates that there are 15 million preventable injuries per year, and this initiative is an attempt to cut that by one-third over the 2-year period December 2006 to December 2008.

The Joint Commission is the principal organization that accredits hospitals and other healthcare organizations in the United States. The commission has increasingly exerted its substantial influence to improve the quality and safety of patient care. With respect to nursing, the Joint Commission has established a national Nursing Advisory Committee, endorsed the NQF voluntary nursing performance standards, produced several reports on the nursing shortage, and conducted national and regional conferences aimed at resolving the current shortage and improving quality of care linked to nurses. In addition, in its hospital accreditation process, the Joint Commission included nursing-sensitive measures that require examination of a minimum of two clinical or service-related indicators and two human resource–related indicators. The clinical indicators can be selected from measures of family complaints, patient complaints, patient falls, adverse drug events, injuries to patients, skin breakdown, pneumonia, postoperative infections, urinary tract infections, upper gastrointestinal bleeding, shock/cardiac arrest, or length of stay. The human resource indicators can be selected from measures of overtime, vacancy rate, staff satisfaction, staff turnover rate, understaffing as compared to the hospital's staffing plan, nursing hours per patient day, injuries on the job, on call or per diem use, and sick time.

Finally, efforts by the RWJF have connected the growing emphasis on improving quality and safety to the resolution of the current nursing shortage and to concerns about the adequacy of the future nursing workforce. In 2005, the RWJF and IHI joined together to develop a multihospital initiative, Transforming Care at the Bedside (TCAB), to create, test, and implement changes to improve care on medical and surgical units and improve staff satisfaction in 13 hospitals. In 2007, the RWJF provided funding to expand the TCAB program to 68 hospitals across the nation. In addition to TCAB, in 2006 the RWJF began a 5-year, $10 million program, The Interdisciplinary Nursing Quality Research Initiative (INQRI), that is aimed at addressing gaps in knowledge about the relationship between nursing and the quality of health care. This program specifically seeks to involve economists, engineers, political scientists, sociologists, and others to work with nurses to generate, disseminate, and translate research findings to improve the quality of care provided in hospitals.

In sum, unlike the circumstances surrounding earlier hospital nursing shortages, the current shortage of RNs has unfolded at the same time that a multifaceted national effort to improve quality and safety was emerging. Increasingly, quality improvement organizations and prominent leaders in the field view the current nursing shortage more in terms of a threat to quality and safety in addition to a serious health workforce problem.

Next we briefly review the key evidence that established the relationship between hospital nurse staffing and patient outcomes and that has contributed to the understanding that nurses are critical to the improvement of quality and the creation of safer patient care environments.

PATIENT OUTCOMES ASSOCIATED WITH HOSPITAL NURSE STAFFING

Interest in the current hospital shortage of RNs grew as an increasing number of studies provided evidence relating low nurse staffing in hospitals to

increased risk of adverse patient outcomes. In particular, just as hospital vacancy rates reached 13% at the end of 2001 and hospitals reported more than
126,000 vacant RN positions (as described in Chapter 11), studies published in
The New England Journal of Medicine (Needleman, Buerhaus, Mattke, Stewart, & Zelevinsky, 2002) and in *The Journal of the American Medical Association* (Aiken, Clarke, Sloane, Sochalski, & Silber, 2002) received extensive media
coverage.[1] These two studies provided strong evidence that inadequate hospital nurse staffing is associated with a number of complications, including death.
Consequently, organizations concerned with improving quality and patient
safety, physicians, and the public began taking greater notice of the current
nursing shortage and expressing concern over its impact. For example, in par-
allel national surveys of physicians and the public about medical errors, 53%
of physicians and 65% of the public identified understaffing of nurses in hospitals as very important causes of medical errors (Blendon, et al., 2002). Moreover, physicians reported only two approaches as very effective in reducing
errors: "requiring hospitals to develop systems to avoid medical errors" (55%)
and "increasing the number of hospital nurses" (51%; Altman, Clancy, &
Blendon, 2004).

Complexity of Studies of Hospital Nurse Staffing and Patient Outcomes

Studies on the relationship between hospital nurse staffing and patient outcomes are complicated because they have used a variety of data sources, different measures of patient outcomes and nurse staffing, and have selected either
the nursing unit level or hospital level as the focus of their analyses. To construct measures of patient outcomes, researchers have used publicly available
and relatively inexpensive administrative data (typically hospital discharge abstracts prepared by medical record departments for billing purposes) that can
yield large samples of cases for analysis. Alternatively, data needed to develop
patient outcome measures can be obtained by reviewing medical charts, which
are not as available, more expensive, and therefore usually result in smaller
samples compared to studies that use administrative data. Samples analyzed in
studies have ranged from less than 100 patients in a single hospital to well over
10 million derived from national samples of hospital patient discharge abstracts.

---

[1] Compared to other healthcare journals, the national media focuses on these two leading weekly
medical journals. Although several important studies had been published in other journals prior to
the studies by Needleman and colleagues and by Aiken and colleagues, these studies generated intense media exposure.

Additionally, some studies have included medical patients only, others included surgical patients only, and a few studies have analyzed both types of patients. Most studies reported in the literature also have excluded pediatrics and inpatient psychiatric units. Published studies have usually obtained data to measure nurse staffing from hospital human resource records or from state and special surveys. Researchers have used different measures of nurse staffing (RN hours per patient days, levels and proportions of staffing by RNs or LPNs and occasionally nursing aides, etc.), applied different criteria to define a full-time equivalent nurse, and they have used different means to overcome the important problem of separating counts of total hospital RNs into those who work in inpatient units from those who work in outpatient units. In addition to these issues, researchers have used very different analytical methods to test for relationships among variables, and they have used different characteristics of hospitals (e.g., teaching, community, level of technology) to control for differences in results that might be attributed to the hospital. Finally, studies have varied greatly in the sophistication with which they have attempted to control for the severity of patients' illnesses.

Summary of Results of Hospital Nurse Staffing Studies and Patient Outcomes

The various issues that arise when conducting research on hospital nurse staffing and patient outcomes illustrate the many challenges that must be overcome in demonstrating an empirical relationship between hospital nurse staffing and patient outcomes. However, the use of different units of analysis, different measures of patient outcomes and nurse staffing, and different analytic methods makes it difficult to directly compare the results of the growing number of studies in this area. For this reason, we provide a summary of the patient outcomes that studies have linked to hospital nurse staffing in **Table 12-2**. These studies show that nurse staffing is linked to important clinical complications and adverse outcomes that, when viewed as a whole, provide some level of confidence in the overall conclusion that nurse staffing in hospitals matters to patients' well-being.[2]

---

[2] It is beyond the scope of this chapter to provide a comprehensive review of studies on the relationship between hospital nurse staffing and quality of nursing care; rather, we focus on the range of patient outcomes that are associated with nurses that have been reported in the literature. An excellent summary of studies can be found in Clarke, S., & Donaldson, N. (2007). Nurse staffing and patient care quality and safety. In R. G. Hughes (Ed.), *Patient safety and quality: An evidence-based handbook for nurses* [AHRQ Publication No. 07-0015]. Rockville, MD: Agency for Healthcare Research and Quality.

Table 12-2   Representative Studies Reporting an Association between Hospital Nurse Staffing and Patient Outcomes

Patient Outcome	Study
Nosocomial infection	Flood & Diers (1988) Giraud, et al. (1993) Archibald, Manning, & Bell (1997)
Sepsis/bloodstream infections	Pronovost, et al. (1999) Amaravaid, Dimick, Pronovost, & Lipsett (2000) Dimick, Swoboda, Pronovost, & Lipsett (2001) Fridkin, Pear, Williamson, Galgiani, & Jarvis (1996) Cimiotti, Hass, Saiman, & Larson (2006)
Pneumonia	Needleman, Buerhaus, Mattke, Stewart, & Zelevinsky (2002) Kovner & Gergen (1998) Pronovost, et al. (1999) Amaravaidi, et al. (2000) Dimick, et al. (2001) Network (2000) Unruh (2003)
Urinary tract infection	Needleman, et al. (2002) Kovner & Gergen (1998) Network (2000) Blegen, Goode, & Reed (1998)
Falls	Blegen & Vaughn (1998) Wan & Shukla (1987) Sovie & Jawad (2001) Langemo, Anderson, & Volden (2002)
Upper gastrointestinal bleeding	Needleman, et al. (2002)
Medication errors	Blegen, et al. (1998) Blegen & Vaughn (1998)
Shock and cardiac arrest	Needleman, et al. (2002)
Pressure ulcers	Network (2000) Unruh (2003) Blegen, et al. (1998)
Longer than expected length of stay	Needleman, et al. (2002) Schultz, van Servellen, Chang, McNeese-Smith, & Waxenberg (1998) Pronovost, et al. (1999) Amaravaidi, et al. (2000) Network (2000) Dimick, et al. (2001) Flood & Diers (1988) Langemo, et al. (2002)

As shown in Table 12-2, studies have found an association between nurse staffing and hospital-acquired nosocomial infections, sepsis, pneumonia, urinary tract infection, patient falls, upper gastrointestinal bleeding, medication errors, shock and cardiac arrest, pressure ulcers, and longer than expected stays in the hospital. Studies have also examined the association of nurse staffing with mortality but have reached mixed conclusions. The study by Needleman et al. (2002) found an association between nurse staffing levels and "failure to rescue," defined in that study as death among patients who had one of five complications (pneumonia, sepsis, shock or cardiac arrest, upper gastrointestinal bleeding, and deep vein thrombosis) in surgical patients and to a lesser extent in medical patients. At least four other studies have found an association between nurse staffing and hospital mortality (Scott, Forrest, & Brown, 1976; Hartz, et al., 1989; Aiken, Smith, & Lake, 1994: Schultz, et al. 1998). With respect to neonatal patient outcomes, one study (Hamilton, Redshaw, Tarnow-Mordi, 2007) found that risk-adjusted mortality was reduced 48% when understaffed neonatal intensive care units increased the ratio of RNs with neonatal qualifications per patients to 1:1. However, other studies have not found an association between nurse staffing and adult patients (Shortell & Hughes, 1988; Al-Haider, & Wan, 1991; Shortell et al., 1994). Thus, the evidence of a relationship between hospital nurse staffing and mortality, while suggestive, remains inconclusive.

One recent study (Needleman, Buerhaus, Mattke, Stewart, & Zelevensky, 2006) sought to determine whether there was a business case for quality in hospitals by investing in nurse staffing. These investigators constructed national estimates of the cost of three options to increase nurse staffing in acute care hospitals and the costs savings of the associated reductions in patient days, deaths, and five adverse outcomes—urinary tract infection, hospital-acquired pneumonia, shock/cardiac arrest, upper gastrointestinal bleeding, and failure to rescue. Only one of the three options for increasing staffing was found to generate net savings to hospitals—raising the proportion of nursing hours provided by RNs without increasing total nursing hours (including LPNs) produced an estimated reduction of nearly 60,000 adverse outcomes, 1.5 million hospital patient days, and 4977 deaths, saving hospitals an estimated $240 million. The other two options for increasing nurse staffing were estimated to cost substantially more, and the incremental costs to hospitals would exceed any savings.

Needleman et al. (2006) argued that policy makers consider more than only the business case and take into account the social case for investing in nurse staffing. They based their argument on the fact that the cost per avoided death estimated for all three staffing options was *below* the value of a statistical life used by federal agencies in their rule making on health and safety. In other words, investing in nurse staffing would save lives at a cost that society would normally view as a bargain. In addition, the investigators did not consider the value to patients and their families of reduced morbidity (decreased pain and suffering and lost days of work), the economic value to hospitals of lower liability and improved reputation and image from reducing adverse nursing-related morbidity and mortality, or the positive effects and cost savings of increased nurse staffing in reducing adverse outcomes not considered in the analysis but which have been reported in other studies (patient falls, blood-borne infections, pressure ulcers, and medication errors). Finally, Needleman et al. (2006) point out that their study did not account for increased patient satisfaction or the benefits of patients achieving higher physical and mental function as a result of increased nurse staffing.

IMPACT OF THE CURRENT SHORTAGE OF HOSPITAL RNs: PERCEPTIONS OF PHYSICIANS, RNs, AND HOSPITAL EXECUTIVES

The delivery of hospital patient care depends on clinicians and administrators working together for the benefit of patients and families. RNs, physicians, and other health professionals provide personal health services and treatments, coordinate the activities of other professionals and support staff, and communicate with various healthcare facilities and health professionals, all of which are critical to the well-being of patients and families. Hospital chief executive officers (CEOs) and hospital chief nursing officers (CNOs) develop strategic plans; build, manage, and continually improve systems of care; and oversee resource allocations all in an effort to ensure that clinicians and support personnel have the resources needed to realize clinical and organizational goals. Of the many stresses that affect hospitals, shortages of nurses are particularly troublesome as they affect clinicians' and executives' ability to do their work and achieve their interrelated goals, potentially endanger the safety and quality of patient care, reduce access to care, and increase costs.

Most of the studies that have provided evidence of a relationship between hospital nurse staffing and patient complications were based on administrative data and were conducted prior to the onset of the current shortage of hospital RNs. Consequently, there is little empirical data directly linking the current shortage to harming the quality of patient care or decreasing safety. There is also little documentation of clinicians' and executives' perceptions of the prevalence of the RN shortage beyond reported vacancy rates, or of the impact of the current hospital RN shortage on dimensions of patient care that are not captured by administrative or other data. In this concluding section we report the results of independent national random sample surveys of RNs, physicians, and hospital

CEOs and CNOs that were conducted in the midst of the current shortage. The surveys were designed to elicit perceptions of the impact of the nursing shortage on care delivery processes, hospitals' capacity, ability of nurses to provide patient care, and the IOM's six aims for high quality healthcare systems (safe, timely, effective, efficient, equitable, and patient centered).[3]

Surveys of RNs, Physicians, Hospital CEOs, and Hospital CNOs

The surveys were conducted only months apart in 2004 and 2005, and although each survey contained items tailored to the particular population studied, several questions included in the surveys were identical. Items assessed in each survey included perceptions of the extent and severity of the current nursing shortage; causes, effects, and hospitals' responses to the nursing shortage; characteristics of the nursing work environment; quality of professional practice and relationships among nurses, physicians, and managers; perceptions of nursing careers; awareness and impact of the Johnson & Johnson Campaign for Nursing's Future; and demographic characteristics of survey respondents.[4]

The national survey of physicians was conducted from January 6 to March 5, 2004. Using the AMA Physician Masterfile, a random sample of physicians was drawn to be representative of primary care and specialist physicians who spend more than 20 hours per week engaged in patient care activities, excluding resident physicians and federal employees. Of 840 physicians who initially received questionnaires, 400 completed and returned the survey for a response rate of 53% based on guidelines established by the American Association for Public Opinion Research (AAPOR, RR1).

[3] This section is adapted from an article published in the health policy journal *Health Affairs*. The article is copyrighted and published by Project HOPE/*Health Affairs* as P. Buerhaus, K. Donelan, C. DesRoches, B. Ulrich, L. Norman, R. Dittus. Impact of the nursing shortage on hospital patient care: Comparative perspectives. *Health Affairs*, May/June 2007; 26(3): 853-852. *The published article is archived and available online at www.healthaffairs.org.*

[4] Funding to conduct each of these surveys was provided by an unrestricted grant from the Johnson & Johnson Campaign for Nursing's Future. The campaign is a national initiative that began in February 2002 and is aimed at increasing nursing recruitment in the United States, retaining nurses in clinical practice, and increasing the capacity of the nation's nursing education programs. The campaign played no role in the design and conduct of the study, analysis and interpretation of the results, and preparation or approval of manuscripts written for publication. Support also was provided by *Nursing Spectrum*. Finally, we wish to acknowledge Sandra Applebaum of Harris Interactive, who administered each of the surveys.

The national survey of RNs was conducted from May 11 to July 12, 2004, shortly after the physician survey. A random sample of 3500 RNs was drawn from a national database compiled from all state board of licensure lists, and 1697 completed surveys were returned for a response rate of 53%. For the analysis reported here, we use a subset of the data that represents all RNs who deliver direct patient care in acute care hospitals (n = 657).

The national survey of hospital CEOs and CNOs was conducted between January 28 and March 11, 2005, from a sample of hospital executives compiled from a list of all U.S. hospitals. Unlike the surveys of RNs and physicians that were conducted by mail, in most cases hospital executives participated by telephone interview. Of 404 eligible CEOs, 142 completed surveys for a response rate of 31%, and 222 out of 443 eligible CNOs completed surveys for a response rate of 50%.

Physician survey data were weighted using the original source AMA Masterfile demographic data to reflect the original random sample of physicians by specialty, region, and year of medical school graduation. Data from the RN survey were weighted to reflect the age and geographic distribution of RNs using the 2000 National Sample Survey of Registered Nurses. Hospital CEO and CNO data were not weighted for analysis because they were deemed to be representative of the national distribution of hospitals in the United States. All surveys are subject to sampling and nonsampling error. For these surveys, there is a 95% certainty that the results are within six percentage points for the physician survey, three percentage points for the RN survey, and nine percentage points for the CEO and CNO survey of what results would be if the entire relevant populations had been surveyed with complete accuracy. Further details on how each of these surveys were conducted are described in Appendix 1-1.

Survey Findings

In this section, we report how RNs, physicians, hospital CEOs and hospital CNOs responded to survey questions regarding their perceptions of the severity of the current nursing shortage, the reasons for the shortage, the impact of the shortage, their expectations for the future, and their beliefs about responsibility for solving the current shortage.

Severity of the Current Hospital RN Shortage

Survey results show that in early 2004 more than 90% of physicians and RNs perceived that the supply of RNs in the United States was less than demand and that a majority of physicians (81%) and RNs (82%) perceived a very or somewhat serious shortage in the hospital where they admitted patients or were employed. Surveys of CEOs and CNOs conducted in early 2005 showed that more than two-thirds of both groups perceived that the supply of RNs in their regions was less than demand; a majority of CNOs (74%) and CEOs (68%) perceived a very or somewhat serious shortage of RNs in the hospitals where they worked. That hospital executives were less likely to perceive a shortage than RNs and physicians (though still a majority) is probably explained by their different positions in the hospital that cause them to observe and experience shortages differently. In addition, because CEOs and CNOs were surveyed 6 to 8 months after physicians and RNs, they might have been surveyed at a time when the impact of the huge growth in RN employment (nearly 185,000 FTEs in 2002 and 2003, as noted in Chapter 6) had been fully absorbed. Unless otherwise noted, the results that are discussed in the following paragraphs are based on survey respondents who had perceived a shortage of RNs in the hospitals where they worked or admitted patients.

Reasons for the Shortage

All survey respondents were asked about the reasons for the current nursing shortage. As shown in **Table 12-3**, RNs were twice as likely to identify salary and benefits as a main reason for the nursing shortage, and they were three times as likely to agree that nursing is not seen as a rewarding career (26%) than CEOs (6%) or CNOs (9%). Physicians were significantly less likely to perceive issues related to the supply of RNs as a main reason for the shortage. Hospital executives were more likely to identify shortages of nursing faculty as a main reason for the shortage. With the exception of CEOs, a little more than one-quarter of all other respondents agreed that heavy workloads and undesirable hours associated with nursing were a main reason for the current nursing shortage.

Impact of the Current Hospital RN Shortage on Care Delivery Processes and Hospital Capacity

All survey respondents were asked, "In the past year, have you observed any of the following as a result of nursing shortages in hospitals?" and were presented with a list of items shown in **Table 12-4**. Overall, the majority of RNs, physicians, CEOs, and CNOs reported that the current shortage had affected three of the four indicators of care delivery process. Substantial majorities of respondents perceived the shortage had resulted in delays in RNs' responses to pages and calls and increased staff communication problems. While three-quarters or more of RNs and physicians perceived that the shortage had increased

Table 12-3   Reasons for the Current Nursing Shortage, 2004 and 2005

Main reasons for the current nursing shortage	RNs 2004 (N=657) Percent	MDs 2004 (N=445) Percent	CNOs 2005 (N=222) Percent	CEOs 2005 (N=142) Percent
More career options for women	32	18*	35	33
Faculty shortages in nursing schools	12	—	20	23
Salary and benefits	41	21*	14	21*
Difficult occupation/high workload/ undesirable hours	28	27	26	17*
Inadequate nursing schools/programs/ seats for students	12	3*	18	17
Nursing not seen as a rewarding career	26	—	6*	9*

— Question not asked
* Statistically significant different from registered nurses (p ≤ 0.05)
Source: National surveys of RNs, Physicians, and hospital executives

patient complaints about nursing care, less than 60% of hospital CNOs and CEOs shared this perception. Significantly more RNs and physicians than hospital executives perceived that the shortage had increased physicians' workload.

The bottom half of Table 12-4 shows that hospitals' capacity had also been affected by the current RN shortage as more than half of all respondents perceived that the current shortage had reduced the number of available hospital beds and delayed patient discharges. Considerable proportions (at least 45%) of all respondents perceived that the shortage had increased patient wait times for surgery or tests. Nearly half of physicians and RNs perceived that the shortage had discontinued or closed patient care programs, whereas significantly fewer CNOs and CEOs (20%) reported this effect.

Impact on Registered Nurses

All survey respondents were asked, "From what you know, how much of a problem do you think the shortage of nurses has been for [the six items shown

Table 12-4   Impact of Nursing Shortage on Processes of Care and Hospital Capacity, 2004 and 2005

In the past year have you observed any of the following as a result of nursing shortages in the hospital?	RNs 2004 (N=657) Percent	MDs 2004 (N=445) Percent	CNOs 2005 (N=222) Percent	CEOs 2005 (N=142) Percent
Impact on Care Delivery Processes				
Nurses' delayed response to pages or calls	82	67*	84	76*
Increased patients' complaints about nursing care	84	74*	58*	55*
Increased staff communication problems	85	71*	72*	69*
Increased workload for physicians	50	55	29*	30*
Impact on Hospital Capacity				
Reduced number of available beds	78	64*	60*	56*
Delayed discharges	69	50*	60*	61
Increased patient wait time for surgery or tests	68	45*	47*	48*
Discontinued/closed patient care programs	44	49	20*	20*

* Statistically significant different from registered nurses ($p \leq 0.05$)

Source: Buerhaus, P., Donelan, K., DesRoches, C., Ulrich, B., Norman, L., & Dittus, R. (2007). Impact of the nursing shortage on hospital patient care: Comparative perspectives. *Health Affairs, 26*(3), 853–862; Exhibit 1: Impact of Nurse Shortage on Processes of Care and Hospital Capacity, 2004–2005. The article is copyrighted and published by Project HOPE/*Health Affairs, The published article is archived and available online at www.healthaffairs.org*

in **Table 12-5**]: A major, minor, or no problem?" Overall, more than half of RNs and CNOs perceived the shortage was a major problem for all items. The majority of physicians agreed with respect to the quality of patient care, nurses' time for

Table 12-5   Impact of Current Nursing Shortage on RNs and Their Ability to Provide Patient Care, Percentage Responding Major Problem, 2004 and 2005

From what you know, how much of a problem do you think the shortage of nurses has been for . . . ? Major, minor, or no problem.	RNs 2004 (N=657) Major Problem Percent	MDs 2004 (N=445) Major Problem Percent	CNOs 2005 (N=222) Major Problem Percent	CEOs 2005 (N=142) Major Problem Percent
Quality of patient care	78	61*	64*	54*
Time for collaboration with teams	55	33*	56	50
Ability of nurses to maintain patient safety	69	21*	62	38*
Early detection of complications	65	44*	60	47*
Nurses' time for patients	91	78*	66*	59*
Quality of nurses' work life	82	59*	76	62*

* Statistically significant different from registered nurses (p ≤ 0.05)

Source: Buerhaus, P., Donelan, K., DesRoches, C., Ulrich, B., Norman, L., & Dittus, R. (2007). Impact of the nursing shortage on hospital patient care: Comparative perspectives. *Health Affairs, 26*(3), 853–862; Exhibit 2: Impact of Nurse Shortage on Nurses and Their Ability to Provide Care, 2004–2005. The article is copyrighted and published by Project HOPE/*Health Affairs, The published article is archived and available online at www.healthaffairs.org*

patients, and the quality of nurses' work life. Compared with RNs, however, significantly fewer physicians and CEOs saw a major impact on patient safety, early detection of patient complications, or time for team collaboration. Across all six items, RNs were significantly more likely than others to report the shortage had been a major problem. Additionally, the responses of CNOs and RNs tended to align on most of these items, and the same can be seen comparing the responses of physicians and CEOs.

When these results are examined more closely, 33% of physicians perceived that the shortage had been a major problem for nurses to collaborate with the care delivery team, compared with at least 50% of RNs, CEOs, and CNOs. Physicians and CEOs were significantly less likely to perceive the shortage had been a major problem for nurses' ability to maintain patient safety; similarly, significantly fewer physicians (44%) and CEOs (47%) perceived that the shortage had been a major problem for the early detection of patient complications by nurses compared to RNs (65%) and CNOs (60%). Data in Table 12-5 reveal not only the effects of the shortage on nurses' ability to provide patient care, but that major differences in perceptions exist between nurses (RNs and CNOs) and physicians and CEOs.

Impact on IOM Aims for High Quality Healthcare Systems

The six aims for high quality healthcare systems advocated by the IOM and the NQF were used to assess the impact of the current hospital shortage of RNs. All respondents were asked "How often (frequently, often, sometimes, or never) would you say the shortage of nurses had an adverse impact on the following aspects of patient care?" As shown in **Table 12-6**, the vast majority of RNs reported that all six aims had been adversely affected, but there was considerable variation in perceptions among physicians, CEOs, and CNOs. RNs and CNOs were significantly more likely than their clinical and administrative counterparts to report each of the six aims had been impacted adversely. Although there were substantial gaps in perceptions between RNs and physicians with respect to safety and equity, these gaps were even greater between RNs and CEOs.

Expectations for the Future

All respondents were asked whether the nursing shortage would lead to higher pay for nurses, the need to substitute other staff for nurses, nurses leaving for nonnursing jobs, more respect for nurses, lower quality care for patients, and improvements in the workplace environment (**Table 12-7**). On nearly every item, RN responses were significantly different from physicians, CEOs, and CNOs. All respondents were in substantial agreement on three items: the need for other staff to provide some nursing care, the likelihood that nurses will leave their jobs, and that the shortage will lower the quality of patient care. There was considerable disagreement on whether the current shortage would lead to more respect for nurses and improvement in the workplace environment. Additionally, only 48% of RNs believe the shortage will lead to higher wages, whereas more than 75% of all other respondents agreed with this perception.

Table 12-6   Impact of Current Nursing Shortage on Institute of Medicine's Six Indicators of High Quality Healthcare Systems, Percent Responding Frequent or Often Adverse Impact, 2004 and 2005

Thinking about the criteria for quality of care established by the Institute of Medicine, how often would you say the shortage of nurses has had an adverse impact on the following aspects of patient care?	RNs 2004 (N=657) Frequently or Often Percent	MDs 2004 (N=445) Frequently or Often Percent	CNOs 2005 (N=222) Frequently or Often Percent	CEOs 2005 (N=142) Frequently Problem Percent
Patient centered	74	61*	44*	44*
Effective	74	58*	34*	28*
Safe	65	36*	26*	17*
Timely	84	72*	50*	41*
Efficient	72	55*	55*	46*
Equitable	63	38*	23*	18*

* Statistically significant different from registered nurses (p ≤ 0.05)

Source: Buerhaus, P., Donelan, K., DesRoches, C., Ulrich, B., Norman, L., & Dittus, R. (2007). Impact of the nursing shortage on hospital patient care: Comparative perspectives. *Health Affairs, 26*(3), 853–862; Exhibit 3: Impact of Nurse Shortage on Institute of Medicine's (IOM's) Six Aims for High-Quality Health Care Systems, 2004–2005. The article is copyrighted and published by Project HOPE/*Health Affairs, The published article is archived and available online at www.healthaffairs.org*

The definitions of each aim for improving the quality of the U.S. healthcare system were provided by the Institute of Medicine. (2001). *Crossing the quality chasm: A new health system for the 21st century.* Committee on Quality Health Care in America, Institute of Medicine. Washington, DC: National Academies Press.

Patient centered: Providing care that is respectful of and responsive to individual patient preferences, needs, and values, and ensuring that patient values guide all clinical decisions. **Effective:** Providing services based on scientific knowledge to all who could benefit and refraining from providing services to those not likely to benefit. **Safe:** Avoiding injuries to patients from the care that is intended to help them. **Timely:** Reducing waits and sometimes harmful delays for both those who receive and those who give care. **Efficient:** Avoiding waste, including waste of equipment, supplies, ideas, and energy. **Equitable:** Providing care that does not vary in quality because of personal characteristics such as gender, ethnicity, geographic location, and socioeconomic status.

Table 12-7   Perceptions of Where the Current Nursing Shortage Will Lead, 2004 and 2005

Regardless of whether a shortage of nurses has impacted your workplace, the problem has been highlighted in the nation in recent years. Do you think the current shortage will lead to . . . ?	RNs 2004 (N=657) Percent	MDs 2004 (N=445) Percent	CNOs 2005 (N=222) Percent	CEOs 2005 (N=142) Percent
Higher pay for nurses	48	78*	86*	94*
Need to have other staff perform some nursing patient care activities	83	92*	81	87
Nurses leaving for nonnursing jobs	91	84*	83*	79*
More respect for nurses	21	44*	36*	59*
Lower quality care for patients	90	83*	71*	69*
Improvements in workplace environment	25	34*	74*	75*

* Statistically significant different from registered nurses (p ≤ 0.05)
Source: Buerhaus, P., Donelan, K., DesRoches, C., Ulrich, B., Norman, L., & Dittus, R. (2007). Impact of the nursing shortage on hospital patient care: Comparative perspectives. *Health Affairs, 26*(3), 853–862; Exhibit 4: Perceptions of Where the Current Nurse Shortage Will Lead, 2004–2005. The article is copyrighted and published by Project HOPE/*Health Affairs, The published article is archived and available online at www.healthaffairs.org*

Responsibility for Solving the Current Nursing Shortage

Finally, all respondents were asked, "If there is a nursing shortage in the United States, how much do you agree or disagree that the following [from the list shown in **Table 12-8**] should be responsible for solving the problem?" Overall, more than 9 in 10 respondents strongly or somewhat agreed that hospitals were responsible, with high percentages also agreeing that nursing professional organizations and the federal government were also responsible for solving the shortage of nurses. Roughly two-thirds or more of all respondents agreed that medical professional associations and private industry are also responsible. Additionally, there was fairly close agreement between physicians and nurses regarding who they perceived is responsible for solving the current shortage of hospital RNs; similarly, hospital CEO and CNO responses closely agreed with each other.

Table 12-8   Responsibility for Solving the Current Shortage of RNs, Percentage Responding Strongly or Somewhat Agree, 2004 and 2005

If there is a nursing shortage in the United States, how much do you agree or disagree that the following should be responsible for solving the problem	RNs 2004 (N=657) Percent	MDs 2004 (N=445) Percent	CNOs 2005 (N=222) Percent	CEOs 2005 (N=142) Percent
Hospitals	93	92	97	97
Nursing professional organizations	78	87	94	96
Medical professional organizations	63	66	71	75
Federal government	78	62	89	86
Private industry	57	64	81	76

* Statistically significant different from registered nurses ($p \leq 0.05$)
Source: National surveys of RNs, physicians, and hospital executives

CHAPTER SUMMARY

At around the same time that the current shortage of hospital RNs developed in the late 1990s, efforts to improve the quality and safety of patient care were beginning to converge into a national movement. These efforts were led by a growing number of researchers, quality improvement specialists, and organizations concerned with quality and safety of patient care. As the current shortage of hospital RNs continued into the 2000s, the IOM, IHI, NQF, and Joint Commission began to incorporate the contributions of nurses more prominently in their activities to identify the sources and frequency of injuries and low quality of care, measure and compare indicators of quality and safety across institutions, and implement actions to prevent injuries and improve quality. The publication of an increasing number of studies providing evidence of the relationship between hospital nurse staffing and various patient complications and adverse clinical outcomes resulted in a growing awareness that shortages of RNs were not only workforce problems but constituted threats to the quality and safety of patient care.

Surveys of RNs, physicians, and hospital executives conducted in 2004 and early 2005 document widely held perceptions that the national shortage of hospital RNs, which had begun in the late 1990s, was continuing. The majority of all groups perceived that the shortage had exerted a negative impact on aspects of patient care delivery processes (nurses' responses to pages and calls, staff communication, and patient complaints about nursing care). The shortage was also perceived to have affected hospital capacity by delaying patient discharges and reducing available hospital beds. RNs, physicians, and executives agreed that the shortage had been a major problem for the quality of patient care, RNs' time for patients, the quality of RNs' work life, and had resulted in adverse impacts on three of the six IOM aims for improving the quality of health care — patient centeredness, efficiency, and timeliness. Additionally, all respondents were concerned about the future if the current shortage continues, with the majority of each group indicating that lower quality of care, the need to shift the work of nurses to other staff, and RNs leaving for other jobs all could result. Virtually all RNs, physicians, and hospital executives believe that hospitals are responsible for solving the nursing shortage, but large majorities also indicate that professional nursing associations and the federal government share in this responsibility.

Results also indicate several areas where there was considerable disagreement among the groups surveyed. The areas in which RNs and CNOs shared common perceptions, but where physicians and CEOs did not, clustered around patient safety and the quality of nurses' work environment. Majorities of RNs and CNOs expressed considerable concern about the impact of the shortage on the early detection of patient complications and the ability of nurses to maintain patient safety, whereas majorities of physicians and CEOs did not agree with this perception. Similarly, clinicians' perceptions cluster around certain survey items where executives' perceptions were in sharp contrast, as most vividly demonstrated by perceptions of the IOM aims for improving the quality of healthcare systems; physicians and RNs perceived that most of the six aims had been negatively impacted far more frequently than did hospital CEOs and CNOs. These divergences in perceptions, while not unexpected, nevertheless identify gaps that could be important barriers to resolving the current nursing shortage, and improving the quality and safety of patient care.

Next, in Chapter 13, we continue our exploration of the current shortage of hospital RNs by turning our attention to the workplace environment of hospital-employed RNs. We examine data from three national surveys of RNs to determine how RNs employed in hospitals perceive their workplace environment and whether there is any evidence indicating that RNs perceive their workplace environment has improved or worsened in recent years.

REFERENCES

Aiken, L., Clarke, S., Sloane, D., Sochalski, J., & Silber, J. (2002). Hospital nurse staffing and patient mortality, nurse burnout, and job dissatisfaction. *Journal of the American Medical Association, 288*(16), 1987–1993.

Aiken, L., Smith, H., & Lake, E. (1994). Lower Medicare mortality among a set of hospitals known for good nursing care. *Medical Care, 32*(8), 771–787.

Al-Haider, A., & Wan, T. (1991). Modeling organizational determinants of hospital mortality. *HSR: Health Services Research, 26*(3), 303–323.

Altman, D., Clancy, C., & Blendon, R. (2004). Improving patient safety—Five years after the IOM report. *The New England Journal of Medicine, 351,* 2041–2043.

Amaravadi, R., Dimick, J., Pronovost, P., & Lipsett, P. (2000). ICU nurse-to-patient ratio is associated with complications and resource use after esophagectomy. *Intensive Care Medicine, 26*(12), 1857–1862.

Archibald, L., Manning, M., & Bell, L. (1997). Patient density, nurse-to-patient ratio and nosocomial infection risk in a pediatric cardiac intensive care unit. *Pediatric Infection Disease Journal, 16,* 1045–1048.

Blegen, M., Goode, C., & Reed, L. (1998). Nurse staffing and patient outcomes. *Nursing Research, 47*(1), 43–49.

Blegen, M., & Vaughn, T. (1998). A multisite study of nurse staffing and patient occurrences. *Nursing Economic$, 16*(4), 196–203.

Blendon, R., DesRoches, C., Brodie, M., Benson, J., Allison, B., Schneider, E., et al. (2002). Patient safety: Views of practicing physicians and the public on medical errors. *The New England Journal of Medicine, 347,* 1933–1940.

Brennan, R., Horwitz, R., Duffy, F., Cassel, C., Goode, L., & Lipner, R. (2004). The role of physician specialty board certification status in the quality movement. *The Journal of the American Medical Association, 292,* 1038–1043.

Brennan, T., Leape, L., Laird, N., Hebert, L., Localio, A., Lawthers, A., et al. (1991). Incidence of adverse events and negligence in hospitalized patients. *The New England Journal of Medicine, 324,* 370–376.

Buchan, J., & Calman, L. (2004). *The global shortage of nurses: An overview of issues and actions.* Geneva, Switzerland: International Council of Nurses.

Buerhaus, P., Staiger, D., & Auerbach, D. (2000). Implications of a rapidly aging registered nurse workforce. *Journal of the American Medical Association, 283*(22), 2948–2954.

Clarke, S., & Donaldson, N. (2007). Nurse staffing and patient care quality and safety. In R. G. Hughes (Ed.), *Patient safety and quality: An evidence-based handbook for nurses* [AHRQ Publication No. 07-0015]. Rockville, MD: Agency for Healthcare Research and Quality.

Cimiotti, J., Haas, J., Saiman, L., & Larson, E. (2006). Impact of staffing on bloodstream infections in the neonatal intensive care unit. *Archives of Pediatric & Adolescent Medicine, 160*(8), 832–836.

Dimick, J., Swoboda, S., Pronovost, P., & Lipsett, P. (2001). Effect of nurse-to-patient ratio in the intensive care unit on pulmonary complications and resource use after hepatectomy. *American Journal of Critical Care, 10*(6), 376–382.

Flood, S., & Diers, D. (1988). Nurse staffing, patient outcome and cost. *Nursing Management, 19*(5), 34–43.

Fridkin, S., Pear, S., Williamson, T., Galgiani, J., & Jarvis, W. (1996). The role of understaffing in central venous catheter-associated bloodstream infections. *Infection Control & Hospital Epidemiology, 17*(3), 150–158.

Giraud, T., Dhainaut, J., Vaxelaire, J., Joseph, T., Journois, D., Bleichner, G., et al. (1993). Iatrogenic complications in adult intensive care units: A prospective two-center study. *Critical Care Medicine, 21*(1), 40–51.

Hamilton, K. E., Redshaw, M. E., & Tarnow-Mordi, W. (2007). Nurse staffing in relation to risk-adjusted mortality in neonatal care. *Archives of Disease in Childhood. Fetal and Neonatal Edition, 92*(2), F99–F103.

Hartz, A., Krakauer, H., Kuhn, E., Young, M., Jacobsen, S., Gay, G., et al. (1989). Hospital characteristics and mortality rates. *The New England Journal of Medicine, 321*(25),1720–1725.

Institute of Medicine. (2000). *To err is human: Building a safer health system.* Washington, DC: National Academies Press.

Institute of Medicine. (2001). *Crossing the quality chasm: A new health system for the 21st century.* Washington, DC: National Academies Press.

Kovner, C., & Gergen, P. (1998). The relationship between nurse staffing level and adverse events following surgery in acute care hospitals. *IMAGE: The Journal of Nursing Scholarship, 30*(4), 315–321.

Langemo, D., Anderson, J., & Volden, C. (2002). Nursing quality outcome indicators. The North Dakota study. *Journal of Nursing Administration, 32*(2),98–105.

Leach, D. (2002). Building and assessing competence: The potential for evidence-based graduate medical education. *Quality Management in Health Care, 11*(1), 39–44.

Leape, L. (1994). Error in medicine. *Journal of the American Medical Association, 272,* 1851–1857.

Leape, L., Bates, D., Cullen, D., Cooper, J., Demonaco, H., Gallivan, T., et al. (1995). Systems analysis of adverse drug events. *The Journal of the American Medical Association, 274,* 35–43.

Leape, L., Brennan, T., Laird, N., Lawthers, A., Localio, A., Barnes, B., et al. (1991). The nature of adverse events in hospitalized patients. *The New England Journal of Medicine, 324,* 377–384.

Leape, L., Lawthers, A., Brennan, T., & Johson, W. (1993). Preventing medical injury. *Quality Review Bulletin, 19,* 144-149.

Needleman, J., Buerhaus, P., Mattke, S., Stewart, M., & Zelevinsky, K. (2002). Nurse staffing and quality of care in hospitals in the United States. *The New England Journal of Medicine, 346*(22), 1715–1722.

Needleman, J., Buerhaus, P., Mattke, S., Stewart, M., & Zelevinsky, K. (2006). Nurse staffing in hospitals: Is there a business case for quality? *Health Affairs, 25*(1), 204–211.

Network. (2000). *Nurse staffing and patient outcomes in the inpatient hospital setting.* Baltimore, MD: American Nurses Association.

Page, A. (Ed.). (2004). Institute of Medicine, Committee on the Work Environment for Nurses and Patient Safety Board on Health Care Services. *Keeping patients safe: Transforming the work environment of nurses.* Washington, DC: National Academies Press.

Pronovost, P., Jenckes, M., Dorman T., Garrett, E., Brewlow, M., Rosenfeld, B., et al. (1999). Organizational characteristics of intensive care units related to outcomes of abdominal aortic surgery. *Journal of the American Medical Association, 281*(14), 1310–1317.

Romano, P. (2005). Improving the quality of hospital care in America. *The New England Journal of Medicine, 353*(3), 302–304.

Schultz, M., van Servellen, G., Chang, B., McNeese-Smith, D., & Waxenberg, E. (1998). The relationship of hospital structural and financial characteristics to mortality and length of stay in acute myocardial infarction patients. *Outcomes Management for Nursing Practice, 2*(3),130–136.

Scott, W., Forrest, W., & Brown, B. (1976). Hospital structure and postoperative mortality and morbidity. In S. Shortell & M. Brown (Eds.), *Organizational research in hospitals* (pp. 72–89). Chicago: Blue Cross.

Shortell, S., & Hughes, E. (1988). The effects of regulation, competition, and ownership on mortality rates among hospital inpatients. *The New England Journal of Medicine, 318*(17), 1100–1107.

Shortell, S., Zimmerman, J., Rousseau, D., Gillies, R., Wagner, D., Draper, E., et al. (1994). The performance of intensive care units: Does good management make a difference? *Medical Care, 32*(5), 508–525.

Sovie, M., & Jawad, A. (2001). Hospital restructuring and its impact on outcomes: Nursing staff regulations are premature. *Journal of Nursing Administration, 31*(12), 588–600.

Wan, T., & Shukla, R. (1987). Contextual and organizational correlates of the quality of hospital nursing care. *Quality Review Bulletin, 13*(2), 61–65.

Unruh, L. (2003). Licensed nurse staffing and adverse events in hospitals. *Medical Care, 1*(1), 142–152.

CHAPTER 13

Registered Nurses' Perceptions of the Hospital Workplace Environment, 2002 to 2006

In the previous chapter, we discussed RNs', physicians', and hospital executives' perceptions of the current hospital RN shortage and how it had impacted the quality and safety of patient care in hospital settings. In this chapter, we turn our focus to how RNs perceive their workplace environment and whether they believe it has improved during recent years, remained about the same, or worsened.

Focusing on the workplace environment is important for at least two reasons. First, as we saw in Chapter 6, RNs consider the satisfaction derived from working when they make short-run labor supply decisions (participation and hours worked) in addition to economic and other factors. For some RNs, in fact, it is the most important factor. If workplace environments are improving (or worsening), then we can expect an increase (or decrease) in the short-run labor supplied by RNs. Second, in Chapter 11 we pointed out that the economic pressures that hospitals experienced during the 1990s (growth of managed care organizations, increasing price competition, market consolidation, and government cost containment policies) affected the hospital work environment negatively in the eyes of many hospital-employed RNs. The bad publicity that this generated negatively influenced the decisions of some people who were considering whether to become RNs and thereby added to the forces discussed in Chapters 8 and 10 that were already at work reducing the long-run supply of RNs.

These complaints about the deterioration in the workplace environment (chiefly, the reduction in support staff, increased volume of patients who were also more acutely ill, and decreased length of stay) were confirmed by a series of high-profile reports. The Institute of Medicine (IOM) 1996 report, *Nursing Staff in Hospitals and Nursing Homes: Is It Adequate?*, emphasized the importance of improving the workplace and studying the impact of RN staffing on the quality of patient care (Wunderlich, Sloan, & Davis, 1996). In 2001, the American Hospital Association's Commission on Workforce for Hospitals and Health Systems published a widely circulated report that provided a sober assessment of the state of the workplace environment (American Hospital

245

Association, 2002). The report urged hospitals to make improvements and offered many examples of how constructive changes could be made and sustained. And finally, in 2004, the IOM issued yet another report (noted in Chapter 12) that focused on quality and safety, *Keeping Patients Safe: Transforming the Work Environment of Nurses*, which contained 17 recommendations aimed at improving the work environment of nurses (Page, 2004). However, this last IOM committee was not charged to, and did not address, the work environment in relation to the current shortage of RNs in the United States. Nonetheless, while there has been much concern about the workplace environment of hospital RNs and considerable effort to understand how the environment impacts patient safety, there is little data indicating whether the hospital nursing workplace has actually improved or worsened in recent years, and in particular how shortages have intereacted with the changing workplace environment.

This chapter seeks to address this gap by examining evidence indicating whether, from RNs' perspective, the workplace environment in hospitals has changed measurably during the current hospital shortage of RNs. We accomplish this task by examining the findings of three national random sample surveys of RNs that were conducted in 2002, 2004, and 2006. After briefly describing these data sources, we report the results of survey items that, when compared over time, reveal areas where RNs' perceive that the quality of the hospital workplace environment has changed.

OVERVIEW OF NATIONAL RN SURVEYS

This section provides a brief overview of the survey themes, data, and characteristics of the RNs who responded to the national random sample surveys. Details of each survey are presented in Chapter 1, Apendix 1-1.

Survey Themes and Data

The surveys were designed to elicit RNs' perceptions in five areas: (1) the extent and severity of the current nursing shortage; (2) causes, effects, and hospitals' responses to the nursing shortage; (3) characteristics of the nursing work environment, including the quality of relationships with nurses, physicians, and managers; (4) satisfaction with current job and the decision to become a nurse; and (5) awareness and impact of the Johnson & Johnson

Campaign for Nursing's Future.[1] The surveys were conducted beginning in 2001 throughout 2006, and many of the questions included in the surveys were identical.[2] In this chapter, we focus mainly on RNs' perceptions of the characteristics of the work environment and satisfaction with their jobs and careers as nurses.

The 2002 national survey of RNs was conducted over the period October 24, 2001, through March 13, 2002. A random sample of 7600 RNs was drawn from a national database compiled from all state board of licensure lists, and 4108 completed surveys were returned for a response rate of 55%. The 2004 national survey of RNs was conducted from May 11 to July 12, 2004. A random sample of 3500 RNs was drawn from a national database compiled from all state board of licensure lists, and 1697 completed surveys were returned for a response rate of 53%. The survey contained many of the same questions used in the earlier 2002 survey, and it included several different questions aimed at exploring new areas and probing certain aspects of the workplace environment in greater depth. The 2006 national survey of RNs was conducted over the period May 24 to July 26, 2006. A random sample of 3436 RNs was drawn from a national database compiled from all state board of licensure lists, and 1392 completed surveys were returned for a response rate of 52%. For the analysis reported in this chapter, a subset of the data from each survey representing only the RNs who delivered direct patient care in acute care hospitals was used, resulting in smaller subsamples for the 2002 survey (n = 1442), the 2004 survey (n = 657), and the 2006 survey (n = 617).

Characteristics of RN Samples

Most hospital-employed RNs providing direct patient care were white and female, and clear majorities were married and worked in hospitals located in urban and suburban areas. Not surprisingly, more than two-thirds were over the

---

[1] This chapter is adapted from an article published in the journal *Nursing Economic$* (Buerhaus, Donelan, Ulrich, DesRoches, & Dittus, 2007).

[2] Funding to conduct the 2002 survey was provided by NurseWeek, a national weekly nursing publication and continuing education company, and by the American Organization of Nurse Executives. Funding for the 2004 and 2006 surveys was provided by an unrestricted grant from the Johnson & Johnson Campaign for Nursing's Future. The campaign is a national initiative that began in February 2002 and is aimed at increasing nursing recruitment in the United States, retaining nurses in clinical practice, and increasing the capacity of the nation's nursing education programs. The campaign played no role in the design and conduct of the study, analysis and interpretation of results, and preparation or approval of manuscripts written for publication. Additional support for the 2004 and 2006 surveys was provided by Nursing Spectrum, which had acquired NurseWeek. Finally, we wish to acknowledge Harris Interactive, and particularly Sandra Applebaum, who administered each of the surveys.

age of 35, and more RNs were between the ages of 35 and 49 years than any other age category. Across the three surveys, approximately 20% rated their health "good," and less than 5% perceived their health was "fair" or "poor." In 2002 and 2004, a little more than one-third (38%) of RNs reported an associate or baccalaureate degree as the highest nursing degree received, and fewer RNs in 2004 (11%) compared to 2002 (19%) reported a diploma certificate as their highest nursing education. In 2006, the mean days worked per week rose slightly to 3.7, and nearly the same proportion of RNs reported that they worked 1–3 days as those who reported that they worked 4–5 days per week.

SURVEY RESULTS

We organize the presentation of survey results into two major areas. First, we compare RNs' perceptions of the nursing shortage and its impact, their views about what the main reasons for the shortage are, and RNs' views about strategies to solve the shortage. Following this, we delve into findings that reveal how RNs perceive a variety of indicators of the hospital work environment. Later, in the chapter summary, we discuss these results with respect to whether and how the workplace environment has improved in the presence of the current nursing shortage.

Prevalence, Severity, and Impact of the Current Hospital RN Shortage

Because we used many of the same identically worded items in each of the three surveys, comparing the results enabled us to determine whether hospital-employed RNs perceived any change in the prevalence and severity of the nursing shortage and whether they had perceived any improvements in the workplace. As discussed in Chapters 6 and 11, hospital vacancy rates were 13% in 2002, 8.1% in 2004, and 8.6% in 2006, suggesting that the current shortage of hospital RNs reached its peak intensity by 2002 but then continued at least through 2006.

Across the years covered by the three surveys, **Figure 13-1** shows that a falling percentage of hospital-employed RNs, but still the majority, perceived that the supply of RNs in their local community was less than demand. In 2002, 87% perceived that the supply of RNs was less than demand (44% "somewhat less" and 43% "much less" than demand), whereas 77% of RNs in 2006 felt that supply was less than demand (44% "somewhat less" and 33% "much less" than demand).

In each of the three surveys, RNs were asked about the severity of the nursing shortage in the past year in the hospital where they had worked the most. The percentage of RNs who perceived a "very serious" or "somewhat serious" shortage decreased significantly from 2002 to 2004, falling from 95% to 82%. Thereafter, the rate of decline slowed as 79% of RNs in 2006 perceived a shortage of nurses (19% perceived a "very serious shortage" and 60% perceived a "somewhat serious shortage") in the hospital where they worked most during the past year.

RNs were asked how much of a problem— a "major problem," "minor problem," or "no problem"—the shortage had been on six aspects of nursing practice. **Figure 13-2**, which shows only the response category "major problem," reveals that across the three surveys, a large proportion of RNs (ranging from 49% to 93%) perceived the shortage had been a major problem for all of the

Figure 13-1   Supply and Demand for Nurses in Local Community, Perceptions of Hospital-Employed RNs Providing Direct Patient Care, 2002–2006

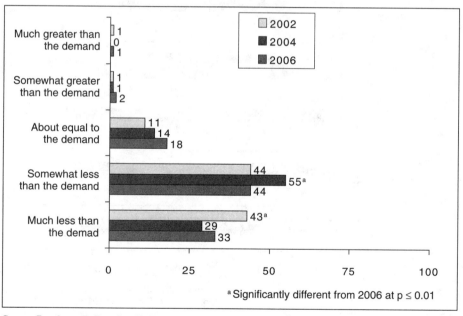

Source: Buerhaus, P., Donelan, K., Ulrich, B., DesRoches, C., & Dittus, R. (2007). Trends in the experiences of hospital-employed registered nurses: Results from three national surveys. *Nursing Economic$, 25*(2), 69–79. Figure 1.

aspects of nursing practice assessed. Nevertheless, over the time covered by the three surveys, RNs perceived the impact had lessened as significantly fewer RNs in 2006 perceived the shortage had been a major problem for five aspects of nursing care: the "early detection of patient complications," "nurses' ability to maintain patient safety," "quality of patient care," "quality of nurses' own work life," and the "time RNs have to spend with patients."

Figure 13-2   Percentage of Hospital-Employed RNs Who Perceived the Shortage Had Been a Major Problem on Nurses' Practice, 2002–2006

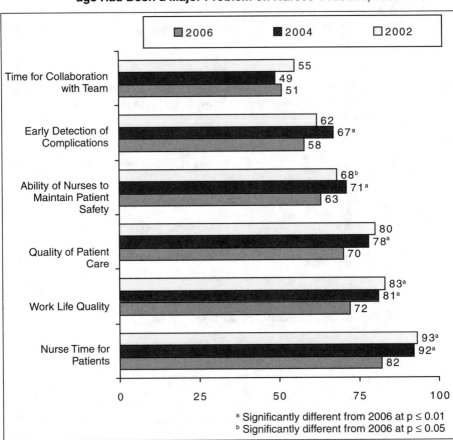

Source: Buerhaus, P., Donelan, K., Ulrich, B., DesRoches, C., & Dittus, R. (2007). Trends in the experiences of hospital-employed registered nurses: Results from three national surveys. *Nursing Economic$*, *25*(2), 69–79. Figure 2.

Causes of the Nursing Shortage and RNs' Views of How to Solve the Shortage

In the 2002 and 2004 surveys, RNs identified the top five reasons for the nursing shortage as "inadequate salary and benefits," "more career options for women," "undesirable hours," a "negative healthcare work environment," and "nursing not seen as a rewarding career" (**Table 13-1**). In the 2006 survey, RNs continued to rank these same reasons as the top five causes of the shortage, although "faculty shortages in nursing schools" increased significantly to become the third highest rated cause. While still a leading factor, the impact of salary decreased significantly over the years covered by the three surveys: In 2002, 58% of RNs agreed that "salary and benefits" were a main cause of the shortage, significantly more than the 41% of RNs in 2004 and nearly twice as many as the 32% of RNs who agreed with this view in 2006. The proportion of RNs who agreed that a "negative perception of the healthcare work environment" was a main

Table 13-1 Main Reasons for the Nursing Shortage, Perceptions of Hospital-Employed RNs Providing Direct Patient Care, 2002–2006

Reasons for the Nursing Shortage	2002 Percent	2004 Percent	2006 Percent
Salary and benefits	58[a]	41[a]	32
More career options for women	44[a]	32	30
Faculty shortages in nursing schools	*	11[a]	26
Undesirable hours	38[a]	27	24
Negative perception of the healthcare work environment	29[a]	15	15
Nursing not seen as a rewarding career	*	26[b]	21
Nursing not a respected profession	*	17	14
Lack of qualified students pursuing nursing as a career	15	12	13
Fewer applicants admitted to nursing schools	7	8[b]	12

Note: *Options not presented to respondent

[a] Significantly different from 2006 at $p \leq 0.01$.
[b] Significantly different from 2006 at $p \leq 0.05$

Source: Buerhaus, P., Donelan, K., Ulrich, B., DesRoches, C., & Dittus, R. (2007). Trends in the experiences of hospital-employed registered nurses: Results from three national surveys. *Nursing Economic$, 25*(2), 69–79. Table 2.

cause of the nursing shortage also dropped significantly, from 29% in 2002 to 15% in 2006. Similarly, the percentage of RNs who ranked undesirable hours and more career options for women as main causes of the shortage also decreased significantly between 2002 and 2006.

When RNs were asked about the strategies they thought would solve the nursing shortage, the data in **Table 13-2** indicate that the vast majority (more than 79%) in all three surveys perceived that "improving the work environment" and "improving wages and benefits" would help a great deal. Compared to 2002, significantly fewer RNs in 2006 (though still a clear majority) agreed that these two strategies were the leading ways to resolve the shortage. Other strategies that more than half of RNs thought would help solve the shortage included "higher status of nurses in the hospital environment" and "better hours." Noticeably fewer RNs thought that "financial aid," "increased capacity to educate

Table 13-2   Strategies to Solve the Shortage, Perceptions of Hospital-Employed RNs Providing Direct Patient Care, 2002–2006

	Percentage who think each strategy would help solve the nursing shortage "a great deal"		
Strategies to Solve Shortage	**2002**	**2004**	**2006**
Improved work environment	89[a]	86[a]	79
Improved wages and benefits	88[a]	85	82
Higher status of nurses in the hospital environment	74	74	71
Better hours	56	58	55
Financial aid	32[a]	40	38
Increased capacity to educate and train nurses	40[a]	47	52
Programs (nonfinancial) to encourage people to enter the field of nursing	20[a]	24	27
Use of support staff for RNs	28	35	32
Recruitment of men and minorities	19[b]	20	24

[a] Significantly different from 2006 at $p \leq 0.01$
[b] Significantly different from 2006 at ≤ 0.01

Source: Buerhaus, P., Donelan, K., Ulrich, B., DesRoches, C., & Dittus, R. (2007). Trends in the experiences of hospital-employed registered nurses: Results from three national surveys. *Nursing Economic$*, *25*(2), 69–79. Table 4.

and train nurses," "nonfinancial programs to encourage people to enter nursing," "use of support staff," and particularly "recruitment of men and minorities" would help solve the shortage a great deal, although a growing number over time thought that these strategies would help.

Characteristics of the Hospital Work Environment

The second major area of the surveys focused on the hospital work environment. Here, we report RNs' perceptions of how they spend their time, the amount and type of overtime hours worked, quality of the work setting and relationships with other professionals, plans to leave their current nursing position, views about collective bargaining, job and career satisfaction, and other areas that help indicate whether the work environment has improved or worsened over the time period covered by the three surveys.

How RNs Spend Their Time

The 2006 RN survey included a new question that asked RNs how much of their time during a typical week of work is spent doing the seven items listed in **Table 13-3**, and they were asked to indicate whether this is "too much," "too little," or "about the right amount of time" spent on each activity. On average, during a typical work week RNs reported spending less than half of their time (41%) providing direct patient care, with 57% indicating this is "too little" time, 36% "about the right amount," and only 2% saying this was "too much" time spent on this activity. Documenting patient-related care consumed nearly one-quarter (23%) of RNs' time during a typical work week, with 30% saying this was "about the right amount" of time, but 56% reported this was "too much" time spent on this activity. On average, RNs spent between 5% and 8% of their time in each of the following: locating supplies and equipment related to patient care; transporting patients; making patient-related telephone calls and obtaining prescriptions, lab results, and referrals; participating in meetings or activities related to quality improvement or patient safety; and spending time in shift changes and other hand-off functions. With the exception of documenting patient-related care and locating supplies and equipment, a much higher percentage of RNs perceived that the amount of time spent in these activities was about the "right amount" of time versus those who felt that time spent was either "too much" or "too little." Only 10% of RNs perceived they spent "too much" time in quality related activities and almost one-quarter (24%) said they spent "too little" time on this activity.

Table 13-3   How Nurses Spend Their Time During a Typical Work Week, Perceptions of Hospital-Employed RNs Providing Direct Patient Care, 2006

| | | Percentage reporting this is ... | | |
| | Percentage of time during | Too little | About the right amount | Too much |
Activities	work week	time	of time	time
Direct patient care, including hands-on care, patient/family teaching, and discharge planning	41	57	36	2
Patient care related notes and documentation	23	8	30	56
Locating supplies and equipment related to patient care	8	2	46	45
Transporting patients	5	3	64	19
Patient-related telephone calls (prescriptions, lab results, referrals)	8	6	59	26
Meetings or activities related to quality improvement or patient safety	7	24	56	10
Shift changes and other hand-off functions	7	5	70	14

Source: Buerhaus, P., Donelan, K., Ulrich, B., DesRoches, C., & Dittus, R. (2007). Trends in the experiences of hospital employed registered nurses: Results from three national surveys. *Nursing Economic$, 25*(2), 69–79. Table 5.

Overtime

Given the concern expressed by many RNs about working overtime hours, RNs were asked in each survey whether, in the past year, overtime hours had increased, decreased, or stayed about the same. Data in **Figure 13-3** shows that across the three surveys, significantly fewer hospital-employed RNs reported that the amount of overtime had increased over the past year: 55% of RNs in 2002, 40% in 2004, and 29% in 2006. The large increase in hospital employment

Figure 13-3   Amount and Type of Overtime Required, Perceptions of Hospital-Employed RNs Providing Direct Patient Care, 2002–2006

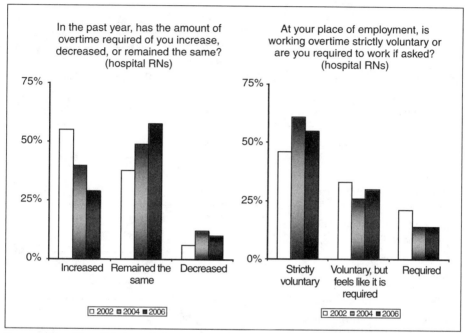

Source: Adapted from Buerhaus, P., Donelan, K., Ulrich, B., DesRoches, C., & Dittus, R. (2007). Trends in the experiences of hospital-employed registered nurses: Results from three national surveys, *Nursing Economic$, 25*(2), 69–79.

that occurred over the 2-year period 2002 to 2003 (discussed in Chapter 6) probably explains this decrease in overtime perceived by RNs, especially in the 2004 survey. In addition, from 2002 to 2006, the percentage of RNs who perceived that overtime was strictly voluntary increased significantly from 46% in 2002 to 55% in 2006, while significantly fewer RNs perceived that overtime was required in the hospitals where they worked (21% in 2002 and 14% in 2006).

Quality of the Work Setting

Across the three surveys, **Table 13-4** shows that many areas of work-related quality of life were rated poorly by RNs employed in hospitals, with fewer than one in four RNs rating them "excellent" or "very good." Those areas are: "opportunities to influence decisions about workplace organization," "recognition of accomplishments and work well done," "opportunities for professional

Table 13-4 Rating the Quality of Current Work Setting, Perceptions of Hospital-Employed RNs Working in Direct-Care Positions, 2002–2006

Characteristics of Work Setting	2002 Excellent or Very Good Percent	2004 Excellent or Very Good Percent	2006 Excellent or Very Good Percent
Your salary and benefits package	16[a]	25	28
Flexibility of scheduling	31[b]	36	36
Opportunities to influence decisions about workplace organization	15	17	17
Recognition of accomplishments and work well done	21	38[a]	18
Opportunities for professional development	17	22	20
Opportunities for professional advancement	17	16	16
Opportunities to influence decisions about patient care	23	25	24
Opportunities to establish relationships with patients and their families	43	46	43

[a] Significantly different from 2006 at p ≤ 0.01
[b] Significantly different from 2006 at p ≤ 0.05
Source: Buerhaus, P., Donelan, K., Ulrich, B., DesRoches, C., & Dittus, R. (2007). Trends in the experiences of hospital-employed registered nurses: Results from three national surveys. *Nursing Economic$, 25*(2), 69–79. Table 7.

development," "opportunities for professional advancement," and "opportunities to influence decisions about patient care." In only two areas was there a significant increase in the percentage of RNs who rated their hospital as "excellent" or "very good." In 2002, 16% of RNs perceived that salary and benefits and 31% perceived that flexibility of scheduling were "excellent" or "very good," whereas in 2006 these percentages increased to 28% and 36% respectively. In all three surveys, less than half of RNs rated "opportunities to establish relationships with patients and their families" as excellent or very good.

When RNs were asked about their agreement with the statement, "My job involves so many nonnursing tasks that little time remains for providing nursing care," RNs were less likely to agree with this statement over time. As shown in **Figure 13-4**, 62% of RNs agreed with this statement in 2002 (24% "strongly agreed" and 38% "agreed"), whereas in 2006 46% agreed with this statement (16% "strongly agreed" and 30% "agreed").

Data in **Table 13-5** show that not much changed over the time covered by the three surveys with respect to RNs' perception of physical safety and mental safety in their workplace environment. Roughly one-third reported they had experienced workplace injuries (back or musculoskeletal injury), and slightly fewer had experienced violence (verbal and physical), with less than 20% reporting sexual harassment or discrimination related to gender, age, or race.

Figure 13-4   Agreement of Hospital-Employed RNs Providing Direct Patient Care to "My Job Involves So Many Nonnursing Tasks that Little Time Remains for Nursing," 2002–2006

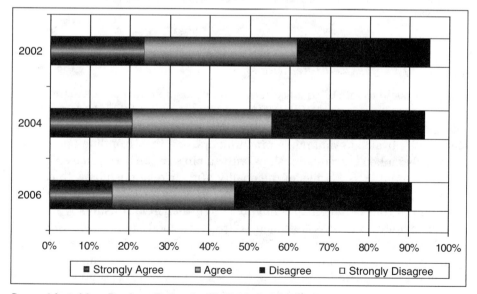

Source: Adapted from Buerhaus, P., Donelan, K., Ulrich, B., DesRoches, C., & Dittus, R. (2007). Trends in the experiences of hospital-employed registered nurses: Results from three national surveys. *Nursing Economic$, 25*(2), 69–79

Table 13-5   Physical and Mental Safety in the Past Year While Working as an RN, 2002–2006

Threats to Physical or Mental Safety	2002 Percent	2004 Percent	2006 Percent
Workplace injury—back or musculoskeletal injury	34	31	33
Violence* Verbal Physical	28	28	48 19
Sexual harassment, hospital work environment	19	16	16
Discrimination—gender, age, race	13	16	16

* In 2006, the question was divided into two parts, one about verbal violence and the second about physical violence
Source: Adapted from Woodring, B. (2001). Lecture is not a four-letter word. In A. J. Lowenstein & M. J. Bradshaw (Eds.), *Fuszard's innovative teaching strategies in nursing* (3rd ed., p. 67). Gaithersburg, MD: Aspen Publishers, Inc.

Quality of Professional Relationships

When asked to rate the quality of their relationships with others in the workplace, hospital-employed RNs in all three surveys assigned their highest overall ratings to their relationships with other RNs, followed next by their relationships with physicians and nurse practitioners, and then frontline nurse managers. RNs ranked their relationships with administration and management the lowest. Overall, RNs' ratings of the quality of their relationships with each of these groups changed little over the years covered by the three surveys. **Figure 13-5** shows that between 20% and 30% rated their relationships with other hospital-employed RNs as "excellent," 40% "very good," about 25% as "good," less than 10% "fair," and less than 5% felt their relationships with other RNs was "poor." With regard to physicians, never more than 12% of RNs rated their relationships as "excellent," approximately 30% said they were "very good," roughly 35% perceived a "good" relationship, a little under 20% said they were "fair," and less than 5% of RNs felt their relationships with physicians were "poor" in each of the three surveys (see **Figure 13-6**). RNs rated their relationships with nurse

Figure 13-5 Quality of Professional Relationships Between Hospital-Employed RNs, 2002–2006

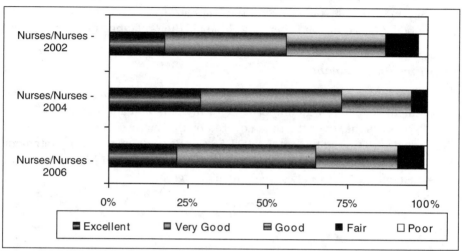

Source: Adapted from Buerhaus, P., Donelan, K., Ulrich, B., DesRoches, C., & Dittus, R. (2007). Trends in the experiences of hospital-employed registered nurses: Results from three national surveys. *Nursing Economic$, 25*(2), 69–79.

Figure 13-6 Quality of Professional Relationships Between Hospital-Employed RNs and Physicians, 2002–2006

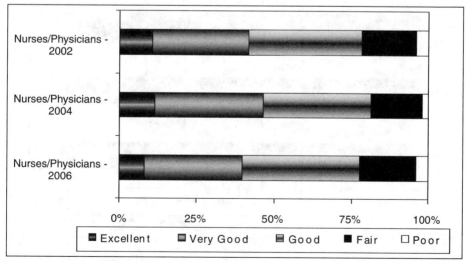

Source: Adapted from Buerhaus, P., Donelan, K., Ulrich, B., DesRoches, C., & Dittus, R. (2007). Trends in the experiences of hospital-employed registered nurses: Results from three national surveys. *Nursing Economic$, 25*(2), 69–79.

practitioners very similarly to their relationships with physicians, and they rated their relationships with frontline nurse managers slightly lower. Finally, RNs perceived their relationships with management and administration poorly in all three surveys: In 2006, only 2% said they had an "excellent" relationship, 14% "very good," 29% "good," 36% "fair," and 18% said their relationships were "poor."

Frontline Management

When RNs were asked about their agreement with the statement "Frontline management recognizes the importance of my personal and family life," **Figure 13-7** shows that over the time covered by the surveys, considerably more RNs agreed with this statement. In 2002, 56% of RNs agreed with this statement (15% "strongly agree" and 41% "agree"), whereas in 2006 70% of RNs agreed with this statement (22% "strongly agree" and 58% "agree").

Figure 13-7   Hospital-Employed RNs Reporting that Frontline Management Recognizes Importance of Personal and Family Life, 2002–2006

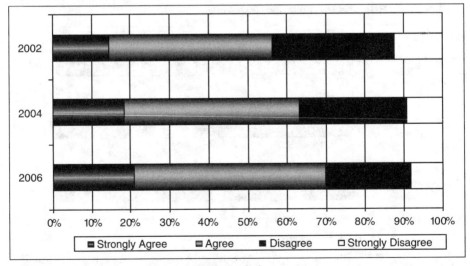

Note: In 2004, "frontline" was added to clarify the level of management.
Source: Adapted from Buerhaus, P., Donelan, K., Ulrich, B., DesRoches, C., & Dittus, R. (2007). Trends in the experiences of hospital-employed registered nurses: Results from three national surveys. *Nursing Economic$, 25*(2), 69–79.

Plans to Leave Current Nursing Position

Results from the three surveys showed little change over time in RNs' plans to stay in or leave their current position. Between 54% and 60% of RNs in each of the three surveys reported that they had "no plans" to leave their current position, 15% to 18% said they planned "to leave within the next 12 months," and 23% to 28% reported they planned to leave their current position "within the next 3 years." Of those in 2006 who planned to leave their position within the next 3 years, 48% said they would take a "different position in clinical patient care," 22% planned to "retire," 17% intended to "work in a nonclinical nursing position in teaching or research," 13% said they intended to "return to school to pursue additional nursing education," 13% would "take time out for family or other personal reasons," and 13% also said they would pursue a job in another profession (RNs were permitted to respond to more than one category).

Union Membership and Effects on Nursing and Patient Care

Across the three surveys, the percentage of RNs who reported they belonged to a union remained fairly stable: 21% of hospital-employed RNs reported in 2002 that they and/or others in their workplace belonged to a union, 25% in 2004, and 23% in 2006. When asked about the effect of unionization on the *nursing profession*, twice as many RNs (54% in 2002, 52% in 2004, and 49% in 2006) perceived the effect was "mostly" or "somewhat" positive versus those who felt the effects of unionization on the nursing profession were "mostly" or "somewhat" negative (23% in 2002, 18% in 2004, and 22% in 2006). With respect to the effect of unionization on the *quality of patient care*, more RNs perceived "mostly" or "somewhat positive" effects (45% in 2002, 42% in 2004, and 51% in 2006) versus those who felt the effects of unionization were "mostly" or "somewhat" negative on the quality of patient care (15% in 2002, 9% in 2004, and 15% in 2006).

Job and Career Satisfaction

Survey results show that most hospital-employed RNs were generally satisfied with their jobs. In fact, as shown in **Figure 13-8**, the percentage who indicated they were "very satisfied" increased from 13% in 2002, to 27% in 2004, and to 29% in the 2006 survey. RNs were also asked, "Independent of your present job, how satisfied are you with being a nurse?" Over the three surveys the percentage indicating they were "very satisfied" increased significantly, from 35% in 2002, to 44% in 2004, and to 55% in 2006.

Figure 13-8   Hospital-Employed RN Satisfaction with Present Job and with the Decision to Become an RN, 2002–2006

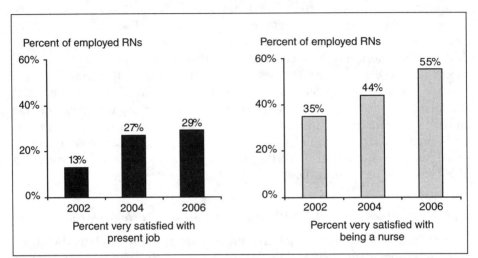

Source: Adapted from Buerhaus, P., Donelan, K., Ulrich, B., DesRoches, C., & Dittus, R. (2007). Trends in the experiences of hospital-employed registered nurses: Results from three national surveys. *Nursing Economic$, 25*(2), 69–79.

Elsewhere Buerhaus et al. (2005) reported results of an additional analysis that was designed to determine the variables that were statistically significant predictors of high and low levels of job satisfaction and career satisfaction, in the 2002 and 2004 surveys (the 2006 survey had not been completed at the time the analysis was done). The increase in job satisfaction was predicted by several factors, namely, RNs who reported that their organizations emphasized the quality of patient care, management recognized the importance of their personal and family lives, satisfaction with salary and benefits, high job security, positive relationships with other nurses and with management, and the age of RNs (older RNs were more satisfied). Decreases in job satisfaction were predicted by feeling stressed to the point of burnout, feeling burdened by too many non-nursing tasks, experiencing an increase in the number of patients assigned, and having a general negative overall view of the healthcare system. With respect to predictors of satisfaction with a nursing career, we found that in addition to the same variables that were correlated with job satisfaction, other factors were also statistically significant predictors of career satisfaction, including opportunities to influence decisions in the workplace, recognition of accomplishments, and overall physical health (healthier RNs reported higher satisfaction).

The same factors that predicted decreased job satisfaction (previously described) also predicted decreased satisfaction with nursing as a career.

Likelihood of Advising a Career in Nursing

The results of the three surveys shown in **Figure 13-9** indicate that hospital-employed RNs who provide direct patient care are increasingly likely to advise a qualified high school or college student to pursue a career in nursing. In 2002, a total of 59% said they would advise nursing (14% "definitely would" and 45% "probably would") but, in 2004, an even larger total (72%) said they would advise nursing (31% "definitely would" and 41% "probably would") to a qualified high school or college student. In the most recent survey, these sentiments increased again; 80% of RNs in 2006 reported they would advise a career in nursing (42% indicated that they "definitely would" and 38% said they "probably would").

Figure 13-9   Hospital-Employed RNs' Likelihood of Advising a Qualified High School or College Student to Pursue a Career in Nursing, 2002–2006

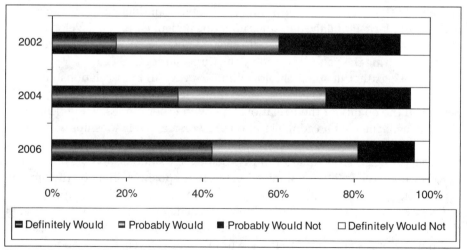

Source: Adapted from Buerhaus, P., Donelan, K., Ulrich, B., DesRoches, C., & Dittus, R. (2007). Trends in the experiences of hospital-employed registered nurses: Results from three national surveys. *Nursing Economic$, 25*(2), 69–79.

CHAPTER SUMMARY

This chapter has focused on comparing the results of three national random sample surveys of RNs conducted in 2002, 2004, and 2006. By using many of the same identically worded questions and administering the surveys every 2 years, these data provide a running snapshot of the experience of hospital-employed RNs since the current hospital RN shortage reached its peak in 2002. Overall, the results suggest that there are areas of the workplace environment where RNs' perceptions have not changed appreciably, areas that seem to be trending positively, and areas where RNs report clear improvements.

With respect to RNs' perceptions that have not changed noticeably since the first national survey was conducted in 2002, survey results document that the vast majority of RNs perceive a nursing shortage in their local communities and in the hospitals where they work. RNs continue to emphasize the causes of the shortage as inadequate wages and benefits as well as factors affecting working conditions, though there appeared to be less emphasis on wages and benefits and growing awareness of the role of faculty shortages by 2006. RNs had observed a variety of hospital recruitment strategies and generally perceived that most were effective. When asked how to resolve the shortage, RNs consistently emphasized economic factors, improving the work environment, and achieving a higher status of nurses in the hospital. Findings also show that fewer than one in four RNs rated any of several characteristics of the hospital work setting assessed in these surveys as "excellent" or "very good." Hospital-employed RNs perceived little change in opportunities for them to influence the organization of the workplace, influence decisions affecting patient care, and develop and advance professionally. Perceptions of physical and mental safety also changed very little during the years covered by the three surveys.

The ratings that hospital-employed nurses gave to their relationships with other professionals changed little over the time covered by the surveys. RNs perceived the quality of their relationships with other nurses as the best overall, with management and administration the worst, and relationships with physicians, nurse practitioners, and frontline nurse managers in between. Across the three surveys, about one-quarter of RNs belonged to unions, and the proportion of RNs who perceived that unionization has had a positive effect on the nursing profession and on the quality of patient care continued to exceed the proportion of RNs who believed the effect of unionization had been negative. A plurality said they did not plan to leave their current position during the next few years; about one-quarter of RNs intended to leave within the next 3 years, with about half of those intending to leave their positions in nursing to find a different position in patient care; and almost a quarter indicated that they would retire.

Significantly *fewer* RNs in the most recent survey reported that the current shortage of nurses in hospitals had been a major problem for the time nurses had for collaboration with teams, early detection of patient complications, ability to maintain patient safety, quality of patient care, work life of nurses, and nurses' time for patients. These results indicate that despite the persistence of a shortage of RNs in hospitals throughout the country, its impact on patient care in 2006 was not as severe in the eyes of the RNs surveyed. A higher percentage of RNs also perceived that salaries and benefits and flexibility of schedules had improved compared to the results of earlier surveys.

RNs report that the amount of required overtime has decreased, and when asked to work overtime, more than half perceived it was strictly voluntary. Fewer RNs agreed that the amount of time they spent performing nonnursing tasks interfered with time for nursing, and more RNs perceived that frontline management recognized the importance of their personal and family life. Over the time covered in these surveys, the percentage of RNs who indicated they were very satisfied with their jobs and with the decision to become a nurse increased noticeably. Additionally, in 2006 far more RNs said they would likely advise a qualified high school or college student to pursue a career in nursing than in 2002.

These national random sample surveys reveal that from the perspective of RNs, much work remains to be done to improve the hospital workplace environment. At the same time, nurses, those concerned with patient safety, and others involved in hospital patient care can be encouraged by the improvements that have been made in recent years, despite a persistent nursing shortage.

Next, in Chapter 14, we begin to pull together the key data and implications of the various chapters of this book. We examine what is likely to occur in the future and discuss the likely impacts of a growing demand for health care and for RNs and an aging RN workforce on hospitals, patients, and nurses.

REFERENCES

American Hospital Association. (2002). Commission on Workforce for Hospitals and Health Systems. *In our hands: How hospital leaders can build a thriving workforce.* Chicago: Author.

Buerhaus, P., Donelan, K., Ulrich, B., DesRoches, C., & Dittus, R. (2007). Trends in the experiences of hospital employed registered nurses: Results from three national surveys. *Nursing Economic$,* *25*(2), 69–79.

Buerhaus, P., Donelan, K., Ulrich, B., Kirby, L., Norman, L., & Dittus, R. (2005). Part two: Registered nurses' perceptions of nursing. *Nursing Economic$, 23,* 110–118, 142.

Page, A. (Ed.). (2004). Institute of Medicine, Committee on the Work Environment for Nurses and Patient Safety Board on Health Care Services. *Keeping patients safe: Transforming the work environment of nurses.* Washington, DC: National Academies Press.

Wunderlich, G., Sloan, F., & Davis, C. (Eds.). (1996). Institute of Medicine, Committee on the Adequacy of Nurse Staffing in Hospitals and Nursing Homes. *Nursing staff in hospitals and nursing homes: Is it adequate?* Washington, DC: National Academies Press.

CHAPTER 14

Long-Term Implications of an Aging RN Workforce

Throughout this book, we have used the framework of supply and demand, as developed in Chapter 3, to better understand trends in earnings and employment and to understand the appearance and disappearance of shortages of RNs. Until recently, shortages have primarily been driven by factors affecting the demand for RNs. As we saw in Chapter 11, the shortages of hospital RNs that developed in the 1970s and 1980s were driven by hospitals' increased demand for RNs. The shortages led to rapid growth in RN wages, which stimulated increases initially in the short-run supply of RNs (via increased participation and hours worked by existing RNs) and later in the long-run supply of RNs (by an increased number of RNs graduating from nursing education programs). A slowdown in demand growth, driven by the growth of managed care, helped to eliminate shortages of RNs and led to stagnant wages and slower employment growth in the 1990s.

The current shortage, in contrast to earlier short-lived, demand-driven shortages, appears to be the leading edge of a long-run shortage that will be driven by a persistent slowdown in the growth of the *supply* of RNs. The initial shortages, which began in 1998, reflected the changing age composition of the RN workforce, with hospital specialty units facing shortages because of a declining number of younger RNs (intensive care and step-down units) and the retirement of older diploma RNs (operating rooms and postanesthesia recovery rooms). More recently, these shortages have spread across all hospital units. Once again, RN wages have risen, which has stimulated increases in the short-run supply of RNs (via an unprecedented number of foreign-born and older RNs entering the workforce) and in the long-run supply of RNs (via increased enrollments in nursing education programs).

The fact that nearly two-thirds of the recent short-run growth in employment was supplied by RNs over the age of 50 reentering the workforce further reflects how significantly the pool of available RNs has aged in recent years. As we discussed in Chapter 10, these recent trends toward an older RN workforce have ominous implications for the future supply of RNs. If current patterns of entry and exit into the workforce continue, the RN workforce will become considerably older over the next 20 years, and shortages as large as 500,000 RNs are likely by 2025. Thus, the impact of recent shortages that were discussed in Chapters 11–13 might be the tip of the iceberg, as the aging of the RN workforce precedes an unprecedented slowdown in supply growth over the next 20 years.

Our purpose in this chapter is to focus on anticipating the long-term implications of the aging RN workforce that is bearing down on the healthcare delivery system. We begin by briefly summarizing the fundamental reasons why RN supply growth is expected to slow, while RN demand growth is expected to continue, leading to a shortage over the next 2 decades. On the supply side, we recap the reasons for the aging of the RN workforce and the impact this will have on the future supply of RNs. On the demand side, we discuss the implications of the inevitable long-term increase in the demand for health care on RNs and what this is likely to mean for RNs with respect to shifts in care delivery settings and in the type of nursing care that will be needed. We follow this by identifying and discussing the impacts these expected trends are likely to have on hospitals; on the quality, safety, and access of care to patients; on nurses themselves; and on nursing education programs.

THE AGING RN WORKFORCE AND ITS IMPACT ON THE FUTURE SUPPLY OF RNs

The RN workforce is aging rapidly because of the inability of recent generations to produce enough RNs to match the large numbers of RNs who were born during the baby boom generation (those born from 1946 to 1964). As described in Chapter 7, in the 1960s and 1970s, when women born in the baby boom generation were entering their 20s, many chose to become RNs. In decades following the baby boom generation, however, smaller numbers of women were born relative to the baby boom generation. Thus, there was a decline in the size of the population aged 20–29, the pool from which nursing education programs traditionally drew students. In addition, societal changes had opened up a greater number of career opportunities to women, further reducing the likelihood that young women would become RNs during the 1980s and 1990s. As a result, the average age of the RN workforce has risen as the baby boom generation of RNs has aged over time and fewer younger RNs have entered the workforce. Although interest in nursing has increased considerably since 2002, and graduations have been rising once again, this trend will not reverse the aging of the workforce until most of the baby boomer nurses have retired. Consequently, in the near future we can expect that the nursing workforce in the United States will continue to grow older. In 2006 the average age of the FTE RN workforce was 43.7, and the largest age group was composed of RNs in their 40s. Our projections from Chapter 10 show that the average age of RNs will reach 44.5 years in 2012, and RNs in their 50s will be the largest age group in the workforce. The average age of the workforce is projected to peak at 44.6 in 2015, before gradually dropping back to 44.2 years by 2025. Thus, for the next 20 years the RN workforce will continue to be considerably older than ever before. In fact, we estimate that in 2025 12% of the RN workforce will be composed of RNs over the age of 60 (just shy of 300,000 FTE RNs).

Short of a sudden and unprecedented surge of younger people becoming RNs, the aging of the RN workforce will eventually begin to affect the size of the RN workforce. As discussed in Chapter 10, we project that the growth in the size of the workforce will begin slowing down when the first of the 1950s RNs approach their 60s after 2010. After growing at an annual rate of nearly 3% per year between 1985 and 2005, the total workforce is projected to grow by only 1.4% per year between 2005 and 2015 as the large 1950s RN cohorts begin retiring, reaching an estimated 2.54 million FTE RNs in 2015. The slowdown will become even more dramatic in the following decade as these largest cohorts exit the workforce entirely, with the total workforce projected to grow by only 0.2% per year between 2015 and 2025, growing to only 2.6 million FTE RNs by 2025. Thus, we expect less growth in the supply of RNs over an entire decade than was typically seen in a single year in the 1980s and 1990s.

THE GROWING DEMAND FOR HEALTH CARE AND ITS IMPACT ON THE FUTURE DEMAND FOR RNs

To appreciate the impact of the aging of the RN workforce on the supply of RNs in the United States, it is important to consider whether the future demand for RNs is expected to grow or slow in the future. If very little new growth in demand is expected, then this would place little pressure on the supply side of the nurse labor market, and any shortages that might develop would not be large or result in any major consequences for nurses, patients, employers, or educators. On the other hand, if the demand for RNs is expected to grow substantially, then we can anticipate that shortages of RNs are likely to develop and result in economic and noneconomic consequences.

Based on our historical analysis of the growth in the healthcare sector (discussed in Chapter 2) and in the factors that are affecting the demand for health care discussed in Chapter 4 (namely, growth in the population, per capita income, and technology), we expect that, barring some unexpected development, the demand for RNs will grow by at least 3% per year during the foreseeable future. From an economic perspective, these factors are expected to continuously shift the annual demand for RNs outward in the United States. This rate of growth reflects a resumption of historic trends in employment growth of RNs prior to the onset of managed care in the 1990s which, as we showed in Chapter 5, slowed the rate of growth by roughly 1% per year during this period. Alternative forecasts of demand for RNs by the Health Resources and Services Administration and Bureau of Labor Statistics that were discussed in Chapter 4 are somewhat more conservative, but they still predict an annual growth rate in demand of about 2% over the coming decades.

We also anticipate that the increasing proportion and number of older people (the aging baby boom generation) in the population will shift the delivery of healthcare services and treatments into community settings, particularly assisted care facilities, home care, retirement communities, hospice, long-term care facilities, and other innovations in older resident living that are likely to be developed. Because older people are likely to have multiple chronic care conditions and diseases, we also anticipate that there will be an increased demand for organizations and healthcare professionals who provide services that respond to these shifting morbidity patterns. Taken together, these developments suggest that not only will the total demand for RNs in the future grow strongly, but there will also be growing demand for RNs who possess education and skills in geriatrics, are able to function efficiently in nonacute care settings, and have expertise in treating and managing multiple chronic conditions.

As has been the case in the past, the future growth in demand for RNs might be affected by major healthcare reforms over the next 2 decades that change the organization and financing of health care. In the past, RNs have been affected by such reform efforts, including the development of Medicare and Medicaid in the 1960s, which increased the demand for RNs; the development of the Medicare prospective payment system in the 1980s, which substantially increased demand for RNs and shifted care to outpatient settings; and the growth of managed care and market competition in the 1990s, which slowed the rate of growth in the demand for RNs and further shifted care to outpatient settings. Given projections of a larger and more expensive healthcare system in the future, new efforts are on the horizon that might reshape the delivery of health care, including changing the tax treatment of employer provided health insurance, stimulating the growth of pay for performance, and expanding the coverage of health insurance at either the state or national level. Some of the most extreme proposals, such as adopting a universal single payer system or eliminating the tax exclusion of employer-provided health insurance, could substantially reduce the growth in demand for health care and, hence, for RNs. On the other hand, given the growing pressure to improve the quality and safety of patient care and the close connection to nursing in achieving these imperatives, it is quite possible that organizations' future demand for RNs could be increased well beyond currently forecasted levels.

Overall, however, even major healthcare reforms are likely to have relatively moderate effects on the growth in demand for RNs over the next 20 years. As we saw with the spread of managed care in the 1990s, such reforms tend to reduce the level of healthcare spending but do little to moderate the long-run factors generating the growth in demand for health care. Thus, as these reforms diffuse throughout the country over many years, they only temporarily moderate the growth in demand for RNs. Even the fairly rapid diffusion of managed care only reduced growth in demand by roughly 1% per year during the 1990s. Thus, while there might be some uncertainty over when and how the healthcare system might be reformed, the impact on the growth in demand for RNs over the next 2 decades is likely to be modest.

THE UNPRECEDENTED SHORTAGE OF RNs THAT IS ON THE HORIZON

When our estimates of future supply growth for RNs are compared to the currently available projections of the future demand for RNs reported by the federal government, a shortage of RNs is expected to develop after 2015 and grow to an estimated deficit of 285,000 FTE RNs in 2020. Although the size of this expected shortage in 2020 is not as large as earlier projected, it will still be nearly three times the size of the current shortage, which has persisted since 1998, is the longest lasting shortage in over 50 years, and resulted in an estimated 126,000 vacant RN positions in the early 2000s. The projected shortage will nearly double in size by 2025, reaching approximately 500,000 FTE RNs.

What will be the impact of such large shortages? Using the simple supply and demand model developed in Chapter 3, the next 20 years can be seen as a period in which the demand curve for RNs is shifting out rapidly while the supply curve for RNs is shifting out slowly or not at all. At current wages, a shortage will develop, which will put upward pressure on RN wages. As RN wages rise, we will see movements along the demand and supply curve until the market reaches balance: increased entry into the workforce (of existing RNs in the short run, and of newly educated RNs in the long run) on the supply side and increased substitution away from using RNs (by healthcare providers) on the demand side. Eventually, wages will rise to the point where shortages are eliminated, and RN employment will lie somewhere in between the current demand and supply projections.

The remainder of this chapter works through the long-term implications of the aging RN workforce in much more detail. This unprecedented shortage of

RNs is expected to develop in the future at the same time the RN workforce will also be growing older. What are the implications of this for hospitals and other employers of RNs; for the quality, safety, and access of care to patients; for nurses themselves; and for nursing education programs?

IMPLICATIONS FOR HOSPITALS AND OTHER EMPLOYERS OF RNs

As the projected gap between demand and supply expands during the latter half of the next decade, we expect the RN shortage to become so large that it will spread beyond hospitals and affect the entire healthcare system. Initially, the response of healthcare organizations and hospitals will be to try to fill these gaps in RN staffing by employing nurses from temporary staffing agencies, providing incentives to RNs for working extra hours, implementing new recruitment and retention initiatives, offering sign-on bonuses, and developing other initiatives designed to increase employment from the existing supply of RNs. Eventually, as the shortage continues, employers will increase real RN wages and nonwage benefits. The increase in RN wages can be expected to induce some RNs to increase their *short-run* supply of labor (participation, hours worked, and delayed retirement). How much the short-run supply of RNs will increase depends on the size of the wage increase, how long it takes for RNs to learn that wages have risen, and how sensitive RNs are to the wage increase (their wage elasticity of supply, which depends on the influence of RNs' level of nonwage income and various noneconomic factors that affect RNs' decisions to work that were discussed in Chapter 6). The wage increase will also exert a positive effect on the *long-run* supply of RNs (the number of RN graduates entering the workforce in future years). For some individuals who are considering nursing but who have not yet made a decision to become a nurse, the wage increase will stimulate them to choose a career in nursing whereas, without the wage increase, they would have been more likely to have selected an alternative profession. Thus, wage increases in the labor market are likely to exert their predictable positive impacts in raising both the short- and long-run supply of RNs, not unlike what occurred in earlier decades.

If, however, the demand for RNs rises faster than the growth in supply, as we expect, then the pressure to increase wages will continue, and it might take a long period of time before the RN labor market reaches a new equilibrium. Higher wages will also attract foreign-born and foreign-educated RNs to the United States. To the extent that these RNs are willing to work for lower earnings and supply a greater number of hours per week than their American RN counterparts, hospitals and other healthcare organizations can be expected to lobby for changes in the law to permit greater immigration. If a large number of foreign-born and foreign-educated RNs enter the United States, the total supply of RNs (and total number of hours worked) will increase and thereby reduce the upward pressure on RN wages.

The substantial increase in employment of foreign-born and foreign-educated RNs, which accounted for one-third of the total hospital employment growth of RNs from 2001 to 2006 (see Chapter 6), demonstrates that RNs from other countries are likely to play an increasingly large role in supplying nursing care in the United States in the years ahead. To be sure, ethical, economic, and other issues related to using foreign nurse graduates to increase the supply of RNs in the U.S. healthcare system will not escape the attention of many interest groups. On the one hand, a policy to increase immigration might be opposed by many groups: unions because of the likely negative impact on wages, patient advocates because of a concern about quality of care, and foreign governments because of the shortages that such a policy might exacerbate in their countries. On the other hand, provider and payer groups are likely to support increasing immigration because it will help reduce labor costs, and foreign-born and foreign-educated RNs are likely to want to enter the United States to live, work, send money home to their families, and acquire new nursing knowledge and skills.

Although increasing wages will stimulate growth in both the short- and long-run supply of RNs, it can be anticipated that it will also induce hospitals and other healthcare organizations to substitute away from RNs (a movement along the demand curve, as discussed in Chapter 3). Because providing health care is labor intensive and the costs associated with labor comprise a large portion of healthcare organizations' budgets, increasing real RN wages will drive up an employer's labor costs. In turn, higher labor costs provide an economic incentive for employers to reduce these costs, primarily by employing *fewer* higher wage RNs and seeking to employ greater numbers of lower wage nursing personnel such as LPNs and nursing aides. This outcome is especially likely if the future shortage is severe and persistent because some organizations will determine that it is quicker and cheaper to seek regulatory changes to expand the tasks and activities that LPNs and aides can legally perform than wait for nursing education programs to expand the output of RNs. By expanding their tasks and scope of practice, these non-RNs can become better and less costly substitutes for higher wage RNs. In addition to stimulating substitution of non-RNs for RNs, raising RN wages will induce some organizations to experiment with new models to reorganize the way nursing care is delivered, modify the content of the work that RNs perform to ensure that the work is necessary and that RNs are spending their time productively, and eliminate costly and inefficient processes and activities that are used to provide nursing care.

Finally, future shortages of RNs, and the response to these shortages as hospitals and other healthcare employers increase RN wages, can be expected to affect the pocketbooks of private and public sector payers. For example, if real wages increase by 20% over the next 2 decades (approximately the cumulative increase that occurred in the late 1980s), the additional cost to employers of RNs would be roughly $30 billion per year, or 1.5% of annual personal healthcare expenditures, with nearly $20 billion of this cost falling on hospitals. Hospitals would seek to pass these costs on to government payers (primarily the Medicare program) by requesting increases in the labor wage index that is included in formulas that are used to determine prospective payment rates. Alternatively, hospitals could lobby for special pass-throughs or payments earmarked to finance the increase in RN wages. If granted, the dollars used to fund such payments would be drawn from the Social Security and Medicare payroll tax paid by employers and employees. Private insurance companies would also feel the effect of higher RN wages and pass the higher costs onto consumers in the form of higher premiums, deductibles, and copayments. Thus, the economic resources of payers and tax-paying citizens will be affected as employers of RNs increase wages in response to future shortages.

Looking ahead, as shortages of RNs continue to grow and hospitals raise wages to increase the short- and long-run supply of RNs, it will take some time before wages, RN supply, and organizations' demand for RNs adjust to the point where the shortage is alleviated. The concern, of course, is the length of time it will take for this adjustment to take place and what will happen during the time the labor market is transitioning to the new market equilibrium where most organizations no longer face shortages of RNs.

IMPLICATIONS FOR QUALITY, SAFETY, AND ACCESS TO CARE

In contrast to the 1970s and 1980s when there were far more RNs in their 20s and 30s than those in the workforce aged 40 and above, in the years ahead most care in hospitals and other healthcare organizations will be provided by older RNs. On the one hand, patients are likely to benefit from receiving nursing care from older members of the RN workforce. These more seasoned RNs possess years of experience, clinical judgment and decision-making abilities, and highly developed technical and interpersonal skills. Such RNs are more likely than younger and less experienced RNs to detect clinical complications early and intervene quickly before complications worsen. As noted in Chapter 12, studies have shown that the failure of RNs to detect patient complications early and intervene effectively is associated with an increased risk of mortality. Having a greater proportion of older RNs practicing in hospitals, therefore, could have a positive impact on improving patient outcomes in the future.

At the same time, should the magnitude of the shortage reach the level forecast and result in several hundred thousand unfilled RN positions, then the benefits of an older RN workforce could be overshadowed by the reduction in staffing levels, thereby jeopardizing safety and quality of patient care. Studies on the relationship between nurse staffing in hospitals and quality of care report that low hospital RN staffing is associated with higher rates of morbidity, mortality, length of stay, and a number of adverse outcomes, including urinary tract and blood stream infections, pneumonia, medication errors, falls, upper gastrointestinal bleeding, pressure ulcers, deep vein thrombosis, shock or cardiac arrest, and failure to prevent and treat patient complications. The development of large shortages of RNs will more than likely result in hospitalized patients experiencing a higher risk of developing one or more of these adverse outcomes. Additionally, based on the perceptions of doctors, RNs, and hospital CEOs and CNOs (also discussed in Chapter 12) of the impact of the current shortage, a much larger future shortage would undoubtedly affect each of the indicators of care delivery processes, hospitals' capacity, and RNs' ability to provide nursing care, as well as substantially affect each of the Institute of Medicine's six aims for improving the quality of healthcare systems: safe, timely, efficient, equitable, effective, and patient centered.

These risks might be offset to some extent by the fact that hospitals will be under growing pressure to avoid poor quality and unsafe patient care. The national effort to improve the safety and quality of care in healthcare organizations, including its focus on systems of care rather than on individuals as being primarily responsible for quality and patient safety lapses and the use of financial incentives to reward organizations that produce the highest quality, will act as a counterbalance to the deterioration in quality and safety resulting from the development of a large nursing shortage. Quality improvement and monitoring organizations and foundations—the National Quality Forum, Institute for Healthcare Improvement, the Joint Commission, and the Robert Wood Johnson Foundation—are developing measures of patient quality and clinical outcomes related to nursing with the idea that hospitals will be held more accountable for improving nursing-sensitive patient outcomes. As the focus on quality of care continues in the years ahead, hospitals and healthcare organizations will have to take into account the relationship between nurse staffing and patient safety, quality of care, and patient and family satisfaction with nursing care. These changes imply that it will be ever more important for hospitals to have enough RNs to maintain (if not improve) the quality and safety of patient care. If they do not, hospitals could squander their reputation as high quality providers, lose their accreditation from regulatory agencies, face reduced payments (if pay for performance or similar payment mechanisms that link payment to quality are adopted), and give up a portion of their share of the patient care market.

Given the growing pressure to improve the quality and safety of patient care, the close connection to nursing in achieving these imperatives, and the lack of good substitutes for RNs, it is likely that organizations' future demand for RNs could be increased well beyond currently forecasted levels. Unfortunately, should this increase in demand develop, it will add to the time required for the nurse labor market to adjust and reach a new equilibrium level. As the time needed for the market to adjust increases, so too will the transitional costs that patients will experience in the form of increased waiting times, postponement of nonemergency surgeries and medical treatments, higher rates of adverse outcomes, lower satisfaction with their care, and increased risk of injury. Hospitals and community-based organizations might not be able to open or staff new facilities and treatment centers. As the nurse labor market takes time to adjust to rising demand, slowly growing supply, and RN shortages, the public will suffer both personally and financially, and social confidence in hospitals and the healthcare system is likely to diminish. Indeed, it is difficult to overstate the seriousness of the implications of an aging and shrinking RN workforce.

IMPLICATIONS FOR RNs THEMSELVES

Beyond the implications discussed thus far, the increasing average age of RNs over the next decade will negatively affect the ability of the RN workforce to perform the physical activities required by their jobs. In the future, many RNs will have spent 10 to 25 years in the workforce and will be experiencing the accumulated effects of the wear and tear on their bodies. Compared to younger RNs, the stress placed on nurses' toes, feet, ankles, knees, hips, back, neck, shoulders, arms, and fingers from years of nursing practice makes older RNs relatively more susceptible to musculoskeletal injuries, as well as a reduced capacity to lift patients, move equipment, and carry out other physical tasks (Rogers, 1996). Studies indicate that nurses have one of the highest incidences of work-related back problems of all occupations (Trinkoff, Brady, & Nielson, 2003). Between 1994 and 2000, nursing occupations ranked as "high risk," with nurse aides ranking second after truck drivers in risks for musculoskeletal injuries. Over three-quarters of a million work days are lost annually as a result of back injuries to nursing personnel, with an estimated 40,000 nurses reporting illnesses from back pain each year (Menzel, Brooks, Bernard, & Nelson, 2004). Because the practice of nursing involves physically challenging work, these stresses and susceptibility to injury will undoubtedly result in some RNs withdrawing from the workplace either temporarily or permanently, thereby reducing the future supply of RNs.

Another implication of future shortages for RNs is that the recent progress that has been made in improving the quality of the hospital nursing workplace could easily be negated. As shown in Chapter 13, RNs have observed improvements in several areas, including increased real wages in 4 of the last 5 years, having more time for patients, greater schedule flexibility, reduction of overtime hours and performance of nonnursing tasks, frontline management recognition of the importance of personal and family life, greater job and career satisfaction, and the nearly twofold increase in RNs' willingness to advise a qualified high school or college student to pursue a career in nursing. These improvements are important to not only enhance the quality of RNs' work life but to provide concrete examples of a positive image of the nursing profession and of the environment where nurses practice, highlight the importance of RNs in improving the quality of care, and demonstrate that the healthcare workplace environment can improve, all of which can help attract more people into the nursing profession. Hospitals and policy makers need only look back at the 1990s to remember how the workplace environment deteriorated during earlier shortages leading to vocal and widespread complaints by RNs that reinforced the decline in the number of people choosing to become RNs. In the future, however, the challenge to improve the workplace will become more complicated because it will be dominated by older RNs whose physical and mental requirements will become even more important to consider than today.

IMPLICATIONS FOR NURSING EDUCATION PROGRAMS

As we saw in Chapter 7, each year between 1995 and 2000, the number of graduates from baccalaureate and associate degree nursing programs decreased substantially. In addition to the negative publicity about the workplace and the decline in real RN wages during much of the 1990s, the decline in graduates from baccalaureate degree programs (which have traditionally attracted younger women and take 4 years to complete) appears to be driven particularly strongly by the same factors that are responsible for the overall aging of the RN workforce: the decrease in the population of younger women (aged 20–29) who were born in decades following the baby boom generation and by the expansion of career opportunities that opened up for women during the 1980s and 1990s. Consequently, fewer younger women graduated from baccalaureate degree nursing programs during the late 1990s compared to earlier decades.

In addition to the workplace and economic factors noted earlier, the decrease in graduates from associate degree programs (which have historically attracted relatively older women and take 2 years to complete) is driven by a different but related set of factors involving the dynamics of the age structure of the U.S. population. During the late 1970s, 1980s, and early 1990s, large numbers of women who were born in the baby boom generation had reached their 30s, the age when many women have changed professions and when some, who have not been working outside of home, decide to enter the labor market or pursue education leading to employment. Given the large number of women passing through their 30s and the economic appeal of a shorter length of education to become an RN offered by community colleges, graduations from 2-year associate degree programs have grown steadily over time (see Chapter 7, Table 7-2). In the mid 1990s, however, many of these women had aged into their 40s, past the time when they were most likely to have embarked on a second career, including nursing. With fewer people behind them entering their 30s, the number of graduates from associate degree programs began to fall.

At the beginning of the current decade, these trends suggested that unless social preferences for a career in nursing became more favorable, the number of graduates from baccalaureate programs would continue to lag behind graduate levels that occurred in the 1970s and 1980s. Additionally, unless associate degree programs could find a way to attract a greater proportion of students from a smaller pool of women in their 30s, these programs could expect further erosion in enrollments and graduations.

In fact, in the ensuing years, several developments occurred that created a new interest in nursing among the cohorts of women (and increasingly men) who were born in the 1970s and early 1980s: In 2001 and 2002, real RN wages increased sharply; the events of 9/11 appear to have stimulated an interest in nursing among some people who desired to have a career that offered them a chance to serve society; and in 2002 the Johnson & Johnson Campaign for Nursing's Future was launched, which began a massive, multiyear national campaign to portray a positive image of nursing and inform the public about the opportunities that a career in nursing offers. Combined, these developments reversed the decline in social preferences for a career in nursing. Enrollments into baccalaureate and associate degree nursing education programs began to increase even though the size of their respective age pools that supply individuals into nursing were smaller than in earlier decades. The increased interest in nursing was so large and developed so fast that nursing education programs began reporting that many thousands of qualified applicants had to be turned away from a nursing education (see Chapter 7) in 2003 and beyond. Most important, renewed interest in nursing and the decision to become an RN by cohorts born in the 1970s largely explain the improved projections of the future supply of RNs in the workforce, at least through 2020 (described in Chapter 10).

Although the apparent improvement in nursing interest is clearly positive, there are two reasons to remain concerned about the ability of education programs to produce the number of RNs that are likely to be required in the future. First, it will be roughly another 10 years before the size of cohorts from which nursing education programs attract students returns to the size last observed in the 1980s. Consequently, during this 10-year period, it will be increasingly difficult to recruit new RNs from the current cohorts despite a renewed interest in nursing. Second, even if it is possible to maintain the level of interest in nursing from the 1970s and 1980s cohorts of women, the capacity constraints affecting nursing education programs (shortages of faculty and clinical and classroom space, described in Chapter 7) will seriously limit the ability to increase the long-run supply of RNs.

Taken together, the trends we expect to develop in the future, described throughout this chapter, imply that nursing education programs will need to become even more flexible and nimble in adjusting their curriculum in an effort to graduate increasing numbers of RNs in the future. Given the constrained size of the population of individuals in the applicant pools over the foreseeable future, education programs will need to lower the time and costs of becoming an RN without diminishing the quality of the education experience or the quality of the RNs they produce. To accommodate the increased number of qualified applicants, nursing education programs will need to expand their capacity; it will do little good to continue efforts to attract people into nursing education programs only to turn them away after these individuals have expended considerable time and effort to apply. Finally, given the increasing numbers of older Americans, nursing education programs can anticipate that students in the future will need the education and skills required to serve the special needs of this population.

CHAPTER SUMMARY

Continuing growth in demand for health care is expected to lead to annual growth in the demand for RNs of at least 2% to 3% annually during the foreseeable future. The location where healthcare services and treatments will be delivered will continue to shift to non-hospital based settings and will require RNs who are prepared in geriatrics, community health care, and the ability to manage older patients who suffer from multiple chronic conditions. As the demand for RNs increases, the RN workforce will become increasingly older and, as large numbers of RNs retire in the years ahead, the future supply of RNs will grow more slowly. Barring some unforeseen event, the gap between demand and supply will eventually result in a long-run shortage that could be at least three times the size of the current shortage of hospital RNs. We anticipate that hospitals will respond to the future shortage using predictable economic and noneconomic strategies they have used in the past, but the magnitude of the shortage will be so great that it will take many years before the nurse labor market adjusts and reaches a new equilibrium that resolves the shortage. During the period of time in which the market is adjusting, we can expect the RN workforce to continue to become older, the number of foreign-born and foreign-educated RNs to increase, and, as real RN earnings increase, some hospitals will attempt to substitute LPNs and nursing assistants for RNs. In addition, during this transition period, patients are likely to bear the costs of the shortage as it lowers nurse staffing levels and results in delays in receiving care, lower quality, decreased safety, and a higher risk of experiencing an adverse outcome.

An older RN workforce will possess years of accumulated nursing knowledge, clinical judgment, and practice skills that can benefit the quality and safety of patient care and help offset the threat to lower quality of care to some extent. At the same time, the physical demands of nursing will place older RNs at increased risk of injury and promote the withdrawal of some RNs from the workforce. Hospitals will be challenged to find ways to provide nursing care using a more mature RN workforce, maintain the recent gains in improving their workplace environment, and ensure that the safety and quality of patient care do not deteriorate to the point where they risk losing their reputation, accreditation, full payment, and market share.

Nursing education programs can anticipate growing pressures to resolve the capacity constraints that are currently causing them to turn away thousands of qualified applicants, which prevents the RN workforce from replacing the large numbers of RNs who will retire in the years ahead. Education programs can also expect to be under pressure to modify their curriculum to better prepare RNs to provide care to a more diverse and older population in an environment that emphasizes quality and safety, while limiting the duration of these degrees to remain attractive to applicants who are increasingly in their late 20s and 30s.

The aging RN workforce and the resulting shortages that can be expected in the future will have impacts on employers, patients, and RNs themselves. Many of the most adverse effects will be more severe if the market fails to anticipate the coming shortage. By accelerating the reaction speed of the nurse labor market, it is possible to reduce the size and impact of the future shortage of RNs and thereby lower the economic and noneconomic costs to patients, nurses, and hospitals. Even after the transition period, when the market has adjusted to the slower growth in RN supply and eliminated shortages, the new long-run market outcome will affect employers, patients, and RNs in important ways. Various policies that could affect the growth in RN supply or in RN demand could moderate these impacts.

Chapter 15, the final chapter of this book, identifies and discusses actions for public and private policy making that are aimed at helping RNs through this transition period, accelerating the nurse labor market's adjustment, and moderating the long-term impacts of an aging RN workforce

REFERENCES

Menzel, N., Brooks, S., Bernard, T., & Nelson, A. (2004). The physical workload of nursing personnel: Association with musculoskeletal discomfort. *International Journal of Nursing Studies, 41*(8), 859-867.

Rogers, B. (1996). Nursing injury, stress, and nursing care. In G. Wunderlich, F. Sloan, & C. Davis (Eds.), *Nursing staff in hospitals and nursing homes. Is it adequate?* Washington, DC: National Academies Press.

Trinkoff, A., Brady, B., & Nielson, K. (2003). Workplace prevention and musculoskeletal injuries in nurses. *Journal of Nursing Administration, 33*(3), 53–58.

Strategies to Ensure a Better Future for the RN Workforce

The most important implication of our analysis is the projected development of a very large shortage of RNs beginning around the middle of the next decade. While the demand for RNs is expected to continue growing at a rate of 2% to 3% per year, as it has done for the last 4 decades, the supply of RNs is expected to grow very little as large numbers of RNs born during the baby boom generation reach retirement age. Our forecasts, discussed in Chapter 10, indicate that a deficit in the number of RNs relative to their expected demand will begin in 2015, grow to an estimated 285,000 FTE RNs by 2020, and reach an unprecedented deficit of roughly one-half million RNs (or 16%) by 2025. The question for policy makers and those interested in developing a strong and well prepared RN workforce is: What can be done to lower the many economic and noneconomic consequences that will be incurred by a future shortage of RNs of this size?

The aging RN workforce and the resulting shortages that are expected in the future will negatively impact employers, patients, and RNs themselves. Unfortunately, it is unlikely that actions undertaken now could prevent the development of the future shortage of RNs. The trend toward greater career equality for women will not be undone, and this was the key development that drew women away from careers as RNs over 20 years ago, resulting in impending shortages. We believe it is more realistic to target policies that, if adopted, could reduce the impact, size, and duration of the future shortage. This chapter builds upon all the data, trends, and implications discussed throughout this book to identify and discuss two sets of policies.

The first set of policies helps the RN workforce *transition* through the period of time it will take before the demand and supply of RNs reaches a long-run equilibrium. Many of the most adverse impacts that were discussed in Chapter 14 will be more severe if the nurse labor market fails to anticipate the coming shortage. By accelerating the reaction of key actors to these impending changes in the nurse labor market, it is possible to reduce the size and impact of the future shortage of RNs and thereby lower the economic and noneconomic costs to patients, RNs, and hospitals. In the first part of this chapter, we identify and discuss a range of public and private policies that are aimed at helping RNs through this transition period and speeding up the nurse labor market's adjustment.

The second set of policies alters the long-run equilibrium in the RN labor market through actions that will affect the long-run supply and demand of RNs. Even after the transition period, when the market has adjusted to the slower growth in RN supply and eliminated shortages, the new long-run market outcome will have to accommodate a lower level of RN supply compared to what we have historically become used to with strong annual growth experienced over the last few decades. As we saw in Chapter 14, this will have lasting and important effects on employers, patients, RNs, and nursing education programs. In the second part of this chapter, we discuss various policies that could affect the long-run growth in RN supply or in RN demand and thereby moderate these long-run impacts.

TRANSITION POLICY STRATEGIES

We first discuss strategies that can help the RN workforce *transition* through the potentially long period of time required before a new equilibrium is reached in the long-run demand and supply of RNs. These strategies are intended to maximize RNs' ability to endure future shortages in the least costly way, ensure that patients receive high quality and safe nursing care, and protect patients from disruptions in access to care even during a period of a prolonged shortage. The strategies discussed here target the factors that impact the demand, supply, and wages of RNs.

Transition Demand Side Strategies

Strategies involving the demand side of the RN workforce assume that there is little that can be done to alter the societal factors (growth in population, increasing per capita income, and adoption of technology) that are driving the demand for health care and, over the next 2 decades, will increase the demand for RNs in hospitals and nonhospital settings. The strategies, therefore, are aimed at increasing the ability of RNs to meet rising demand. Because RNs will become increasingly scarce resources, hospitals should use RNs' time as efficiently as possible so that it is not wasted and patients are more likely to receive the appropriate amount and type of nursing care. By increasing the efficient use of scarce RNs, the productivity (output) of the RN workforce will improve and help keep the costs of nursing as low as possible. In the following paragraphs we describe several strategies to improve the efficiency of the RN workforce through increased use of technology, experimentation with new models of care, management actions, and avoiding regulating nurse staffing levels (see **Table 15-1**). We recognize that many organizations are already beginning to respond in these ways and thus we do not describe specific actions in detail. Rather, our focus is to discuss how these strategies will help RNs pass through the transition period and stress the need to quickly put into practice actions designed to implement these strategies.

Technology Development and Effective Use of Nonprofessional Nursing Personnel

RNs can be helped through the transition period—the time it will take for the nurse labor market to reach an eventual equilibrium in the long-run demand and supply of RNs—by speeding up the design, testing, and implementation of

Table 15-1   Transition Policy and Strategies

Strategies	Transition Policy
	Goal: Anticipate and prepare the nurse labor market for impending shortages, thereby reducing their duration and impact and lowering the economic and noneconomic costs to patients, nurses, and hospitals.
Demand Strategies	• Speed up development and adoption of technology and use nonprofessional nursing personnel more effectively • Remove barriers to efficiency and redesign the work content and organization of nursing care • Strengthen management decision making • Avoid regulating nurse staffing
Supply Strategies	• Accommodate an older RN workforce • Accelerate improvements in working conditions • Expand the capacity of nursing education programs • Continue to inform the public about opportunities in nursing
Wage Strategies	• Assist hospitals and other healthcare employers in financing needed RN wage increases • Avoid imposing controls on RN wages

information and patient care technologies that explicitly recognize the reality that RNs in the future will be practicing under shortage conditions. Better ways to provide basic nursing services by using labor-saving technology need to be developed and evaluated. Medical device manufacturers, pharmaceutical firms, and developers of health information and bioinformatics technology should recognize their long-run economic interests in having enough RNs available so that hospitals and other healthcare delivery organizations will thrive financially and thereby have the resources needed to purchase their services and products in the future. These firms can become more deeply involved in developing technology to eliminate or at least reduce unnecessary demands on RNs' time, make accomplishing their jobs easier and more efficient, and also enable non-RNs to perform activities that have traditionally required RNs.

More efficient ways to provide basic nursing services using other care providers, particularly unlicensed assistive personnel, also need to be developed and evaluated. Because studies have established the association between hospital nurse staffing and a range of adverse outcomes (skin pressure ulcers, falls that cause injury, urinary tract infections, pneumonia, deep vein thrombosis, detection of clinical complications early before they worsen, etc.), the jobs of nursing aides and other support staff could be oriented more toward preventing adverse outcomes and improving patient safety. Taking full advantage of technology and nonprofessional nursing personnel will enable increasingly scarce RNs (and the organizations that employ them) to better prepare for and deal with the challenge of maintaining high quality even in the presence of nursing shortages.

Efficiency, Work Redesign, and Systems Improvement

As we saw in Chapter 13, RNs spend more than half their time carrying out functions other than providing patient care. Awkward and outdated communication systems, excessive paperwork, the need to hunt and find supplies, archaic patterns of care delivery, cumbersome physician and nursing order entry systems, and various other difficulties contribute to wasting RNs' time, lowering job satisfaction, and promoting a frustrating workplace environment. These problems are not new and yet they continue as barriers that prevent the current RN workforce from providing more efficient and appropriate nursing care. Given the outlook for the future, it is important to step up the pace of activity aimed at overhauling the delivery of hospital-based nursing care and eliminate these costly impediments. The lessons from Transforming Care at the Bedside, which was discussed in Chapter 12 (the national project that is creating, testing, and implementing changes to improve care on medical and surgical units and improve staff satisfaction in hospitals), are expected to provide guidance in how to make such changes quickly and successfully.

Helping RNs through the transition period will also require redesigning the way that nursing care is currently organized in many hospitals. Because changing the work and organization of nursing care is not easy and is likely to be threatening, hospital executive and clinical nursing leaders will need to work together to build trust and to understand each other's perspectives while working closely with nursing managers and staff nurses throughout the change process. Initially, it is important to identify new care delivery models that are likely to work within an organization's culture and that will support the values and objectives of all stakeholders. Parties affected by changing the work of RNs and reorganizing nursing care systems must explicitly understand what will be required to ensure successful implementation, including needed resources and support from physicians (and others, including pharmacy, human resources, etc.) who will be affected by such changes. It also will be important to avoid repeating the mistakes made during the hospital restructuring era in the mid-1990s that led to so much job dissatisfaction and nurse burnout. During that time, many hospitals used external consultants to design and implement change, focused heavily on cost cutting, often failed to include physicians, labor unions, and nurses themselves in redesigning the work and organization of nursing, and did not evaluate the results of their efforts or carry through in sustaining a relationship built on trust and mutual respect.

Improve Management Decision Making

Improving management decision making in areas that benefit RNs is required to aid the nursing workforce through the transition period. Changing hospital admission and discharge policies is one of the most important areas where management can make important improvements. In far too many hospitals, nursing units are bombarded with a flood of patients who frequently arrive on the unit at the same time to be admitted. This influx of patients causes RNs to take on time-consuming tasks, including assessing the condition of the patient, developing a plan of nursing care, implementing the medical plan (assuming one is already developed; often it is not), and prioritizing these demands in the context of their current assignment of patients who continue to require care while new patients are being admitted. RNs are forced to make trade-offs between responding to the needs of their current patients and the uncertain needs of newly admitted patients. Predictably, RNs often shortchange their current patients by not providing them with enough of their time, and some patients might even fail to receive needed services and treatments (feeding, turning, medications, dressing changes, ambulation, etc.).

To add to the difficulty of this situation, at the same time patients are arriving on the unit waiting to be admitted, RNs are often discharging other patients and ensuring that they and their families are prepared for transfer to home or to some other facility, all of which is complicated and time consuming. To accommodate these competing demands, RNs scramble to maximize the time they have with all of their patients and defer completing paperwork and nonessential care activities until their shifts are completed. The resulting overtime hours spent completing required paperwork and other activities not only increases the hospitals' total labor costs, but it increases RNs' time and aggravation costs, which for many RNs exceeds the value of the additional money earned by working overtime.

The Management of Variability Program (Boston University Health Policy Institute) and the Institute for Healthcare Improvement (Boston) have documented the substantial and avoidable burdens these common admission and discharge policies place on RNs, the threat to patient care, and how they contribute to costly emergency room backups and diversions. Admission and discharge policies are under management's discretion and appear to reflect historic patterns aimed at satisfying the demands of revenue-producing physicians whose interests are not always aligned with maximizing the hospital's overall productivity or minimizing the burdens on RNs. We believe that in this one area alone, management could diagnose the degree to which admission and discharge policies impact RNs and make appropriate adjustments that, from the RNs' perspective, would smooth out the peaks and valleys of demand on their time and thereby reduce the chance that patients will experience an adverse outcome.

Avoid Regulating Nurse Staffing

We believe that flexibility in nurse staffing will help RNs adjust to changing situations that will characterize the transition period during which the future long-run supply of RNs is catching up to the steadily rising future demand for RNs. Regulating nurse staffing by imposing mandated nurse-to-patient ratios (as is currently being done in California) increases inefficiency, increases labor costs, and does not fix the underlying problems that proponents of regulations feel need to be addressed through regulation. Rather than helping RNs and hospitals adjust to rapidly changing conditions, staffing regulations retard the ability to make the very adjustments that will help RNs through the expected transition period. Barring some unexpected decrease in the demand for RNs or some unanticipated large increase in the supply of RNs, it is inevitable that there will be some reduction in nurse staffing levels and nurse-to-patient ratios. Thus, we believe the issue to focus on is how to minimize the impact of staffing reductions on patient safety and quality of care, while avoiding dangerously low staffing levels. Rather than expanding regulation of nurse staffing, efforts could be more productively directed toward fixing the underlying problems that motivate the regulatory approach, monitoring hospitals that reduce nurse staffing excessively, and making staffing levels publicly available so that consumers, employers, politicians, media, and health plans are aware of these conditions.

Transition Supply Side Strategies

Implementing supply side strategies can also help RNs transition through the potentially long period of time it might take for the long-run supply of RNs to catch up to the rising demand for RNs. We believe that four strategies will be particularly helpful: accommodating the needs of the existing supply of older RNs; maximizing the short-run output (participation and hours) of existing RNs by improving working conditions; expanding the capacity of nursing education programs; and continuing to inform the public about the future employment opportunities and economic rewards of the nursing profession (see Table 15-1). Again, we recognize that some organizations have already implemented actions that exemplify these strategies and, therefore, we do not elaborate on specifics but rather emphasize how these supply side strategies are capable of helping RNs through the transition period.

Accommodate an Older RN Workforce

In the coming years, healthcare organizations will face the formidable challenge of finding ways to minimize the number of RNs who retire from the workforce. If policies to increase the flow of people into nursing are not effective and the flow into the labor market is slower than the flow out, it is possible to help offset the difference by extending the work life of RNs. With very large cohorts reaching retirement age in the near future (RNs in their 50s will be the largest age group in the workforce by 2012), even having a small percentage of RNs work a few more years could have a relatively large impact. As noted in Chapter 14, because of their clinical experience, nursing knowledge, and critical decision-making ability, older RNs are more likely to detect or prevent patient complications following surgery and initiate timely interventions that protect patients and improve clinical outcomes. At the same time, however, older RNs are more susceptible to developing musculoskeletal injuries and, when injured, they take longer to heal. Hospitals, therefore, need to quickly improve the ergonomic environment of the nursing workplace to promote re-tention of older RNs.

The rising numbers of obese Americans will not only increase the demand for health care as a consequence of the negative health effects of obesity, but overweight patients will increase RNs' risk of injury. RNs lift, transfer, and am-bulate patients, often using outdated or malfunctioning equipment. RNs reach over and around patients, bend over repeatedly to reach awkwardly placed elec-trical outlets and switches on machines, and contend with a wide variety of physical obstacles in the course of carrying out daily activities. Problems such as these can be addressed to make the workplace environment more ergonom-ically sensitive and minimize the development of injuries. Failure to take into ac-count the ergonomic needs of an aging RN workforce is likely to induce many RNs to leave the workforce altogether or seek employment in institutions that provide a more ergonomically friendly workplace. Making ergonomic improve-ments should become a priority of nursing managers, plant operations and en-vironmental engineers, and hospital executive leadership. In addition, taking the time to identify and fix ergonomic problems is an excellent way for man-agement to communicate to nurses that they are valued and respected.

In addition to making ergonomic improvements, hospitals and other health-care delivery organizations could offer more favorable work schedules to older RNs, redesign or modify the content of their work, provide access to exercise and strength training facilities, adjust retirement benefits, and use economic in-centives to delay retirement. Hospitals should experiment with new roles for older RNs, perhaps by offering positions in which they could act as preceptors and counselors to new graduates or as in-house consultants to other less senior RNs or nursing students rotating throughout the institution. Finally, because older RNs are less likely to accept unreasonable restrictions on their autonomy and control over nursing practice or tolerate a workplace in which they experi-ence lack of respect from physicians, administrators, and others (including other nurses), organizations should act to minimize such behaviors.

Accelerate Improvements in Working Conditions

As discussed in Chapter 6, some RNs attach greater importance to working conditions offered by employers than to economic factors when deciding to par-ticipate in the labor market and the number of hours they are willing to work. Thus, the time between now and 2015 (when we expect the transition period to begin) provides time for hospitals to continue making significant improvements and build off the gains that they have recently accomplished as reported in the national surveys of RNs that were conducted in 2002, 2004, and 2006: decreases in overtime, increases in job and career satisfaction, decreases in time spent on nonnursing tasks, managers' recognition of the importance of personal and family life, etc. Among the major problems that need to be addressed, according to these surveys, are: the decrease in RNs' time with patients, RNs' inability to detect complications early due to short staffing, decreased time to collaborate with teams and communicate with staff, and inadequate opportunities to influence decisions on how the workplace is organized and how patient care is delivered. That so few RNs report they have an excellent or very good relationship with physicians and hospital management, both of whom are integrally involved in creating and maintaining the kind of environment that fosters high quality and safe patient care, also warrants priority attention by hospitals.

Key to improving the workplace environment is understanding and responding to the way RNs feel about themselves and the ways they perceive they are viewed and treated by others, namely managers, physicians, support staff, patients, and other clinical disciplines. Hospitals should conduct focus groups or survey their nursing staff to determine the most important changes that need to be made to improve the workplace climate, and they should elicit suggestions on how these changes can be made and who should be involved in making them. Because the history and culture of every organization is unique, each organization should conduct its own assessment of its workplace, unit by unit, to guide their improvement efforts rather than rely solely on the shortcomings that we described via national surveys.

Prepare for Increased Enrollment in Nursing Education Programs

Rapidly increasing the flow of new RNs into the workforce is essential to replacing the large number of soon to be retiring RNs and expanding the long-run supply of RNs. Unfortunately, as noted in Chapters 7 and 9, the sudden increase in the number of people who have applied to nursing education programs in the past few years has been met by an inadequate capacity of nursing education programs with the result that thousands of qualified applicants have been turned away by schools of nursing. The factors that seem to be constraining educational capacity involve shortages of faculty, classroom space, and sites for students to obtain hands-on clinical education and skill development. While most of the funding for nursing education programs comes from local and state sources, the benefits from training additional RNs will spill over to other regions through migration and lower RN wages at the national level. Thus, states and localities will tend to underinvest in additional educational capacity, and the federal government might have to become involved in providing incentives and subsidies for the expansion of RN education programs.

Inadequate educational capacity has two important consequences. First, it will slow the rate of increase in the long-run supply of RNs and thereby prolong the time required to complete the transition to a new long-run equilibrium and eliminate the shortage; RNs will practice in an environment characterized by large shortages for a longer period of time. Second, until the capacity of education programs is increased, the rising demand for RNs will be met by responses from the short-run labor supply of RNs, which we know from Chapter 6 is not very sensitive to wage increases. Hence, the very large wage increases needed to increase the output of the short-run supply of RNs will drive the costs to hospitals and taxpayers much higher than would be the case if educational capacity were adequate to educate all those interested in becoming an RN.

For these reasons, it is important to quickly expand the capacity of the nation's nursing education programs. To guide this expansion, we believe that an independent study (perhaps conducted by the Institute of Medicine) could be undertaken that would determine the following: the prevalence and magnitude of each of the factors that are reported to be constraining educational capacity; the fastest and least costly options to eliminate each of these capacity constraints; and whether options to eliminate the capacity constraints can be accomplished more quickly and cheaply by either the public or private sector. A study addressing these issues need not take a long period of time, would help clarify the best options to expand capacity, and would stress the importance of expanding educational capacity as soon as possible.

With this information, policy makers would know how best to design and target policies to expand capacity in the fastest, least costly manner. Assuming that some of the funding for this expansion would come from the federal government, we believe that there might be ways to increase the benefits to taxpayers who will finance them. Specifically, we believe that the magnitude of subsidies to nursing education programs should be explicitly linked to adopting policies, discussed elsewhere in this section, that are intended to moderate the impacts of the impending nurse shortage, such as: (1) rapidly revising the nursing curriculum to incorporate greater knowledge in the theory and implementation of quality improvement, creating safe patient environments, and developing opportunities where students who are learning to become nurses, physicians, pharmacists, hospital administrators, and others learn in an interdisciplinary and team-based fashion; (2) expanding the number of men and Hispanics who complete their nursing education and pass nurse licensure examinations; and (3) developing programs to assess the quality of foreign nurse graduates, offering ongoing continuing education programs to help ensure they adapt successfully to the U.S. healthcare system, and providing programs aimed at helping these RNs overcome language or cultural barriers that might impede their ability to provide high quality and safe patient care. Tying the size of any subsidy to performance on these criteria will help assure that the goal of the subsidy (raising the long-run supply of RNs) is achieved at the same time that the productivity and level of social contributions of the RN workforce are increased.

Continue Informing the Public About the Nursing Profession

As shortages of RNs develop over the next 2 decades, we can expect RN wages to rise significantly. It is important that the public understands this so that cohorts currently choosing an occupation will be more likely to choose a career as an RN and so that other stakeholders are able to anticipate and prepare for the effects of the coming shortage. Without the knowledge that there will be large shortages in the near future, entry into RN education programs would be delayed until large shortages actually appear, at which point it would take years before the increase in long-run supply would be felt in the RN workforce. Similarly, other stakeholders would be more likely to delay necessary preparations until the shortage is upon them, at which point adapting to a lower supply of RNs will be more difficult.

Indeed, one of the most unique aspects of the current shortage is the amount of attention that the profession attracted from the media and the sustained private sector involvement in helping to inform the public about the shortage. As discussed in earlier chapters, a wide range of initiatives have documented effects on the public's knowledge and appreciation of RNs. Since 2002, the Johnson & Johnson Campaign for Nursing's Future has spent $50 million to help increase nursing recruitment in the United States, retain nurses in clinical practice, and increase the capacity of the nation's nursing education programs.[1] Studies have shown this campaign is widely recognized and viewed positively by the public, teenagers and their parents, nurses, nursing students, doctors, and hospital executives—all of whom exert important influences on the decisions of individuals to choose a career in nursing. Other initiatives by nursing organizations (e.g., Sigma Theta Tau International) and foundations (e.g., Robert Wood Johnson Foundation) have similarly implemented important national initiatives that have provided positive images of nurses to the public, provided information about the employment opportunities and earnings of RNs, and conveyed the personal satisfaction and rewards of a nursing career (among other things). These and other private sector initiatives have contributed substantially to the recent increase in interest in nursing among college freshmen and in the number of applicants into nursing education programs that we have discussed in previous chapters.

---

[1] Dr. Buerhaus has received funding to conduct studies on the effectiveness of the campaign. The Johnson & Johnson Campaign for Nursing's Future has played no role whatsoever in the development, preparation, or review of this book.

It is important to continue to inform the public about the nursing profession and the very strong outlook for job security and earnings growth. By stimulating interest in nursing, the demand to increase the capacity of education programs will increase not only from qualified applicants but from hospitals, health care organizations, and others who have an interest in increasing the long-run supply of RNs. In turn, hospitals and other organizations will be more likely to provide resources to eliminate the factors that are constraining capacity. Most important, providing information on the bright future of nursing careers will ensure that the long-run increase in the supply of RNs materializes sooner, thereby decreasing the time it takes to transition to a new equilibrium in the long-run demand and supply of RNs.

Transition Policies Involving RN Wages

Ensuring that RN wages are not prevented from increasing is the final strategy that will help RNs pass through and shorten the transition period needed to reach a long-run equilibrium in the demand and supply of RNs (see Table 15-1). As we have seen throughout this book, increasing RN wages exerts a critically important influence on the short-run labor supply decisions of existing RNs to participate in the labor market, increases their hours worked, and delays retirement. A rising wage also increases the long-run supply of RNs by influencing the number of people who decide to become RNs. In Chapter 11, we discussed instances when hospitals raised real RN wages and how this resolved the nursing shortages in the 1960s, 1980s, and early 1990s, as well as how sharp wage increases in 2002 and 2003 led to the unprecedented 2-year increase in hospital RN employment of just under 185,000 FTE RNs. We also described how hospital RN shortages developed when real RN wages were *not* allowed to increase through the apparent collusion of hospitals in the early 1960s and by wage controls imposed by the federal government in the 1970s. Moreover, when wages were not allowed to rise to the equilibrium wage level, the resulting shortage of RNs induced hospitals to substitute non-RNs for RNs and increase employment of foreign-educated RNs.

Given the projected increased demand for RNs and the expected inability of the long-run supply of RNs to match this growth in demand, hospitals will face strong pressures to raise RN wages for many years to come. Because of the large costs that continuous wage increases will involve, it is reasonable to expect hospitals to seek ways to keep wages from increasing as fast as market conditions indicate. However, if wages are not allowed to increase, this will only delay the time when the RN labor market is brought into equilibrium and hence prolong the transition period for RNs currently in the workplace. Unfortunately, many hospitals might be in such a weak financial condition that increasing RN wages over an extended period of time could cause serious financial distress. The Medicare and Medicaid programs and private payers could help hospitals (and other healthcare delivery organizations that rely on RNs) finance these wage increases, not unlike what was done in the mid-1960s when Medicare helped hospitals resolve a severe nursing shortage by providing them "cost plus 2%" to help them increase RN wages. Today, the formula used by the Medicare program to determine prospective hospital payments incorporates a labor wage index that can be adjusted as needed to help hospitals meet higher payroll costs.

A different threat to ensuring that real RN wages are allowed to increase might arise from provisions (implicit or explicit) contained in national healthcare reform proposals that might be developed in the future. It is conceivable, for example, that some proposals to reorganize the healthcare delivery system could assert that controlling RN wages would be an appropriate means to lower healthcare costs. As RN wages and pressures to reform the healthcare system continue to increase over time, the appeal of imposing wage controls might become more politically palatable. If implemented, however, the effect would be to extend indefinitely the time RNs spend in shortage conditions because the labor market will not be allowed to reach its long-run equilibrium wage level.

LONG-RUN POLICIES

Thus far in this chapter we have discussed policies aimed at helping RNs through the period it will take for the labor market to transition to the point where the long-run demand and supply are in balance. In the long run, shortages of RNs have been eliminated through a combination of higher wages, rising entry of new and existing RNs into the workforce, and substitution by healthcare providers away from employing RNs. This transition period could take many years given the projections of the growing demand for RNs and the impact of the aging of the RN workforce in slowing the growth in the long-run supply of RNs. In this section we discuss a different set of policies that are targeted at changing the underlying long-run growth rates in the demand and supply of RNs

From an economic perspective, there is a predisposition to allow markets (consumer, labor, housing, equity, debt, etc.) to adjust by themselves to long-run changes in supply and demand. This view reflects the belief that when left alone, markets will more efficiently determine the correct price and quantity of goods and services compared to when governments or firms interfere with the adjustment process. In fact, one of the most important results in economics is the First Welfare Theorem, which states that a competitive market equilibrium leads to an efficient allocation of resources, that is, one in which there is no way that government could intervene and reallocate resources in a way that makes everyone better off.

This theorem, of course, does not imply that economists think that governments should never intervene in markets. Instead, it highlights that resources will *not* be allocated efficiently when the conditions for competitive market equilibrium are unmet, and in these circumstances, government intervention might be justified. There are two common circumstances in which most economists would agree it is appropriate to intervene in markets: when the market is not competitive (for example, firms face barriers to enter into an industry); and when there are externalities (benefits or costs that accrue to others in society) that are not being properly valued by private decision makers in the market. Thus, from an economic point of view, there are good reasons to intervene in the RN labor market to solve problems that either restrict or retard entry into the nursing profession or cause the contributions of RNs to be improperly valued.

Reducing Barriers to Enter the Nursing Profession in the United States

The first set of policies aimed at increasing the underlying long-run growth rate in the supply of RNs involves the barriers to entering the nursing profession (see **Table 15-2**). These barriers apply to two groups: RNs educated in other countries and citizens of the United States who are not choosing to become professional nurses.

Table 15-2   Long-Run Policy and Strategies

Strategies	Long-Run Policy
	Goals: Expand employment of RNs in the long run by eliminating barriers causing inadequate supply of RNs and by appropriately valuing the contributions of RNs.
Supply Strategies	• Remove barriers to hiring foreign-educated RNs • Remove stigmas and barriers facing men and Hispanics
Demand Strategies	• Reinforce development of pay-for-performance systems • Increase the number of nurse-sensitive outcomes included in pay-for-performance systems

RNs Educated in Other Countries

The expected future increase in real RN wages will provide a strong incentive for foreign-educated RNs to immigrate to the United States. If large numbers of foreign-educated RNs enter the country, the long-run supply of RNs could be rapidly increased. This, in turn, would decrease the long-run pressures on hospitals to raise wages and spare taxpayers from financing these higher wages. Regardless of opinions about the desirability of using foreign-educated RNs to supply the U.S. nurse labor market, we anticipate the labor market for RNs will become a global market. Thus, in a global market, free of entry barriers, RNs would be able to move freely to countries that offer the most attractive wages, benefits, and working conditions.

We recognize that relying on foreign-educated RNs might have unintended consequences possibly involving lower quality of care, worsening shortages in other parts of the world, and depressed domestic RN wages, to name a few. Clearly, the political process has taken the social costs and benefits of immigration into account in determining the existing barriers on immigration, and it is unclear whether the benefits of expanding the supply of RNs through increased immigration offset these potential social costs and potential political costs of doing so. To avoid these costs, we believe it might be better to focus on removing other existing barriers to becoming RNs faced by U.S. citizens: barriers that discourage men and Hispanics from entering nursing.

Men and Hispanics

As we observed in Chapter 2, over the past 25 years, the number of men and Hispanics in the RN workforce has grown slowly. Of the estimated 2.24 million RNs in the RN workforce in 2006, 200,000 or 8% were estimated to be men, and 100,000 or about 4% were estimated to be Hispanic or Latino. While the proportion of the RN workforce that was male or Hispanic has roughly doubled since 1983, both groups continue to be underrepresented relative to their presence in the population (49% men and 15% Hispanic) or in the workforce (54% men and 14% Hispanic). In contrast, while African Americans were underrepresented in the nursing workforce in the 1980s, they now account for roughly 11% of the RN workforce, which is equal to their proportion in the overall workforce (Asians have not been underrepresented in the RN workforce).

Because men and Hispanics together comprise over half of the working age population, they represent an important untapped pool that could potentially be drawn into the nursing profession. Furthermore, Hispanics are the fastest growing demographic group in the United States, and they are expected to account for 24% of the population by 2050. As we have seen in prior chapters, attracting ever more white women into the RN workforce will be an uphill struggle as the population aged 20–39 continues to grow slowly and women continue to be attracted to other professions. In contrast, some simple calculations suggest that even modest increases in the propensity of men and Hispanics to become RNs could contribute substantially to filling the future RN shortage.

For example, data from the CPS estimates that roughly 3% of all white women in the United States aged 21–65 were working as RNs in 2006. In contrast, less than 1% of Hispanic women and one-quarter of 1% of men were working as RNs. If Hispanic women worked as RNs at the same rate as white women by 2025, more than 300,000 additional RNs would have entered the workforce, eliminating over half of the projected shortage in that year. Similarly, if men doubled their participation rates in the RN workforce from one-quarter to one-half of 1% by 2025, an additional 200,000 RNs would be supplied.

Alternatively, suppose that we could encourage men and Hispanics from cohorts born since 1983 (those who were age 23 or younger in 2006) to enter RN education programs at the same rate as white women. This would roughly double the number of RNs that these cohorts would supply to the labor market. Our estimates from Chapter 10 suggest that such an increase in the propensity of recent cohorts to become RNs would be enough to eliminate the projected shortages through 2025 and beyond. Furthermore, from Chapter 6, we learned that men and minorities have higher labor force participation rates and also work more hours per year than their white RN counterparts. Thus, attracting more Hispanics and men into nursing will increase not only the number of RNs significantly, but it will have an even greater impact on workforce FTEs through higher participation and hours worked.

A number of barriers might help to explain why nursing is a less attractive career for men and Hispanics than it is for white women (American Association of Colleges of Nursing, 2001; Sullivan Commission, 2004). The stigma of being in a traditionally female-dominated profession is generally believed to be one of the primary factors discouraging men from becoming RNs. The stereotype of RNs as white women might also discourage minority women from choosing a nursing career. Moreover, the fact that the current RN workforce (and faculty in nursing education programs) includes few men and Hispanics might result in a lack of role models and mentors for younger people who are considering nursing as a career. Educational and financial barriers might further discourage Hispanics from becoming RNs because Hispanics are roughly four times more likely than whites not to complete high school or to live in poverty. However, educational preparation is not the sole factor, because even among high school graduates, whites are nearly three times more likely than Hispanics to become RNs.

The long period of time in which men and Hispanics have remained underrepresented in the nursing profession suggests that they might face persistent barriers to entry into the RN workforce that are difficult to overcome. On the other hand, the progress made by African Americans over the last 20 years, to the point where they are now represented in the RN workforce in nearly the same proportion as in the labor market as a whole, suggests that the barriers facing minority groups are not insurmountable. Recently, the Sullivan Commission (2004) proposed a wide range of policies that aim to remove many of the perceived barriers. Their recommendations include public awareness campaigns; partnerships of healthcare employers with public schools and communities to promote opportunities for men and minorities in nursing and encourage necessary academic preparation; increased support services, such as mentoring; increased representation of men and minorities in faculty and leadership positions; and increased tuition assistance and student loans to reduce the debt burden for students from underrepresented groups. In the past, these strategies have been viewed primarily as a means to promote diversity of the workforce as an end in itself. With large RN shortages on the horizon, these strategies should be an even higher priority because they have the potential to greatly expand the number of people entering the profession.

Today, men and Hispanics are still far less interested in nursing compared to white women. Whether this is due to social stigma attached to the nursing profession, lack of mentors and role models, or other reasons, some type of barrier is making the profession less attractive to those who are not white women. If the root cause of the barriers facing men and Hispanics can be identified, actions could then be taken to remove them. If this were done, and men and Hispanics began entering nursing at the same rate as white women, then the size of the future shortage of RNs projected in Chapter 10 could be reduced significantly and possibly even prevented from developing in the first place. Therefore, identifying and eliminating the barriers to recruiting more men and Hispanics into nursing is perhaps the most important opportunity to increase the long-run supply of RNs.

Nursing as an Undervalued Social Benefit

Other than in cases where there are entry barriers, a second reason that justifies intervention into market performance is when there are externalities—either benefits or costs that accrue to others in society—that are being improperly valued by private decision makers. Market intervention is not uncommon. For example, the government subsidizes education because a more educated population is thought to benefit society as a whole, and cigarettes are taxed because smoking imposes a cost on others through second hand smoke and medical costs borne by society. Similarly, the federal government has helped many key industries whose performance affects others in the economy: bailing out automobile companies to prevent large-scale unemployment; intervening in the savings and loans scandal that threatened the collapse of the banking industry and the loss of individuals' homes; and recently the Federal Reserve injected billions of dollars to provide liquidity into the tightening credit market in the summer of 2007 as a means of preventing the subprime loan crises from affecting the larger economy. With respect to intervening in the nurse labor market, is there any justification for intervention? To intervene, we must make the case that there are external benefits attached to the output produced by RNs that are not being properly valued.

Redefining the Social Contribution of RNs

Many studies have demonstrated the association of hospital nurse staffing with a growing number of patient complications and adverse outcomes, including mortality. The study by Needleman, Buerhaus, Mattke, Stewart, & Zelevinsky (2006), discussed in Chapter 12, explicitly sought to determine the business and social case for investing in hospital nurse staffing. Recall that this study estimated that increasing all U.S. hospital nurse staffing to the 75th percentile would result in 6754 fewer hospital deaths annually and reduce five adverse outcomes by 60,000 to 70,000 cases. Approximately three-quarters of these deaths and 85% of the adverse outcomes could be achieved by simply raising the proportion of nursing personnel who are RNs (without raising the total numbers of nursing personnel), which is the only option that would pay for itself. That is, the cost savings associated with decreasing the five adverse outcomes, lowering patient length of stay, and decreasing the number of deaths would offset the cost of increasing RN staffing, thereby saving hospitals an estimated $242 million in the short run and $1.8 billion in the long run after hospitals fully adjust their fixed costs. The cost per avoided death estimated in this study for all three staffing options that were modeled was below the value of a statistical life used by federal agencies in their rule making on health and safety. This evidence suggests that the contributions of RNs are currently being undervalued by hospitals; even from the point of view of private financial benefits, a good case can be made for hiring more RNs.

It is important to recall that the Needleman et al. (2006) study did not consider the value to patients and their families of reduced morbidity (decreased pain and suffering and lost days of work), the economic value to hospitals of lower liability and improved reputation and image from reducing adverse nursing-related morbidity and mortality, or the positive effects and cost savings of increased nurse staffing from reducing adverse outcomes not considered in the analysis but which have been reported in other studies (patient falls, blood-borne infections, pressure ulcers, and medication errors). In addition, the study did not account for increased patient satisfaction or patients achieving higher physical and mental function as a result of nursing care. Combining these unmeasured but real economic and noneconomic benefits, many of which accrue to others and are unlikely to be considered by hospitals, with the value of reduced mortality obtained by increasing RN staffing only strengthens the argument that current efforts to recognize the contributions of RNs are lacking and are highly likely to undervalue the true social benefit of RNs.

The apparent undervaluation of the social benefit of RNs suggests that even when the long-run demand and supply of RNs are eventually brought into equilibrium, the number of RNs employed in hospitals will be inadequate and not reflective of their true social value. This suggests that *one goal of intervening in the nurse labor market should be to expand the number of RNs in the future beyond the equilibrium quantity of RNs that would otherwise be achieved by the nurse labor market.* We therefore conclude this chapter by discussing strategies designed to intervene on the *demand* side of the nurse labor market.

Intervening to Increase the Labor Market's Demand for RNs

The goal of demand-side intervention is to actually *expand the future demand* for RNs (shifting the demand curve for RNs outward and to the right, as discussed in Chapter 3). As demand expands, more RNs will be working in the labor market and in hospitals at any given wage level compared to when the demand was lower. Equivalently, as demand expands, healthcare employers are willing to pay a higher wage to attract a given number of RNs because they value the contribution of RNs more highly. Thus, policy makers need to determine how to increase the valuation that healthcare employers place on the contribution of RNs, thereby shifting out the long-run demand for RNs.

Fortunately, two budding changes in hospital payment policies offer promise. The first is the decision of the Centers for Medicare & Medicaid Services to stop compensating hospitals for treating certain reasonably preventable conditions that are hospital acquired. The change, scheduled to begin in October 2008, means that hospitals would not get paid for injuries from patient falls, pressure ulcers, urinary tract infections, vascular-catheter-associated infections and mediastinitis, as well as several "never events" including blood incompatibility. Some of these conditions are associated with low nurse staffing levels (as discussed in Chapter 12) and therefore represent an economic incentive for hospitals to increase RN staffing to prevent these conditions. Expanding the number of these conditions to include additional nurse-sensitive outcomes will give hospitals added economic incentive to increase their demand for RNs.

The second strategy is the closely related and nascent pay-for-performance system being adopted by private sector payers of hospital services. Again, policy makers could attempt to include nurse-sensitive outcomes on the list of payable hospital outcomes, which would give hospitals an incentive to expand their demand for RNs. Having more RNs will increase the likelihood that the pay-for-performance system will reward hospitals for their investment in nurse staffing. Taken together, these payment policies, if properly modified to include a greater number of nurse-sensitive outcomes, will raise the economic value of nurses and achieve a greater long-run increase in the number of RNs in the workforce and hence provide greater social benefits to patients and the broader society than what could be reasonably expected if the nurse labor market was left alone.

CHAPTER SUMMARY

This chapter has focused on discussing policies aimed at helping RNs through what is likely to be an extended transition period until the long-run demand and supply of RNs adjusts to reach a new equilibrium in which the future shortage is eventually resolved. RNs can be helped through this transition by speeding up the development and adoption of technology and use of nonprofessional nursing personnel, removing barriers to efficiency and redesigning the work content and organization of nursing care, improving management decision making, and avoiding regulating nurse staffing. On the supply side, transition strategies should focus on accommodating an older RN workforce, accelerating improvements in working conditions, expanding the capacity of nursing education programs, and continuing to inform the public about the opportunities in nursing. Beyond these strategies, there is a critical need to assure that RN wages are flexible (avoiding wage controls) so that the nurse labor market can adjust to the long-run equilibrium as rapidly as possible.

Beyond transition policies, we believe that policy makers will need to consider long-run strategies aimed at expanding the number of RNs in the labor market. Removing barriers to entry into the nursing profession for men and Hispanics could be especially helpful to quickly increase the long-run supply of RNs and help offset pressures to expand the number of foreign nurse graduates entering the U.S. nurse labor market. Additionally, revaluing the social contributions of RNs and thereby increasing their long-run demand could be achieved by stimulating the development of pay-for-performance systems and increasing the number of nurse-sensitive outcomes included in these systems.

The seriousness of the challenges facing the nursing profession and the broader healthcare delivery system cannot be overstated. Leaders of the nursing profession, healthcare organizations, and the nation's political institutions must recognize that the magnitude and momentum of the demographic and social forces underpinning the aging RN workforce are so powerful that it will be impossible for the nursing profession alone to address the expected shortage that will be of unprecedented size, duration, and impact. Assistance is needed from hospitals, physicians, policy makers, media, politicians, unions, corporations, and the public to bring the problems confronting nurses higher on the national social policy agenda. Hopefully, policies along the lines discussed in this chapter can be implemented to ensure a strong and well-prepared professional RN workforce for years to come.

REFERENCES

American Association of Colleges of Nursing. (2001). *Effective strategies for increasing diversity in nursing programs.* Retrieved December 11, 2007, from http://www.aacn.nche.edu/Publications/issues/dec01.htm

Needleman, J., Buerhaus, P., Mattke, S., Stewart, M., & Zelevinsky, K. (2006). Nurse staffing in hospitals: Is there a business case for quality? *Health Affairs, 25*(1), 204–211.

Sullivan Commission. (2004). *Missing persons: Minorities in the health professions.* Retrieved December 11, 2007, from http://www.aacn.nche.edu/Media/pdf/SullivanReport.pdf

Index